Bottom Line's
HEALTH
BREAKTHROUGHS
2005

Bottom Line
Books
www.BottomLineSecrets.com

First Edition

10 9 8 7 6 5 4 3 2 1

ISBN 0-88723-332-5

HealthDay

Articles in this book were written by reporters for HealthDay, an award-winning international daily consumer health news service, headquartered in Norwalk, Connecticut.

The articles were selected and edited by HealthDay Editor-in-Chief Barry Hoffman and Managing Editor Jean Patman. The staff at Bottom Line Books reviewed and edited all content.

The editors would like to acknowledge and thank the following veteran journalists who crafted the articles specifically for this book:
Adam Marcus; Anne Thompson; Dennis Thompson

Bottom Line® Books is a registered trademark of Boardroom® Inc.
281 Tresser Boulevard, Stamford, CT 06901

Printed in the United States of America

Contents

8 • EMOTIONAL WELL-BEING

9 • FAMILY HEALTH

10 • HEART DISEASE

11 • NATURAL REMEDIES

12 • NUTRITION, DIET & FITNESS

13 • PAIN TREATMENTS

14 • RESEARCH NEWS

1

Aging & Senior Health

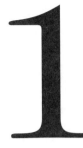

Three Common Viruses Increase Risk of Dementia

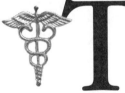

Three fairly common viruses appear to increase the risk that elderly people will get dementia, according to a study. People with a history of infection with at least two of the viruses—two strains of herpes and a microbe called cytomegalovirus—were approximately twice as likely to show significant mental decline during the one-year study as those infected with one or none of the pathogens.

THE VIRUSES

Herpes and cytomegalovirus are known to damage brain cells, so infection with either or both viruses could lead to the loss of neurons, and eventually dementia, according to the researchers.

In theory, drugs to treat existing infections or vaccines to prevent infections could prevent dementia, they add.

THE INFLAMMATION CONNECTION

Scientists are beginning to recognize that a variety of brain diseases, from Alzheimer's to Parkinson's, have at least some connection to inflammation.

In elderly patients, inflammation from a localized infection in another part of the body can undermine the integrity of the blood-brain barrier, allowing harmful molecules to pass into the brain that normally wouldn't be able to, says Dr. Howard Gendelman, director of the Center for Neurovirology and Neurodegenerative Disorders at the University of Nebraska Medical Center in Omaha.

This process can damage neurons and lead to dementia. It often does so in HIV patients, for example, he says.

Yet not all dementia results from infection, and not all infections lead to dementia. Genetics,

Howard E. Gendelman, MD, director, Center for Neurovirology and Neurodegenerative Disorders, University of Nebraska Medical Center, Omaha.

Larry Goldstein, MD, professor, medicine, and director, stroke center, Duke University Medical Center, Durham, NC.

Stroke.

nutrition and other factors likely affect a person's susceptibility to brain inflammation, Gendelman says.

THE STUDY

In the study, Dr. Timo Strandberg, of the University of Helsinki in Finland, and his colleagues followed up 383 elderly men and women with varying stages of blood vessel disease. More than 80% of the study participants had a history of heart disease and 37% had had at least one stroke.

The researchers looked for signs of infection with three common viruses: Herpes simplex 1, which causes cold sores; a related sexually transmitted virus, herpes simplex 2; and cytomegalovirus, which can be harmful to babies in the womb but typically causes no problems for healthy adults.

Blood tests revealed that 48 people had evidence, in the form of proteins called antibodies, of one or none of the viruses; 229 had antibodies to two of the microbes; and 106 had signs of infection with all three viruses.

At the beginning of the study, 58 people (15%) had cognitive trouble on a standard psychological exam.

Subjects with antibodies to three viruses were 2.5 times more likely to fall into this group than people with fewer or no infections.

The greater the level of antibodies (that is, the greater the number of infections), the more severe the dementia.

During the following 12 months, 150 of the subjects lost ground on the cognitive test. Again, history of infection was strongly linked to the likelihood of mental decline.

CAUTION URGED

Dr. Larry Goldstein, director of Duke University Stroke Center and a spokesman for the American Stroke Association, cautions that the Finnish findings may not translate to other groups of people. Not only did all the subjects have some form of vessel disease, but Finland is far more ethnically homogenous than the United States. The study "is not applicable to the general population. It's limited to that narrow group of folks," he says.

info For more on dementia, visit the National Library of Medicine at *www.nlm.nih.gov* or the Alzheimer's Association at *www.alz.org*.

Stress Linked to Memory Loss

Robert S. Wilson, PhD, professor, neurophysiology, Rush University Medical Center, Chicago.
John C. S. Breitner, MD, director, Geriatric Research, Education and Clinical Center, VA Puget Sound Health Care System, Seattle.
Neurology.

People who are easily stressed are more likely to suffer memory loss later in life, a study has found.

There was "an extraordinary decline in memory" among the older people who tested highest on a standardized scale of susceptibility to stress, says study leader Robert S. Wilson, a professor of neurophysiology at Rush University Medical Center in Chicago.

The finding raises the possibility that treating stress-prone people, perhaps with antidepressants, can help prevent memory loss, Wilson says. But that is still a distant prospect.

"It is too early for us to start treating people on that basis, but it is not too early to do tests," he says.

"In animal studies, antidepressant therapy does have some effect. Also, there is some indication that physical exercise might block the effects of stressful experience," Wilson adds.

THE STUDY

This finding comes out of the Religious Orders Study, which has followed up nearly 800 Catholic nuns, priests and lay brothers. The average age of the people in this study was 75 years when the study began.

The participants' vulnerability to stress was measured using a rating scale that evaluated their responses to such statements as *I am not a worrier* and *I often feel tense and jittery.* Within five years of the testing, people who scored in the top 10% of susceptibility to stress were twice as likely to develop memory loss, compared with those in the bottom 10%, the researchers say.

SURPRISING RESULT

One unexpected finding came from anatomical studies of the brains of the 141 participants who died during the study.

The brains of those who suffered memory loss did not contain the plaques and nerve cell tangles that are well-known abnormalities of Alzheimer's disease.

"The interesting thing is that stress proneness does not predict the pathology of Alzheimer's disease," says Dr. John C. S. Breitner, director of the Geriatric Research, Education and Clinical Center at the Veterans Administration Puget Sound Health Care System in Seattle. "What it predicts is how those brain centers get expressed in terms of dementia."

Preventive treatments might be difficult because vulnerability to stress is "a stable aspect of personality" that is not easily changed, Breitner says. But, he says, treatment could be possible if depression eventually is found to be a major factor in susceptibility to stress.

"Depression is an archetypical treatable disorder," Breitner says. "And a lot of depression doesn't get recognized."

Another question, according to Wilson, is when treatment should begin. "We really aren't sure at what point in lifespan [the onset of memory loss] occurs," he says. "We could be seeing it in old age because it takes many years to occur. We really need to understand how it works."

More studies are needed of larger and different groups of people to verify the finding, Wilson says. But there are some "really exciting" possibilities if the results are proved to be valid, he says.

A WORD TO THE WISE

Meanwhile, Wilson adds, it is helpful to remember that "people have known for a long time that trying to take life less seriously is a good thing."

info For tips on stress management, visit the Web site of the College of Saint Benedict, Saint John's University, at *www.csbsju.edu.*

New Ways for Seniors to Remember More

Neuropsychological Rehabilitation.
Wake Forest University, Winston-Salem, NC, news release.

A new memory training technique may help older adults improve their memory of recent events and information.

This memory training approach involves gradually increasing the delay intervals during memory training. This can help older adults successfully recall information across increasingly longer delays.

The new technique was tested on a group of older adults, whose average age was 73 years. After seven days of training for approximately 45 minutes a day, the adults performed 14 times better overall on a memory task.

THE STUDY

During the training sessions, the people in the study were shown lists of words. Participants were asked to remember the words that had already appeared on the list. After each correct trial, the number of intervening items between the repeated words was gradually increased.

Initially, accurate identification of the words occurred with only two intervening items. However, after six hours of training, accurate identification occurred with as many as 28 intervening items.

This form of memory training, which is best done with professional assistance, is meant to improve overall memory function rather than teach recall tricks that are specific to a single memory task.

"Many efforts to improve memory function in adults have focused on teaching strategies rather than improving cognitive processes," according to Wake Forest psychologist, Janine Jennings.

"In the current study, we tested the efficacy of a memory training technique with older adults that is based on the theory that memory consists of two processes—an automatic process, which is known as familiarity, and a consciously controlled process referred to as recollection," Jennings says.

For example, the automatic process informs you that someone you see is familiar. The recollection process then provides information about why the person is familiar or when you last saw them.

The primary goal of this new memory training technique is to try to strengthen the recollection process.

Although it delivered impressive results in the laboratory setting, the next step is to determine whether it works outside the lab and can help older adults' daily memory function and stave off dementia.

DEMENTIA VS. DEPRESSION

Dementia, or the debilitating loss of brain function as people age, is a common problem among the elderly. Alzheimer's disease, a brain tumor or a head injury can all cause dementia.

Many times, depression in the elderly is mistaken for dementia. But unlike dementia, mood problems can be successfully reversed with a variety of therapies, including medication and counseling.

info You can find out more information about age-related memory loss from the Web site *http://familydoctor.org.*

Watch Out! These Memory-Building Drugs Could Backfire

Amy F.T. Arnsten, PhD, associate professor and director, graduate studies in neurobiology, Yale University School of Medicine, New Haven, CT.

Paula Bickford, PhD, professor, neurosurgery, University of South Florida Center for Aging and Brain Repair, Tampa, and past president, American Aging Association.

Bill Thies, PhD, vice president, medical and scientific affairs, Alzheimer's Association, Chicago.

Neuron online.

Experimental drugs designed to preserve memory function lost to age or brain disease may do so at the expense of other forms of recall.

Researchers believe that regional differences in the brain could undercut the effectiveness of drugs that are being developed to enhance memory in people with Alzheimer's disease and other age-related dementia.

UNDERSTANDING MEMORY

Two areas of the brain are associated with different types of memory. The hippocampus has been associated with long-term memory formation, while the prefrontal cortex has been associated with working or functional memory (such as remembering the phone number of your babysitter or holding onto a phone number long enough to dial it).

In a healthy individual, the two brain systems work together. When a person gets older, however, both forms of memory can be adversely affected.

The prefrontal cortex—the working memory—naturally flags with normal aging, "so it's particularly important to see what this cortex loses, and give it back," says study author Amy F.T. Arnsten, an associate professor and director of graduate studies in neurobiology at Yale University School of Medicine.

"There's some deterioration in the hippocampus [the long-term memory function] with normal aging, but what really erodes the hippocampus is Alzheimer's."

Experts believe that increasing the activity of an enzyme called *protein kinase A* (PKA) in the hippocampus may improve memory and other cognitive deficits. There are drugs in development that may accomplish that.

THE PROBLEM WITH DRUGS

The problem, according to Arnsten and her colleagues at Yale, is that a particular drug can have vastly different effects on different parts of the brain.

Their study found that drugs that might benefit the hippocampus might have deleterious effects on the prefrontal cortex.

"Different regions of the brain that control various kinds of learning and memory may be affected differently by drugs that are targeted at improving cognition," explains Paula Bickford, a professor of neurosurgery at the

University of South Florida Center for Aging and Brain Repair in Tampa and a past president of the American Aging Association.

"They may improve one kind of cognition but impair a different type of cognition," according to Bickford.

THE STUDY

The researchers did a series of tests in rats and monkeys using drugs to increase or decrease PKA activity.

Inhibiting PKA in the hippocampus actually improved functioning in the prefrontal cortex. PKA activation in the hippocampus impaired functioning in the prefrontal cortex.

In other words, opposite processes seem to be at work in the hippocampus and in the prefrontal cortex.

RESEARCH IMPLICATIONS

As people age, PKA activity declines in the hippocampus but increases in the prefrontal cortex, suggesting that different measures are needed to improve the situation in each area of the brain.

"A drug that would correct one would hinder the other," Arnsten says. "That's why this is so tough."

Right now, no pharmaceutical memory enhancers are effective in people in any "significant way," says Bill Thies, vice president of medical and scientific affairs at the Alzheimer's Association.

The current research may not necessarily be a setback. "It just makes the direction we need to go in more clear. It helps clarify what may or may not work," Bickford says.

"Unfortunately, it is the reality of our world. It's never quite as simple as we thought it was," Bickford adds.

"Different brain regions have developed different chemical pathways, and that's how you get specificity within the brain. But it then makes it more difficult to design pharmaceuticals that are memory-enhancing," Bickford explains.

info For more on memory and aging, visit UCLA's Memory and Aging Research Center Web site at *www.memory.ucla.edu.*

Lower Blood Pressure Boosts Memory

J. Richard Jennings, PhD, professor, psychiatry and psychology, University of Pittsburgh, PA.

Daniel C. Fisher, MD, clinical assistant professor, medicine, New York University, New York City.

American Heart Association's 57th Annual High Blood Pressure Research Conference, Washington, DC.

Remembering to take blood pressure medication might help older people remember many other things, according to a study.

The study found that blood flow in the brain and memory skills are different in individuals who are older. The difference in blood flow depends on whether their blood pressure is under the recommended level.

THE STUDY

The study, led by J. Richard Jennings, a professor of psychiatry and psychology at the University of Pittsburgh, enlisted 59 volunteers (*average age:* 60 years) who had blood pressure below the then-recommended 140/90 reading, and another 37 volunteers (*average age:* 61), with blood pressure in the hypertension region—an average reading of 144/84. Current guidelines classify blood pressure readings between 120/80 and 139/89 as prehypertension. Optimal blood pressure is now considered to be below 120/80.

Participants were given tests to measure baseline memory and reasoning abilities and they underwent ultrasound imaging of the carotid arteries, the vessels in the neck that supply blood to the brain.

They performed a series of everyday memory tests while scans recorded activity in parts of the brain involved in memory.

Example: A participant would be asked to look up a phone number, walk to another room and dial that number. That's the kind of short-term memory task that often troubles older people, Jennings says.

THE RESULTS

Sure enough, "blood flow wasn't as rapidly or as fully available among people with high blood pressure as it was in the nonhypertensive volunteers," he says.

In addition, a lower performance level accompanied that diminished blood flow, according to Jennings.

The finding supports the theory that "the brain protects itself when you have high blood pressure by expanding blood vessels in different parts of the brain," he says.

Some blood pressure medications have a greater effect than others on blood flow in the brain, Jennings says. He is studying those differences.

WIDER IMPLICATIONS

"As we age from 45 to 75, we all probably suffer some decline in cognitive function," Jennings says.

"It isn't clear whether that is due to aging alone, or to the chronic diseases that develop as we get older, such as atherosclerosis or diabetes," says Jennings.

So someday, he says, this line of research could determine "whether we would all have perfectly normal mental function at age 75 if we are perfectly healthy."

ANOTHER REASON TO CONTROL BLOOD PRESSURE

Jennings' findings will have to be verified by a larger study, says Dr. Daniel C. Fisher, a clinical assistant professor of medicine at New York University and a spokesman for the American Heart Association, but they add another facet to the importance of controlling blood pressure.

"This is one more reason why we need to focus on blood pressure as a risk factor not only for heart disease but also other problems in older people," Fisher says.

"Keeping blood pressure under control also helps prevent stroke and other cardiovascular problems. The possible effect on memory would be an added benefit."

info Medications and other ways to control blood pressure are described by the National Heart, Lung, and Blood Institute at *www.nhlbi.nih.gov.*

Memory Zappers: High Blood Pressure and These Common Diseases

David Madden, PhD, professor, medical psychology, Duke University Medical Center, Durham, NC.
Aging, Neuropsychology and Cognition.

The effects of high blood pressure on mental function in older people are more complex than previously believed, according to a recent study.

The study included people who were otherwise healthy but who had uncontrolled high blood pressure.

This research highlights the importance of other conditions, such as diabetes or heart disease, on mental function, according to study author David Madden, who is also a professor of medical psychology at Duke University Medical Center.

COMPLEX INTERACTION IS AT WORK

"This challenges the conventional wisdom that high blood pressure and aging interact to affect cognitive function," Madden says.

"They do interact, but in much more complex ways than we currently understand."

"Although the changes in cognitive performance associated with elevated blood pressure seen in our experiments were statistically significant, they are unlikely to interfere with the mental functioning during everyday life," Madden adds.

"However, the changes that we recorded in the laboratory may represent a situation that could become clinically significant when various other diseases, especially those that are cardiovascular in nature, are included," according to Madden.

THE STUDY

The Duke experiment included 96 volunteers. Half of the study participants had high blood pressure for which they were not taking medication and the other half of the subjects had blood pressure that was brought down to healthy levels by medication.

The volunteers did a visual search test on a computer in which they were shown a pair of letters and then had to tell whether those letters were present in another, larger display. A different sequence of letter displays was used to test their memory.

THE RESULTS

Looking at the results by age group, Madden and his colleagues found that high blood pressure slowed mental function only in participants aged 40 to 59.

High blood pressure did not dim the performance of the oldest participants, who were aged 60 to 79.

Most similar studies have looked only at people with high blood pressure who had other illnesses, Madden notes.

"Our goal was to determine if there was an effect of elevated blood pressure on the natural course of healthy people," he says.

SURPRISING FINDING

The results do not support the classical belief that high blood pressure causes deterioration of mental function in all older people, he says. "You must consider both a person's age and disease condition."

However, the laboratory results do not mean that older individuals can disregard their high blood pressure, Madden says, because "it is relatively rare to have high blood pressure by itself."

Even if uncontrolled high blood pressure does not affect an individual's thinking ability, it is a major risk factor for heart disease and stroke, he says.

Madden is continuing to research the complex effects of high blood pressure on thinking ability.

"The significance of these cognitive effects will become clearer as additional evidence is obtained regarding the changes in brain structure," the report says.

info The Minnesota Humanities Commission's Web site has information on how to enhance your mental abilities as you age at *www.minnesotahumanities.org*.

Big Bonus! Blood Pressure Pill Slows Bone Loss

Bruno H.Ch. Stricker, PhD, professor, Erasmus University Medical Center, Rotterdam, The Netherlands.

Felicia Cosman, MD, clinical director, National Osteoporosis Foundation and associate professor, clinical medicine, Columbia University, New York, NY.

Annals of Internal Medicine.

Thiazide diuretics that control high blood pressure can also reduce age-related bone loss and the resulting fractures, but the protection vanishes once the drugs are stopped, researchers say.

Osteoporosis, which can sometimes lead to hip fractures, is a common problem in older men and women, as bones become thinner and weaker during the normal aging process.

Studies have shown that thiazides slow calcium loss and may be a factor in preventing age-related bone erosion.

Now, Dutch investigators have clearly shown that thiazides significantly reduce the risk of hip fractures.

In a large population of elderly patients, the use of a thiazide medication "offered a substantial protection from hip fracture," says lead researcher Dr. Bruno H.Ch. Stricker, a professor at Erasmus University Medical Center located in Rotterdam.

THE STUDY

In their study, the researchers collected data on hip fractures among 7,891 men and women older than 55.

They classified patients as those who had never used a thiazide, those who had used a thiazide for a short time, and those who had used a thiazide for a year or more.

They also looked at individuals who had stopped using a thiazide for a short period and those who had stopped the medication for six months or more.

RISK REDUCED BY HALF

During up to nine years of follow-up study, Stricker and his team found that compared with patients who had never taken a thiazide diuretic, those who had taken a thiazide for more than one year had about a 50% lower risk of hip fracture.

However, this lower risk disappeared within four months after the medication was stopped, the research team says.

WHAT THE RESEARCH IMPLICATIONS ARE

Because thiazide diuretics are relatively safe drugs, Stricker believes that they might be useful for treating older patients who have high blood pressure and who are also at risk for hip fracture.

"But I do not advise using thiazides primarily to protect against hip fracture if you do not have hypertension—not until a clinical trial has demonstrated that it is truly effective and how big that effect is," he cautions.

According to Stricker, based on the current study's findings, "it is reasonable to treat an older woman with hypertension who is also liable to hip fracture with a thiazide as a first medication."

FINDINGS SUPPORT OTHER STUDIES

Dr. Felicia Cosman, clinical director of the National Osteoporosis Foundation as well as an associate professor of clinical medicine at Columbia University in New York City, comments that these findings are consistent with those of other studies.

According to Cosman, it is not surprising that the protective effect of thiazide medications wears off after use of the drug is discontinued. This is a common occurrence that is also found with numerous other medications, she explains.

"We still need to follow the same preventive measures for osteoporosis. People need to maximize their calcium and vitamin D intake, exercise regularly and reduce any possible risk factors," she advises.

info To learn more about how to prevent osteoporosis, visit the National Osteoporosis Foundation at *www.nof.org*.

One Third of Falls in Elderly Women Linked to These Three Diseases

Debbie Lawlor, MD, PhD, senior lecturer, epidemiology, Department of Social Medicine, University of Bristol, United Kingdom.

Gerard Varlotta, DO, associate professor, rehabilitation medicine, New York University/Rusk Institute, New York City.

British Medical Journal.

A study has found that elderly women who had chronic conditions, such as arthritis or depression, are at a higher risk of falling, and that these conditions may actually account for approximately one third of their falls.

WHY OLDER PEOPLE ARE LIKELY TO FALL

Previously, doctors believed that taking multiple medications was an important factor in the risk of falling.

"In other words, the more tablets you take, the more likely you are to fall," says study author Dr. Debbie Lawlor, who is also a senior lecturer in epidemiology at the University of Bristol in Britain. "But we found that it is the disease processes, rather than the drugs, that are responsible."

Older people are prone to falls, some of them with devastating consequences, because a number of different processes can interfere with balance.

One condition, *peripheral neuropathy,* happens when damage occurs to the peripheral nerves. Vertigo, inner ear disorders and visual disturbances also play a part.

"A number of senses come into play when we talk about why someone falls. Muscle strength is also a critical factor," says Dr. Gerard Varlotta, an associate professor of rehabilitation medicine at New York University/ Rusk Institute in New York City. "Those are processes that deteriorate as we get older, and that's why the elderly are more susceptible to falling."

Many medications also cause dizziness or low blood pressure, and it has been thought that these drugs can contribute to falls as well. What's interesting about the current study, Varlotta says, is that it is the diseases rather than the medications treating them seem to be implicated.

THE STUDY

The study authors asked 4,050 British women aged between 60 and 79 years how many times they had fallen during the past year and whether they received medical attention for those falls.

The authors also collected information on the patients' chronic diseases and took their drug histories.

Approximately 75% of the women studied had been diagnosed with at least one chronic disease and more than 70% were taking at least one drug.

The authors found that one third of all the falls in elderly women were caused by having at least one chronic disease.

Each additional chronic disease diagnosis was associated with an approximately 40% increased risk of falling.

Chronic diseases also increased the risk of frequent falls and severe falls.

THE BREAKDOWN OF FALLS

Of all total falls, 17.4% occur in people with arthritis, 9.4% in people with depression, 8% in people with chronic obstructive pulmonary disease, 6.2% occur in those people who have coronary heart disease and 6.2% in people with a circulatory disease.

Only two types of drugs—sedatives and antidepressants—were associated with an increased risk of falling.

Each raised the odds by approximately 50%. In total, 2% to 5% of all falls happened in people who were taking these medications.

The findings suggest prevention and treatment of chronic disease may be the right strategy for preventing falls.

info For more on falling and the elderly, visit the *Journal of the American Medical Association* patient page at *www.hmc. psu.edu/healthinfo/articles/aging/falling.pdf*.

Coronary Bypass Can Often Improve The Quality of Life

John Spertus, MD, director, cardiovascular outcomes research, Mid America Heart Institute at Saint Luke's Hospital, and professor, medicine, University of Missouri, Kansas City, MO.

Stephen Siegel, MD, cardiologist, New York University Medical Center, and clinical assistant professor, medicine, New York University School of Medicine, New York City.

Journal of the American College of Cardiology.

Age should not deter a person from having life-improving surgery. A study shows that coronary artery bypass surgery offers people older than 75 years as much improvement in their quality of life as it does younger people.

WHY AGE IS NOT A FACTOR

"Age used to be a more important indicator of the risks and benefits of procedures than it is today," says study author Dr. John Spertus, a professor of medicine at the University of Missouri in Kansas City.

In coronary artery bypass surgery, a piece of a healthy blood vessel is used to make a detour around the blocked portion of a coronary artery.

"While older patients did have a slower pace of recovering physical function, relief of [their chest pain] was just as brisk as it was for the younger patients and the quality of life improvements were just as dramatic," adds Spertus, who is also director of cardiovascular outcomes research at the Mid America Heart Institute of Saint Luke's Hospital in Kansas City, Missouri.

THE STUDY

Spertus and his colleagues conducted their study by asking 690 people who were undergoing coronary bypass surgery to complete a questionnaire. The questionnaire was created to assess their quality of life and physical functioning before the surgery and one year later. Of the 690 study subjects, 156 were older than 75 years.

The mortality rate during surgery was slightly higher for the group older than 75, and that group was more likely to die in the year following surgery.

But, in symptom relief, the group of older people fared equally as well as the group of younger people.

"There's a sense that doing a very invasive, open procedure like bypass surgery on older patients subjects them to a lot of risk and potential pain, so one would want to be sure that there were benefits to offset the risk," Spertus says.

"What we found [from this study] was that compared with younger patients, older patients got just as much benefit in terms of quality of life," he says.

STUDY SUPPORTS CURRENT STANDARD OF CARE

Dr. Stephen Siegel, a cardiologist at New York University Medical Center, says this is a very helpful study that supports the current standard of care.

"It's clear that older patients take longer to recover, but when they do they can have a very good quality of life and enjoy life," he says.

"I don't see any reason why we should be more concerned about adding five years of life to a 60-year-old than to an 80-year-old," Siegel says.

This study did not assess who is a good candidate for surgery. Those patients included in the study already were chosen by surgeons to be good candidates for surgery, which could have affected the results.

Coronary bypass procedures substantially improve symptoms in more than 90% of patients who undergo the treatment.

The procedure also helps to prolong life in people with either left main coronary disease or blockages in several of the major vessels, especially if the pumping action of the heart is also reduced.

info To learn more about coronary bypass surgery, visit the Carolina Regional Heart Center at *http://carolinaregionalheart center.com.*

We're Living Longer— But Not as Healthy

Amy Bernstein, ScD, acting chief, analytical studies branch, National Center for Health Statistics, Centers for Disease Control and Prevention, Hyattsville, MD.
Health, United States, 2003.

The US government has announced the results of the nation's latest checkup, and there's good news and bad news.

First, the good news: Americans are living longer than they ever have before and the disparity between the longevity of blacks and whites is narrowing.

Now, the bad news: We're living longer with chronic diseases like diabetes that are the result of our sedentary ways. More Americans are also overweight and obese than ever before, and fewer of us get regular exercise.

Few of the findings are particularly surprising. "It's to be expected," says Amy Bernstein, director of the report and acting chief of the analytical studies branch at the National Center for Health Statistics in Hyattsville, Maryland. "As the population ages, the prevalence of chronic disease is almost inevitably going to go up."

LIVING LONGER

In 2001, average life expectancy hit an all-time high of 77.2 years, adding almost two years since estimates made in 1990. Women's life expectancy increased one year to 79.8 years, and men's increased two years to 74.4 years.

Although African-American people still lagged behind Caucasians in life expectancy, the gully narrowed from 5.7 years in 2000 to 5.5 years in 2001. That's a considerable improvement from the numbers that were recorded in 1990, when Caucasians lived an average of seven years longer than African-Americans.

BETTER CARE

There's also good news on the preventive-care front. The number of adult women having Pap tests is now 81%, up from 78% in 1987.

Seventy-eight percent of infants received complete childhood vaccinations, and two-thirds of elderly citizens followed recommendations and got their flu shots.

"We find that, in general, people are taking advantage of more preventive services, and that's a positive trend," Bernstein says.

MORE TROUBLING TRENDS

The number of people who smoked declined only slightly, to 25% of men and 20% of women, in 2002. Twenty-nine percent of high school students reported smoking cigarettes in the month before they were surveyed. Illicit drug use among 12- to 17-year-olds increased from 1% to 11%.

In addition, the nation is getting fatter. Almost one in three (31%) people is now obese, which is double the rate of 30 years ago. Two thirds of adults aged 20 to 74 years were overweight or obese in 1999-2000. Among children, the prevalence of those who are overweight more than doubled, from 7% to 15% in 20 years. Among adolescents, the rate more than tripled, from 5% to 16%.

Americans also proved themselves to be sedentary: 38% of female high school students and 24% of male high school students did not do the recommended amounts of exercise in 2001. The problem got worse as people got older. Nearly one fifth of men aged 65 and older and more than one quarter of women aged 65 and older were inactive.

DIABETES EPIDEMIC

Not surprisingly, all of this presages the skyrocketing diabetes rate. In 2002, 6.5% of American adults were diagnosed with diabetes, versus 5.1% in 1997. The health care associated with the disease has also increased. "One in five hospitalizations now has a diagnosis of diabetes associated with it," Bernstein says.

"People don't seem to be getting the message about diet and exercise as much as we had hoped they would," Bernstein adds. "As people get older and have the opportunity to live longer and take advantage of all the great new innovations in medical care, they also have to be responsible for some aspect of their own health care."

info *Health, United States, 2003,* is available online at the National Center for Health Statistics at *www.cdc.gov/nchs*.

The Longevity Gene— Do You Have It?

Nir Barzilai, MD, director, Institute for Aging Research, Albert Einstein College of Medicine, New York City.
Winifred K. Rossi, special assistant, planning, Geriatrics and Clinical Gerontology Program, National Institute on Aging, Bethesda, MD.
Journal of the American Medical Association.

S cientists have discovered a gene that may explain why having a long life runs in some families.

THE GENE THAT MAY BE RESPONSIBLE

The gene that may let people live into their 90s and even past 100 leads to the production of larger high-density lipoprotein (HDL) and low-density lipoprotein (LDL) molecules.

Apparently, these larger molecules protect people from the many diseases that are associated with aging, including heart disease, stroke and diabetes.

"This is the first gene that was associated with longevity," says Dr. Nir Barzilai, lead author of the study that discovered the gene. "I think there will be more."

AVOIDING THE MAJOR DISEASES

"We know that centenarians, in many cases, seem to miss getting the major diseases that kill a lot of other people at much younger ages," says Winifred K. Rossi, special assistant for planning at the National Institute on Aging, which helped fund the study.

"The question is what are the protective factors that help them get away from those major diseases," Rossi says.

THE STUDY

For the study, Barzilai and his colleagues examined blood samples that were taken from 213 Jewish men and women of Ashkenazi descent and from 216 of their children, all of whom were living in America at the time of the study.

The age of the parents ranged from 95 to 107 years, with an average age of 98 years; almost half were older than 100. The children had an average age of approximately 68 years.

WHY THE SUBJECTS WERE CHOSEN

Ashkenazi Jews, who are of Eastern European descent, are very homogenous in their genetic makeup, making them ideal subjects for studies that are looking to find single genetic mutations.

The Ashkenazi elders and their offspring were three times more likely than a control group to have a DNA alteration in a gene that helps regulate the size and blood levels of HDL and LDL molecules. The mutation resulted in increased levels of HDL and larger HDL and LDL molecules.

Although almost all the people that Barzilai has studied had larger-size molecules, only 25% had that specific genetic mutation.

"There are other genes that are probably doing the same thing," he says.

GOOD GENES BETTER THAN GOOD HABITS?

The study participants also seemed to prove that genes can override the environment.

One 103-year-old woman, for example, just celebrated 95 years of smoking two packs of cigarettes every day.

"We know that we should exercise and diet and not be overweight, but those guys could do whatever they wanted," Barzilai says.

Of 300 elders that Barzilai and his colleagues interviewed (some after this study was completed), 30% were overweight.

And Barzilai and his team of researchers cannot find a single lifestyle factor that would explain their longevity. The primary thing that these individuals had in common was parents who had lived a long time.

THE NEXT STEP

Now that the gene mutation has been discovered, the next logical step would be for a pharmaceutical company to find a drug that replicates the effect of that gene.

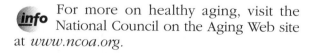 For more on healthy aging, visit the National Council on the Aging Web site at *www.ncoa.org.*

Testosterone Isn't The Way to Fight Aging

Teleconference with Dan Blazer, MD, professor of psychiatry and behavioral sciences, Duke University Medical Center, Durham, NC.

E. Darracott Vaughan Jr., MD, chairman emeritus, department of urology, Weill Medical College of Cornell University, NY.

Deborah Grady, MD, professor, School of Medicine, University of California, San Francisco.

National Institute on Aging statement.

Institute of Medicine report, *Testosterone and Aging: Clinical Research Directions.*

Although some older men believe it's a good way to fight the effects of aging, there is not enough scientific evidence to support testosterone therapy.

A recent Institute of Medicine (IOM) report stresses the need for more clinical studies on the use of the hormone, particularly in men 65 years and older.

FEW STUDIES, SKYROCKETING USAGE

To date, there have been only 31 small, short-term trials of testosterone supplementation in that age group, and most of those studies had fewer than 50 participants; only one trial lasted more than one year.

Yet the IOM report also points out that there has been a 170% increase in the number of prescriptions for testosterone since 1999. No doubt that number will be even higher for this year, notes Dr. Dan Blazer, chair of the committee that wrote the report. Blazer also is a professor of psychiatry and behavioral sciences at Duke University Medical Center in Durham, North Carolina.

"We live in a society where many people are really looking for an antiaging drug, and [testosterone] is a very popular candidate," Blazer says.

"We think the scientific community and individuals who are receiving these products need to be thinking more carefully about it," he adds.

There is a certain logic to viewing testosterone as a possible fountain of youth. Levels of the hormone decrease with aging and the possible benefits of supplementation include improvements in strength, cognitive functioning and sexual function. Potential problems, however, include an increased risk of clotting and prostate cancer.

LIMITED APPROVED USAGES

The US Food and Drug Administration has approved the hormone only for a limited number of conditions, notably hypogonadism, a condition marked by inadequate production of testosterone.

The increase in the use of testosterone as an antiaging product is also fueled by the many more ways it is now dispensed.

In the past, a monthly intramuscular injection was the only way to administer the hormone. Today, gels and patches, which are also more efficient at maintaining levels, are available, says Dr. E. Darracott Vaughan Jr., chairman emeritus of the department of urology at Weill Medical College of Cornell University in New York City and a member of the committee.

FUTURE STUDIES

The IOM report recommends that new studies should start by looking at the potential benefit of this type of supplement.

"We are interested in both the benefits and risk of testosterone therapy. But it's not worth putting up with any risk if there's absolutely no benefit, so our approach was to first try to prove there were some benefits," says Dr. Deborah Grady, another committee member and a professor at the School of Medicine of the University of California San Francisco.

It's easiest to see a benefit if you start with the group that is most likely to benefit: Men 65 years and older who have documented low testosterone levels and who are also experiencing symptoms that might be related to those low levels.

The report also recommended looking at testosterone as a therapy rather than as a preventive measure, because the evidence of any preventive benefit "is almost nil," according to Blazer.

info To access the full report on testosterone and aging, visit the National Academies Press at *www.nap.edu.*

Move Over, Botox®? New Ways to Erase Wrinkles

Neil Sadick, MD, clinical professor, dermatology, Weill Medical College, Cornell University, New York City.

Tewodros Gedebou, MD, director, plastic and reconstructive surgery/trauma, Cedars-Sinai Medical Center, Los Angeles.

Move over, Botox®. Step to the side, collagen injections. A new type of injectable antiaging treatments are coming forward to return your weathered, baby-boomer face to a kinder, gentler time.

Among the most promising are volume fillers—compounds that promise to replace those laugh lines and angry wrinkles with smooth skin.

"These are various compounds that are injected just under the skin and work to fill out the indentations that appear as age lines and wrinkles," says Dr. Neil Sadick, professor of dermatology at Weill Medical Center of Cornell University in New York City.

Unlike Botox® injections, which get rid of wrinkles by paralyzing the tiny muscles that help form the line, the new volume fillers work more like the original bovine collagen shots first popularized more than 20 years ago. They simply plump up the tissue that lies just under the surface of the wrinkle.

NEW AND IMPROVED?

The big differences between then and now? The new compounds are longer lasting and, many dermatologists believe, safer for a greater number of people.

"One to two percent of people have an allergy to bovine collagen—you don't see that with these newer treatments," says Sadick. In addition, most of the newer treatments last twice as long as collagen's three-month stay, and some last even longer than that.

Some dermatologists, however, warn the new treatments may pose potential risks, such as an allergic skin reaction or eczema.

The new volume-filler treatments generating the loudest beauty buzz include…

•**Artecoll,** an injection that combines 75% collagen with 25% microbeads of a synthetic material similar to Plexiglas.

•**Restylane,** a gentle treatment that is derived from hyaluronic acid, a fluid found naturally in human joints.

•**Radiance,** composed of tiny particles derived from calcium.

•**Hylaform,** a slightly different form of hyaluronic acid derived from rooster combs.

IS NEWER BETTER?

As intriguing as the new options are, some doctors continue to believe the tried-and-true bovine collagen injections remain the gold standard for antiaging care.

"Collagen has a safety profile that goes back more than 20 years," says Dr. Tewodros Gedebou, director of plastic and reconstructive surgery/trauma at Cedars-Sinai Medical Center in Los Angeles.

"And with the proper pretreatment testing to rule out allergic reactions, it offers both predictable results and few, if any, complications. And I don't think we can say that about these newer treatments," he says.

info For more information on a variety of antiaging treatments, visit The American Academy of Dermatology's AgingSkinNet at *www.skincarephysicians.com.*

Amazing Gadget Smoothes Sagging Necklines

Arvind Prabhat, MD, Central Jersey Otolaryngology, Shrewsbury, NJ.
Keith A. LaFerriere, Facial Plastic Surgery Center, Springfield, MO.
Archives of Facial Plastic Surgery.

A plastic implant can provide long-term improvement for the sagging neckline commonly known as "turkey neck."

The device, an under-the-skin sling stretching from earlobe to earlobe, got a nod of approval from more than 90% of patients who lived with it for three years or more, according to a recent report.

"This is a new technique that builds on existing techniques, such as removal of fat and tightening of the skin," says Dr. Arvind Prabhat, a co-author of the report. He began working on the sling technique as a fellow at Emory University School of Medicine under the supervision of Dr. Wallace K. Dyer, II, the man who pioneered the technique.

The sling can be used in combination with other plastic surgery methods, such as a facelift and liposuction, he says.

THE PROCEDURE

The sling is made of Gore-Tex®, a material widely used in medicine as well as in clothing, and is inserted using local anesthesia. The recipients take antibiotics daily for a week after the procedure. Two of the 100 patients described in the report had infections that led to removal of the sling. Two other patients had swelling caused by an accumulation of fluid that had to be drained for more than a week.

OTHER TREATMENTS SAG WITH TIME

Other techniques to improve appearance of the neck almost inevitably begin to lose their effect over time, Prabhat says. That can also happen with the sling procedure, but there is a quick fix for a slackened sling. Nine of the 100 patients in Prabhat's study needed a tightening operation, an average of 14 months after the initial procedure.

"It's a simple procedure," he says. "You go in behind the ear, find the band and tighten it. It takes about 20 minutes."

It's noteworthy that the sling recipients in the study were followed for at least three years, Prabhat says. "Most studies have just a one-year follow-up," he says.

Sling insertion is not difficult to learn, Prabhat says. "Any surgeon who has the ability to do a neck lift and face-lift can add the technique to the repertoire," he says.

The sling "has the potential to significantly improve our ability to reverse certain signs of aging in the neck," says Dr. Keith A. LaFerriere, director of the Facial Plastic Surgery Center in Springfield, Missouri.

Inflammation is a possible problem because "you're using a plastic substance where we don't usually use it," LaFerriere says. But Gore-Tex® usually causes inflammation only when it is placed close to the surface of the skin, and the sling is implanted deep enough to avoid that problem, he says.

If You're 75 or Older, You May Not Need Prostate Cancer Screening

Journal of the National Cancer Institute.
Journal of the National Cancer Institute news release.

Older men may be receiving unnecessary prostate cancer screening, a recent study suggests.

The study found doctors frequently recommend *prostate-specific antigen* (PSA) screening to men 75 years and older, even though there is general agreement that routine cancer screening of men in this age group has little benefit.

Prostate tumors typically grow slowly, so early detection is thought to improve the chances of survival. But statistics demonstrate that the mortality of men 75 years and older isn't affected by the disease.

Men between the ages of 55 and 74 are considered good candidates for prostate cancer screening. However, the latest study indicates that many men beyond the upper limit of the guidelines are undergoing testing. Screening may find a cancer in these men, but treating it will not increase life expectancy and may cause side effects.

THE STUDY

Researchers analyzed data from 7,889 men who took part in a National Health Interview Survey. Approximately 32.5% of men 75 years or older reported undergoing a PSA screening test during the previous year. On a national level, that percentage represents approximately 1.47 million American men.

Among the elderly men who reported having a PSA screening test, 88.4% said that their doctor first suggested screening.

Screening those people who are unlikely to benefit may deplete health-care resources, potentially harm patients and cause unnecessary anxiety, the authors suggest.

"Ultimately, decisions regarding the appropriateness of PSA screening in elderly men and the allocation of health-care resources will have to be made by patients, physicians and society working together," the authors write.

Age Not a Factor In Donated Kidneys

JAMA/Archives Journals news release.

People who receive kidneys from donors over the age of 55 years seem to have outcomes that are as good as people who receive kidneys from younger donors, researchers have found.

The study, conducted by scientists at Brown Medical School, notes that the percentage of deceased kidney donors aged 55 and older in the United States has increased during the last decade. That's a result of the lower death rates in people who are aged 18 to 35 and increased acceptance of kidneys from older, deceased donors.

THE STUDY

Researchers studied data from 324 people who received a kidney from a donor aged 18 years or older. The recipients were divided into groups based on donor status (living or deceased) and donor age. One group received kidneys from donors aged 54 years or younger; the other group from donors aged 55 years and older.

People who received kidneys from donors 55 years and older were older themselves (*average age:* 53.6 years) compared with the people who received kidneys from younger donors (*average age:* 43.6 years).

The study found that 12.7% of the transplants from donors 55 years and older failed, compared with a 15.2% failure rate in people who received kidneys from younger donors. Kidney function following transplant was acceptable in all groups, but was better in people who received kidneys from younger donors.

The survival rate of both groups did not differ at one, two and three years after the transplant was performed.

"Older donor kidneys provide good [graft] function in most recipients," the authors conclude. "After proper evaluation, kidneys from older deceased or living donors are appropriate for selected candidates, including older patients awaiting transplantation and those with limited life expectancy based on their severity of illness."

Each year, approximately 9,000 Americans have kidney transplants, making the operation the second most common graft procedure after corneal transplants, according to the National Institutes of Health (NIH).

Transplants are generally successful, at least in the short term—between 80% and 90% of transplants are still working within two years of the operation, the NIH says.

info For more information on kidney transplants, visit the National Kidney Foundation Web site at *www.kidney.org*.

Best Way to Beat the Flu— Vaccines

Michael B. Rothberg, MD, MPH, internist, Baystate Medical Center, Springfield, MA.

Carolyn Bridges, MD, medical epidemiologist, National Immunization Program, US Centers for Disease Control and Prevention, Atlanta.

Annals of Internal Medicine.

Giving seniors drugs to fight influenza can cut treatment costs, as well as the risk of complications and hospitalization, but vaccination remains the best strategy for this age group, according to a recent study.

Flu sends about 114,000 Americans to hospitals and kills about 36,000 people each year, the US Centers for Disease Control and Prevention (CDC) says. More than 90% of the deaths occur among people 65 years and older.

THE STUDY

Vaccination decreases the likelihood of getting the flu and reduces hospitalization by one third and mortality by half, according to the researchers.

Their study looked at published information and computer models to compare strategies for caring for patients older than 65 with influenza-like illness.

To determine the cost-effectiveness of treating older patients, the researchers weighed direct medical costs, including doctor visits, diagnostic tests, medications and hospitalization.

The researchers found treatment with the flu drug *oseltamivir* (Tamiflu) proved cost-effective for patients older than 65 who had flu-like symptoms during flu season but who had not been vaccinated or were considered at high risk for complications, including those with heart or lung disease.

But during flu season, patients who have been vaccinated and are considered at low risk for complications should be tested for flu, then given medication only if flu is detected, the study recommends.

Study author Dr. Michael B. Rothberg says complications from the flu, such as pneumonia, typically lead to hospitalization, and flu drugs can reduce such complications.

Doctors often are hesitant to prescribe flu drugs because they're expensive and won't work if the patient has a virus other than influenza, Rothberg says. He also notes that flu medication works only if taken within 48 hours of the first symptoms.

VACCINATIONS VITAL

Despite the benefits of flu medication, Rothberg stresses the vital importance of vaccinations for those who are older than 65. Vaccines cost less and are more effective than treatment, he says, and vaccinated patients live longer and incur fewer expenses than non-vaccinated patients.

But only about two thirds of Americans 65 and older have gotten annual flu vaccinations in the past three years, says Dr. Carolyn Bridges, a medical epidemiologist in the CDC's National Immunization Program.

■■■■

Who Needs a Flu Vaccination?

The CDC *strongly* recommends flu vaccines for anyone six months or older who is at increased risk for complications from influenza. This includes all people 65 and older. *Vaccines also are recommended for...*

•**People with chronic, long-term health problems** such as heart or lung disease, kidney problems, diabetes, asthma, anemia, HIV infection, AIDS or any other illness that suppresses the immune system.

•**People aged 50 to 64 years** because this group tends to have more high-risk conditions.

•**Health-care workers** and others in close contact with those at high risk, to reduce the possibility of transmitting the flu.

•**Children aged 6 to 23 months old,** their household contacts and caregivers.

Flu season typically runs from November through March or beyond. The flu season has peaked in January or later during 22 of the past 26 flu seasons, the CDC says.

info For more information on the flu, visit the National Foundation for Infectious Diseases at *www.nfid.org/library/influenza*.

The Vitamins that May Save Your Eyesight

Johanna M. Seddon, MD, ScM, director, epidemiology unit and surgeon in ophthalmology, Massachusetts Eye and Ear Infirmary, Harvard Medical School, and associate professor, Harvard School of Public Health, Boston.
Lee Jampol, MD, professor, ophthalmology, Northwestern University, Evanston, IL.
Archives of Ophthalmology.

If you're one of the millions of older people who are at risk of losing your vision to age-related macular degeneration, a simple regimen of antioxidants and zinc may save your eyesight.

If all people at risk took the antioxidants, hundreds of thousands of them would preserve their vision, according to a recent study.

The Macular Degeneration Partnership calls age-related macular degeneration "the number one cause of vision loss and legal blindness in adults over 60 in the US." It is the fastest-growing type of macular degeneration, a progressive eye disease that attacks the macula of the eye, where the sharpest central vision occurs. The condition affects 15 million people in the United States and millions more around the world.

The disease rarely causes complete blindness, but it steals all but the outermost, peripheral vision, leaving just dim images or black holes at the center of sight.

Previously, the researchers from the Age-Related Eye Disease Study (AREDS) showed that people can reduce their risk of advanced age-related macular degeneration by taking high-doses of antioxidants, including vitamin C, vitamin E and beta-carotene, plus zinc either alone or as zinc oxide.

At that time, the researchers recommended that people who had early stages of macular degeneration consider taking these vitamin supplements.

"If the AREDS recommendations were followed, more than 300,000 people with moderate to severe age-related macular degeneration could have their vision saved over the next five years," says co-researcher Johanna Seddon, an associate professor at the Harvard School of Public Health.

Since the initial findings, more physicians and patients are using the AREDS vitamin regimen, according to Seddon. Physicians should be aware of the danger of age-related macular degeneration and determine if their older patients have a family history of the condition, she says.

EYE EXAMS CRITICAL

In addition, patients older than 55 need to have regular eye exams to be sure there are no signs of age-related macular degeneration, Seddon says. Patients should also make it a point to ask their eye doctor if they notice any sign of the disease.

Seddon notes that it is becoming more apparent that nutrition plays an important role in maintaining eyesight.

"You should eat a healthful, low-fat diet with lots of fruits and vegetables and watch your cholesterol intake. Such a diet can help ward off eye disease, as well as heart disease. If necessary you can add the AREDS vitamin regimen," she says.

MANY PATIENTS NEGLECTING EYE-SAVING REGIMEN

Lee Jampol, a professor of ophthalmology at Northwestern University, comments, "It is very difficult to get elderly people to understand that they need to take the proper doses of these vitamins at the proper time." More than half his patients fail to follow the regimen, he says.

Jampol says that this problem arises partly because patients do not understand how the AREDS regimen works and partly because of the cost of the vitamins.

"Many patients are hesitant to spend money, even on medication that might save their vision," he adds.

"It is very important that ophthalmologists go over the treatment with their patients at every visit to make sure they are taking their proper doses," Jampol says.

But he cautions that patients who do not meet the criteria for age-related macular degeneration should not be on the AREDS regimen, because it will not make a difference in preserving eyesight.

"These are not multivitamins. The doses are big, and they should only be taken if you have the proper indications, as determined by your physician," Jampol says.

■ ■ ■ ■

The Difference Between The Two Types Of Macular Degeneration

The National Eye Institute explains the difference between wet and dry age-related macular degeneration (AMD)…

●**Wet AMD** occurs when abnormal blood vessels behind the retina start to grow under the macula. These new blood vessels tend to be very fragile and often leak blood and fluid, raising the macula from its normal place at the back of the eye. Wet AMD is more severe than the dry form because when this type of damage occurs, the loss of central vision happens quickly.

An early symptom of the wet form of AMD is that straight lines appear wavy. If you notice this condition or other changes to your vision, contact your eye care professional at once.

●**Dry AMD** occurs when the light-sensitive cells in the macula slowly break down, gradually blurring central vision. As dry AMD progresses, a person may see a blurred spot in the center of their vision. Over time, as less of the macula functions, central vision in the affected eye can be lost gradually.

One of the most common early signs of dry AMD is drusen—yellow deposits under the retina. Often found in people over age 60, your eye care professional can detect drusen during a comprehensive dilated eye exam.

Dry AMD has three stages, all of which may occur in one or both eyes…

●**Early AMD.** People who have early AMD have either several small drusen or a few medium-sized drusen. At this stage, there are no symptoms and no vision loss.

●**Intermediate AMD.** People who have intermediate AMD have either many medium-sized drusen or one or more large drusen. Some people see a blurred spot in the center of their vision. More light may be needed for reading and other tasks.

●**Advanced AMD.** In addition to drusen, people with advanced AMD see the blurred spot in the center of their vision getting bigger and darker, taking more of the central vision. People may have difficulty reading or recognizing faces until they are very close.

If you have vision loss from dry AMD in one eye only, you may not notice any changes in your overall vision. With the other eye seeing clearly, you still can drive, read, and see fine details. You may notice changes in your vision only if AMD affects both eyes.

info To learn more about macular degeneration, visit The Macular Degeneration Partnership at *www.amd.org*.

Great News! Multivitamins Could Cut Medicare Costs

The Lewin Group, *Study of the Cost Effects of Daily Multivitamins for Older Adults.*

There may be a new soldier in the fight against rising health-care costs for older Americans—multivitamins.

An economic impact study by The Lewin Group, a national health-care consulting firm, determined that increased daily intake of a multivitamin by older adults could save Medicare more than $1.6 billion over five years.

"The available evidence most strongly supports the beneficial effects of multivitamins in improved immune functioning and a reduction in the relative risk of heart disease," the report concludes.

Sources of potential savings, say the researchers, would include fewer hospitalizations for infection and heart attacks, a reduction in Medicare nursing home stays for infection, and a reduction in home health care associated with infection (pneumonia).

The authors analyzed 128 clinical studies and concluded that older adults who take a daily multivitamin can reduce their risk of cardiovascular disease by 24% and improve their immune system function.

THE SAVINGS

The results show that in 2004 it would cost approximately $149 million to provide each American older than 65 years with a daily multivitamin. However, the health benefits offered by multivitamins would reduce the costs of nursing home stays, hospitalizations and home health care associated with pneumonia, sepsis and other infections by about $83 million. And there would be another $215 million in savings because of lower hospital admissions from cardiac disease, including heart attacks, the study says.

Over five years, the total savings in Medicare costs were estimated to be $1.6 billion.

Only about one third of Americans currently take a daily multivitamin. And many fall as much as 50% short of getting the daily dosage of vitamins recommended by the American Dietetic Association, the study notes.

■ ■ ■ ■

Know Your Vitamins

There are two types of vitamins—fat-soluble and water-soluble. When you eat foods that contain fat-soluble vitamins, the vitamins are stored in the fat tissues in your body and in your liver. They wait in your body fat until your body needs them. Then, when it's time for them to be used, special carriers in your body take them to where they're needed. Vitamins A, D, E and K are all fat-soluble vitamins.

Water-soluble vitamins are not stored in your body. Instead, they travel through your bloodstream, and whatever your body doesn't use comes out when you urinate. This group of vitamins includes vitamin C and the B vitamins—B-1 (thiamin), B-2 (riboflavin), niacin, B-6 (pyridoxine), folic acid, B-12 (cobalamine), biotin and pantothenic acid.

info You can learn more about vitamins from the Harvard School of Public Health's Web site at *www.hsph.harvard.edu/nutritionsource.*

Hidden Threats to Older Adults

Carol Colleran, national director, older adult services, Hanley-Hazelden Center, West Palm Beach, FL, which provides abstinence-based recovery services for those with substance abuse problems.
Bottom Line/Health.

Most people don't think of a silver-haired retiree as a substance abuser, but it happens all too often.

According to a report from the Substance Abuse and Mental Health Services Administration (SAMHSA), a federal agency, one in six American adults aged 60 or older are believed to use alcohol or prescription drugs in destructive, uncontrolled ways.

When addiction takes hold in anybody, considerable health hazards may accompany it. These health hazards include hypertension, brain damage, liver ailments, secondary diabetes, memory loss and stroke.

WHY IT HAPPENS

Although many older people who abuse alcohol and drugs have had substance abuse problems all their lives, for a rising proportion —approximately one third—difficulties with alcohol and drugs start after age 50.

Perhaps the single most common contributing factor in late-onset substance abuse is a loss of a sense of purpose, which frequently occurs when an older adult enters retirement or finishes raising a family.

This is a real danger for people who may have given considerable thought to financial planning, but little to the "emotional retirement" that occurs when work is left behind.

In one's personal life, the death of a spouse brings not only the ache of bereavement, but also a terrible sense that the survivor is no longer needed.

ACCIDENTAL ADDICTION

Drug or alcohol problems can sneak up on people who have no idea they're engaging in risky behavior. *Here's how...*

●**Alcohol.** As we age, the changes that occur in our bodies dramatically affect how we respond to alcohol.

For example, the water content of the body decreases and the fat content increases, which slows the rate at which some substances are metabolized. This can result in quicker intoxication and greater damage to the liver, kidneys and other organs.

A slowdown in the liver, stomach and kidneys also reduces the rate at which alcohol is broken down and processed. *Result:* Even when you consume small amounts, it builds up and the effects last longer.

Women become intoxicated faster than men from small amounts of alcohol. In general, women have less body water than men of similar body weight, so women achieve higher concentrations of alcohol in the blood after drinking equivalent amounts.

Result: Many people who continue drinking the same modest quantities that they have for years—or even less than they used to— start running into difficulties.

To protect yourself: Limit your alcohol intake to no more than two drinks a day for older men, and one drink a day for women. (One drink equals one five-ounce glass of wine, one 12-ounce wine cooler, 1.5 ounces of hard liquor or one 12-ounce glass of beer.)

●**Drugs.** Most older adults don't intend to get high. But they can become dependent on medications that their doctors prescribed for medical reasons.

Most common offenders: Opiate painkillers, including *codeine, oxycodone* (OxyContin) and *acetaminophen* and *oxycodone* (Percocet)...and anxiety-quelling benzodiazepines, such as *diazepam* (Valium) and *alprazolam* (Xanax).

Caution: Do *not* discontinue any medication without first consulting your doctor.

Problem: Most drugs are tested only on younger people, and doctors fail to adjust the dose to take into account the slower metabolism of older adults.

Most of these drugs are stored in body fat. Because the aging body has a higher proportion of fatty tissue, more of the drug remains in the fat, lessening its effect on the body. This often causes the person to take more of the drug.

Also: Doctors frequently fail to follow the guidelines advising that these medications be used only for limited periods. It's not unusual, for example, to see older adults who have been taking Valium regularly for 20 years.

To protect yourself: Whenever you are prescribed a drug, ask your doctor why you are taking it...how long it should be used... and whether it's known to cause addiction.

TREATING A HIDDEN EPIDEMIC

Substance abuse problems in older adults often go undetected. That's partially because many red flags that would arouse attention in a younger person are dismissed as simply the effects of aging. These red flags include shaky hands…balance problems…erratic driving… and loss of memory.

If a problem is identified, treatment typically includes a medical evaluation, nutritional plan and counseling. Whenever possible, older adults should undergo treatment with people of the same age, studies have found.

Twelve-step programs, such as Alcoholics Anonymous or Narcotics Anonymous, are excellent resources for older adults.

info To find additional help, contact the Substance Abuse and Mental Health Services Administration at *www.findtreatment. samhsa.gov.*

Once-a-Week Resistance Training Keeps Older Folks on Their Feet

Interview, Colin Milner, president, International Council on Active Aging.
Journal of Gerontology: Biological Sciences.
Ball State University, Muncie, IN news release.

Older adults can maintain their muscle strength by doing resistance training just once a week, a study says.

Sarcopenia, a condition that is characterized by the loss of muscle mass and strength, is commonly associated with aging. Sarcopenia-related problems, such as falls, can cause injuries and the loss of independence for older adults and result in millions of dollars in health-care costs.

Researchers at Ball State University examined a group of 10 men, with an average age of 70 years, who had spent three months building up muscle strength by training with resistance equipment three times a week. The strength increases experienced by the men in that time ranged from 20% to 90%.

Over the following six months, half of the men continued to do their resistance training once a week and they maintained their muscle size and strength. The other five men returned to their previous routines of no regular

physical exercise and they lost muscle strength and mass.

"Engaging in a once-a-week resistance training program seems to be effective to prevent the advancement of sarcopenia. Older adults could engage in a low-volume, high-intensity program and still maintain independence and reduce their chances for falls and injuries," says Scott Trappe, director of Ball State University's Human Performance Laboratory in Muncie, Indiana.

It can be difficult for older people who are interested in exercise to find a way to start a program because most exercise facilities and programs are aimed at younger people, says Colin Milner, head of the International Council on Active Aging, a trade association of more than 3,500 organizations that specializes in senior fitness.

"While many organizations are trying to accommodate an older crowd—such as YMCAs, hospital wellness centers and retirement communities with trained staffs—the vast majority of health centers are still very youth-oriented," he says. "The fitness industry has portrayed exercise as an activity for younger people, and the message turns off the elderly."

■■■■

Getting Started

The International Council on Active Aging provides some guidelines to help seniors increase their physical activity…

•**Get a checkup** to find out if there are any physical modifications you have to incorporate into an exercise plan.

•**Find your baseline of activity** by keeping a diary of your physical movement, tracking how much time you are sedentary (watching television, sitting at a desk) and active (walking to your car, preparing a meal, doing chores around the house).

•**Think about the most enjoyable way for you to exercise.**

•**Check out any facility before you join.** If you want to join a gym, visit it to see if it feels comfortable and if the staff is friendly and trained in the type of exercise that accommodates your needs.

•**Make a date to exercise.** Once you've figured out what you'd like to do, put it into your schedule.

•**Set specific short- and long-term goals.** Decide how many times a week you will do your activity.

•**Increase your activity in your daily life.** Move around when you're talking on the phone, stand up and move during television commercials, do your own yard and house work, and walk as much as possible to local stores by parking your car in the back of the parking lot.

•**Don't quit.**

info You can learn more about exercise for seniors from a National Institutes of Health Web site at *http://health.nih.gov.*

■ ■ ■ ■

Strength Exercises for Older People

Just because you're getting older, you don't have to lose your muscle tone or strength. *The National Institute on Aging suggests these strengthening exercises as part of its senior fitness program…*

HOW MUCH, HOW OFTEN?

Perform strength exercises for all your major muscle groups at least twice a week. Don't do strength exercises for the same muscle group two days in a row. Depending on how fit you are, you might need to start out with 1- or 2-pound weights, or no weight at all, to allow your body to adapt to strength exercises.

ARM RAISES STRENGTHEN SHOULDER MUSCLES

1. Sit in a chair with your back straight.

2. Keep feet flat on the floor, even with your shoulders.

3. Hold hand weights straight down at your sides with palms facing toward your body. (You can substitute cans of soup or start without weights.)

4. Raise both arms to sides, shoulder height.

5. Hold the position for 1 second.

6. Slowly lower arms to the sides. Pause.

7. Repeat 8 to 15 times.

8. Rest. Do another set of 8 to 15 repetitions.

CHAIR STANDS STRENGTHEN STOMACH AND THIGH MUSCLES

1. Place pillows against the back of chair.

2. Sit in the middle or toward front of chair, knees bent, feet flat on floor.

3. Lean back on the pillows in half-reclining position, keeping your back and shoulders straight.

4. Raise the upper body forward until sitting upright, using hands as little as possible —or not at all, if you can. Your back should no longer be leaning against the pillows.

5. Slowly stand up, again, using hands as little as possible.

6. Slowly sit back down. Keep back and shoulders straight throughout the exercise.

7. Repeat 8 to 15 times.

8. Rest. Then repeat 8 to 15 times more.

BICEP CURLS STRENGTHEN UPPER-ARM MUSCLES

1. Sit in an armless chair. Keep feet flat on the floor and even with shoulders.

2. Hold hand weights straight down at your sides with palms facing toward your body.

3. Slowly bend one elbow, lifting the weight toward the chest. Be sure to rotate the palm to face the shoulder while lifting weight.

4. Hold this position for 1 second. Slowly lower arm to starting position.

5. Repeat with the other arm. Alternate until you have repeated the exercise 8 to 15 times on each side.

6. Rest. Then do another set of 8 to 15 alternating repetitions.

TRICEPS EXTENSIONS STRENGTHEN MUSCLES IN THE BACK OF THE ARM

1. Sit near the front edge of a chair, feet flat on the floor and even with shoulders.

2. Hold a weight in one hand, raise that arm straight toward the ceiling, palm facing in.

3. Support the arm below the elbow with the other hand.

4. Slowly bend the raised arm at elbow, bringing the hand weight down toward the same shoulder.

5. Slowly restraighten the arm toward ceiling. Hold this position for 1 second.

6. Slowly bend the arm toward the shoulder again.

7. Pause, and then repeat the bending and straightening until you have done the exercise 8 to 15 times. Repeat 8 to 15 times with the other arm.

8. Rest. Then repeat another set of 8 to 15 repetitions on each side.

KNEE FLEXING STRENGTHENS MUSCLES IN THE BACK OF THE THIGH

1. Stand straight, holding onto a table or chair for balance.

2. Slowly bend one knee as far as possible, lifting the foot up behind you. Don't move your upper leg at all; bend your knee only.

3. Hold this position.

4. Slowly lower the foot down to the floor.

5. Repeat with the other leg.

6. Alternate legs until you perform 8 to 15 repetitions with each leg.

7. Rest. Then do another set of 8 to 15 alternating repetitions.

■ ■ ■ ■

Brisk Walking Builds Bone Mass

According to Katarina T. Borer, professor of movement science at the Center for Exercise Research at the University of Michigan, postmenopausal women who walked three miles fast enough to become winded, five days a week for 15 weeks, increased their bone mineral density by 0.4%. This can be compared with a 1% bone-density loss in those who walked at a slower, less challenging pace.

Theory: Intense exercise triggers greater secretion of hormones that may increase bone mineralization.

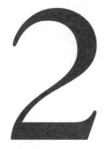

2

Alzheimer's Disease

Inflammation and the Alzheimer's Connection

Inflammation—the protective reaction of the body's tissue to injury or infection—may be a leading culprit in the loss of mental agility with age, researchers are finding. And a recent study adds weight to the hypothesis that inflammatory processes in the body play a role in several age-related diseases, including Alzheimer's. "There has been a lot of [medical] literature suggesting that inflammation may contribute to Alzheimer's disease and other disorders of aging," says study author Dr. Kristen Yaffe, an assistant professor of psychiatry, neurology and epidemiology at the University of California, San Francisco.

THE STUDY

Yaffe and her colleagues studied 3,031 men and women with an average age of 74 years. The scientists looked at the blood levels of three known markers of inflammation—C-reactive protein, interleukin-6 (IL-6) and tumor necrosis factor. They repeated the tests two years later. They also gave a battery of mental tests to evaluate concentration, memory, language and other measures of cognitive functioning, both at the start of the study and two years later.

THE RESULTS

After adjusting for age and other factors, the researchers found that those who had the highest levels of inflammation had more cognitive decline than those whose levels of those substances were in the lowest third.

ANTI-INFLAMMATORY DRUGS PROBED

Researchers are now looking at whether preventing inflammation with medication makes any difference in cognitive function. But

Kristen Yaffe, MD, assistant professor, psychiatry, neurology and epidemiology, University of California, San Francisco, and chief, geriatric psychiatry, San Francisco VA Medical Center.

Joseph Quinn, MD, neurologist, Portland VA Medical Center, and assistant professor, neurology, Oregon Health & Science University, Portland.

Neurology.

Yaffe says it's too soon to recommend taking drugs to ward off age-related cognitive decline.

To date, the results of research indicate anti-inflammatory drugs show more promise as a preventive option, rather than as a treatment.

Adds another expert, Dr. Joseph Quinn, a neurologist at the Portland (Oregon) VA Medical Center, "There are only two other studies that have suggested that inflammatory markers predict future cognitive abilities. And this one is different because it includes multiple markers of inflammation and includes large numbers of African-Americans."

"It is a very solid study," Quinn says. *But he adds a caveat:* "It is also important to note that these results do not mean that people should start taking anti-inflammatory medicines for the prevention of Alzheimer's."

■ ■ ■ ■

Warning Signs

An estimated 4.5 million Americans have Alzheimer's disease, according to the Alzheimer's Association.

The condition, which has no cure, is the nation's leading cause of dementia, the umbrella term for the loss of mental skills like memory, judgment and the ability to carry out routine tasks of daily life.

Although Alzheimer's disease cannot be stopped, drugs can delay the progression of symptoms by a matter of months. Ultimately, however, the disorder destroys so much of the brain that it is uniformly deadly.

The early signs of Alzheimer's are difficult to distinguish from the normal lapses of memory and mental function that nearly everyone experiences at one time or another. *But the Alzheimer's Association offers the following 10 warning signs...*

1. Memory loss. People who have dementia forget addresses, phone numbers and other information more often than what is considered normal. And, unlike normal forgetting, they won't remember these facts later.

2. Difficulty performing familiar tasks. People who have dementia often have trouble with everyday tasks that most of us find to be second nature. A person with Alzheimer's may forget how to use a can opener or how to perform their lifelong hobby.

3. Problems with language. Everyone has trouble finding the right word sometimes, but a person who has Alzheimer's disease often forgets simple words or substitutes unusual words.

4. Disorientation to time and place. People who have Alzheimer's disease can become lost on the street where they live, forget where they are and how they got there and not know how to get home.

5. Poor or decreased judgment. Individuals who have Alzheimer's disease may dress without considering the weather, wearing very little clothing in cold weather, for example. They may show poor judgment about money, giving away large amounts of money to telemarketers or paying for home repairs they don't need.

6. Problems with abstract thinking. Balancing a checkbook is difficult for many people, but for someone with Alzheimer's disease, it may become totally impossible. They could completely forget what the numbers are and what needs to be done with them.

7. Misplacing things. Anyone can temporarily misplace his/her wallet or key. *A person with Alzheimer's disease may put things in unusual places:* an iron in the freezer or a wristwatch in the sugar bowl.

8. Changes in mood or behavior. Everyone can become sad or moody from time to time. Someone with Alzheimer's disease can show rapid mood swings—from calm to tears to anger—for no apparent reason.

9. Changes in personality. People's personalities ordinarily change somewhat with age. But a person with Alzheimer's disease can change a lot, becoming extremely confused, suspicious, fearful or dependent on a family member.

10. Loss of initiative. It's normal to tire of housework, business activities or social obligations at times. The person with Alzheimer's disease may become very passive, sitting in front of the television for hours, sleeping more than usual or not wanting to do usual activities.

Everyday Painkillers
May Block Memory Loss!

Lon Schneider, MD, professor, psychiatry, neurology and gerontology, Keck School of Medicine, University of Southern California, Los Angeles.

Theo Palmer, PhD, assistant professor, neurosurgery, Stanford University, Palo Alto, CA.

John C. Morris, MD, professor, neurology, and director, Alzheimer's Disease Research Center, Washington University School of Medicine, St. Louis, MO.

Science.

Two studies indicate that nonsteroidal anti-inflammatory drugs (NSAIDs), including aspirin and other aspirin-like drugs such as ibuprofen, can restore brain cell (neuron) production and decrease harmful levels of amyloid beta proteins by reducing inflammation.

Amyloid beta proteins form clumps in the brains of people who have Alzheimer's, and those clumps are suspected to cause or at least contribute to the disease. The buildup of amyloid beta-42 seems to be the most harmful form of these proteins.

The results of these two studies suggest that memory and learning problems in conditions such as Alzheimer's and other types of dementias, stroke and traumatic brain injury might be helped by a simple drug, a researcher says.

THE FIRST STUDY

In one study, Dr. Steven Paul and researchers from the drug maker Eli Lilly and Co. report that anti-inflammatory drugs can reduce the production of amyloid beta proteins, including amyloid beta-42.

These results support the notion that NSAIDs have a protective effect against future neurodegeneration, says Dr. Lon Schneider, a professor of psychiatry, neurology and gerontology at the University of Southern California.

Schneider believes trials are needed to see which NSAIDs might prevent dementia and treat head injury and stroke.

THE SECOND STUDY

In another study, a team led by Theo Palmer, an assistant professor of neurosurgery at Stanford University, experimented with rats to see if reducing brain inflammation might have an effect on neuron production.

"The dogma for many decades has been that the brain doesn't replace neurons, but that is not true. There are regions of the brain that continue to make neurons throughout life. These new neurons are made by stem cells called precursors," Palmer says.

These new neurons may be important for memory and learning, he adds.

The team found that in rats with brain inflammation, the production of new neurons stopped. However, when they treated the rats with the anti-inflammatory drug indomethacin, the production of neurons was completely restored.

These results suggest that people with Alzheimer's, stroke and brain injury might benefit from a simple drug such as indomethacin, Palmer says.

Dr. John Morris, director of the Alzheimer's Disease Research Center at Washington University School of Medicine, comments, "These reports suggest that commonly used anti-inflammatory drugs may lessen the toxic effects of brain inflammation believed to be important in Alzheimer's disease."

"However, neither study involved human subjects. Whether the positive effects shown in these experimental models translate to actual patients is far from clear," Morris says.

info Get an explanation of how NSAIDs reduce inflammation at the American Academy of Orthopaedic Surgeons Web site, *www.orthoinfo.aaos.org.*

■ ■ ■ ■

History of Alzheimer's

According to the National Institute on Aging, Alzheimer's disease is named after Dr. Alois Alzheimer, a German doctor. In 1906, Dr. Alzheimer noticed changes in the brain tissue of a woman who had died of an unusual mental illness. He found abnormal clumps and tangled bundles of fibers, today considered one of the signs of Alzheimer's disease.

Scientists also have found other brain changes in people with the disease. Nerve cells die in areas of the brain that are vital to memory and other mental abilities. Researchers also believe the disease may reduce the levels of some brain chemicals that carry messages between nerve cells.

The disease usually begins after age 60 years, and the risk of getting it increases with age. Approximately 5% of men and women ages 65 to 74 years have the disease, and nearly half of those age 85 and older suffer from it.

info The National Institute on Aging has more information at their Alzheimer's Disease Education and Referral Center (ADEAR) at *www.alzheimers.org.*

Antibiotics May Ease Alzheimer's Disease

Mark B. Loeb, MD, MSc, associate professor, pathology and molecular medicine, McMaster University, Hamilton, Ontario, Canada.

Bill Thies, PhD, vice president, medical and scientific affairs, Alzheimer's Association, Chicago.

Presentation, Infectious Diseases Society of America annual meeting, San Diego.

Two common antibiotics, when taken together, may improve the symptoms of Alzheimer's disease, according to a new Canadian study.

But the lead researcher says the concept needs more study before it is recommended, and the Alzheimer's Association urges caution about the results.

"It's not ready for prime time," says Dr. Mark B. Loeb, an associate professor in the pathology and molecular medicine department at McMaster University in Hamilton, Ontario.

THE STUDY

In the study, Loeb's group decided to focus on antibiotic treatment because one theory suggests the bacterium *Chlamydia pneumoniae* may play a role in causing Alzheimer's.

However, in the study, the antibiotics did not cause a drop in the levels of the bacteria as greatly as would be expected. Loeb speculates the antibiotics may work instead by interfering

with the accumulation of protein plaques around the brain's neurons, which are associated with the disease. "Or it could be a local anti-inflammatory effect," he says.

Researchers looked at 101 patients who had "probable" Alzheimer's and mild-to-moderate dementia. The team randomly assigned them to one of two groups. One group received 200 milligrams (mg) of the antibiotic doxycycline and 300 mg of rifampin daily for three months. The other group, the control group, received a placebo.

The researchers evaluated the patients before the study using a standard Alzheimer's test to determine mental functioning, and repeated the test after six months with the patients who remained in the study—43 remained in the antibiotic group and 39 remained in the placebo group.

THE RESULTS

The mental functioning scores of participants in the control group declined on average by 2.75 more points on a 70-point scale than did those in the treated group. At 12 months there still was a difference in function, but it was not a significant one.

"The magnitude of the difference was similar to the effects seen with therapy with cholinesterase inhibitors," Loeb says. Cholinesterase inhibitors, which are approved by the US Food and Drug Administration to treat cognitive Alzheimer's symptoms, are meant to boost memory and other cognitive functions by influencing certain chemical activities in the brain.

However, caution in using antibiotic treatment for Alzheimer's was urged by Bill Thies, vice president of medical and scientific affairs for the Alzheimer's Association. "It's a relatively small study, with a relatively short follow-up," he says. Although the idea definitely deserves more research attention, Thies says, "It's not a clarion call to put large parts of the population on antibiotic therapy."

And, Thies notes, the number of Alzheimer's experts who think the Chlamydia pneumoniae bacteria play a role in the onset of the disease is small. But, he is quick to add, "That doesn't mean [the concept] isn't right."

info For more information about Alzheimer's disease, visit the National Institutes of Health SeniorHealth Web site at *http://nih seniorhealth.gov.*

Cancer Drug Helps Conquer Alzheimer's

William Netzer, PhD, research associate, Fisher Center for Research on Alzheimer's Disease, Rockefeller University, New York City.
Proceedings of the National Academy of Sciences.

The cancer-fighting drug Gleevec shows some promise in the treatment of Alzheimer's disease, researchers say.

Gleevec has been tested only in guinea pigs and cells in a dish, and researchers don't yet know if it will work in humans. But a study showed that Gleevec significantly reduced the buildup of harmful proteins in brain cells that have been linked to Alzheimer's.

Chiefly used against chronic myeloid leukemia, Gleevec has been so effective against the blood cancer that it has been called a cure for the disease.

One of Gleevec's effects is to compete for proteins in cells that bind with *adenosine triphosphate,* or ATP, the chemical energy courier in living things. ATP plays a role in the formation of amyloid beta, the protein many researchers believe is to blame for the brain cell damage in Alzheimer's disease, because ATP improves the efficiency of an enzyme called gamma-secretase which helps cells produce amyloid beta.

Preventing the production or buildup of amyloid beta is one of the central aims of Alzheimer's research. However, blocking ATP is dangerous—done carelessly, it kills cells and the bodies they comprise. Intrigued, William Netzer, an Alzheimer's expert at the Rockefeller University in New York City, and his colleagues sought to learn if Gleevec could suppress amyloid beta production with minimal side effects.

"We had lots of ATP inhibitors, but they're all very toxic," Netzer says. "We felt that if we could inhibit ATP without killing the organism we might be able to inhibit gamma-secretase and inhibit amyloid beta."

Netzer and his colleagues, including Nobel Prize winner Paul Greengard, tested the cancer drug in brain cells harvested from rat fetuses, against human amyloid beta proteins in the laboratory, and also in live albino guinea pigs, whose amyloid beta is similar to what humans produce.

In each case, amyloid beta levels dropped in cells exposed to Gleevec. The effect increased as the dose of the drug rose—an important measure of genuine effect—to as much as a 50% reduction compared with untreated cells.

There is at least one catch. Gleevec doesn't reach the brain particularly well, barred at the door by the blood-brain barrier, a molecular gate that locks large molecules out of the brain.

"Most important," Netzer says, "We do not yet know whether Gleevec or related compounds will actually help human Alzheimer's patients or whether they will be safe when introduced into the brain."

The researchers' next step is to uncover what protein or proteins Gleevec tweaks that ultimately allow it to block amyloid beta buildup. Learning its mechanics could lead to more treatments for Alzheimer's disease, Netzer says.

New Alzheimer's Drug Shows Promise

Paul Aisen, MD, professor, neurology and medicine, and director, Memory Disorders Program, Georgetown University Medical Center, Washington, DC.
Steven Ferris, PhD, director, Alzheimer's Disease Center, Silberstein Institute for Aging and Dementia, New York University Medical Center, New York City.
Presentations, 15th International Conference on Alzheimer's Disease and Related Disorders, Philadelphia.

A study has found that a drug to treat Alzheimer's was "safe and well-tolerated" in 58 patients.

It is widely agreed that the cause of Alzheimer's, or at least its symptoms, are a result of the accumulation of protein called amyloid beta in the brain.

To combat Alzheimer's, scientists have been trying various approaches: Clearing away the accumulations, or "plaques," after they have developed; preventing the protein pieces from forming plaques; and stopping the formation of the protein in the first place.

The new drug, called Alzhemed, works by interfering with the ability of these proteins to stick together.

"We were able to establish that the drug is safe, that it gets into the brain and also that it reduces amyloid levels, so the results are very encouraging," says study author Dr. Paul Aisen, a professor of neurology and medicine and director of the Memory Disorders Program at Georgetown University Medical Center in Washington, DC.

Ideally, the drug would be used to treat people in the extremely preliminary stages of the disease to prevent progression into full-blown Alzheimer's, Aisen says.

The current study, while important, is small and of short duration, warns Steven Ferris, director of the Alzheimer's Disease Center at the Silberstein Institute for Aging and Dementia at New York University Medical Center. "There's a hint that it's doing what it's supposed to do, but it's not a big enough study or a long enough study where you would expect to see any clinical effect," he says.

Found! The Missing Molecule that Protects Against Alzheimer's

Kun Ping Lu, MD, PhD, associate professor, medicine, Harvard Medical School, Boston.
Bill Thies, PhD, vice president, medical and scientific affairs, Alzheimer's Association, Chicago.
Nature.

Alzheimer's disease, a neurodegenerative condition that affects people as they age, is marked by a progressive loss of mental function.

The brains of people with Alzheimer's have been shown to possess two distinctive characteristics: "Tangles" in the brain's neurons and "plaques" made up of amyloid protein.

According to new research, a missing enzyme may be responsible for these tangles of proteins that form in the brains of people with Alzheimer's disease. That enzyme, called *Pin1,* may therefore play a protective role in the aging brain.

To date, more research on the disease has focused on plaques rather than on tangles, says Bill Thies, vice president of medical and scientific affairs for the Alzheimer's Association.

UNRAVELING TANGLES

The brain tangles are made up of amyloid beta, a protein that is also present in normal cells. Its function is to assemble and maintain the cell's structure that links one end of a nerve cell to another and transports nutrients and structural components, explains Dr. Kun Ping Lu, the author of the study, who is also an associate professor of medicine at Harvard Medical School.

In people with Alzheimer's disease, this protein changes shape and collects into these tangles, which destroy neurons in that area of the brain.

In research facilities, tangles have been overlooked compared with plaques, and scientists have tended to focus on the overexpression of genes rather than the underexpression, says Lu. "We went in a completely different direction: how to protect the neuron from undergoing age-dependent degeneration," he says. "We identified Pin1, an enzyme which changes the shape of the protein in the neuron. This suggests that Pin1 may play an important role in protecting neurons."

To test the hypothesis, the researchers conducted two experiments.

THE STUDY

First they compared Pin1 levels in different regions of the brains of both healthy people and of people who had died of Alzheimer's. "There was a striking difference in levels of the enzyme in different regions of brains," Lu reports. Areas in the brain that had been injured by Alzheimer's tended to have very low levels of Pin1. "That suggests Pin1 may help protect against neurodegeneration," he says.

Next, the researchers looked at mice that had had the gene for Pin1 removed. All of these mice went on to develop age-related neurodegeneration changes, including tangle formation and loss of neurons that occur in patients with age-dependent Alzheimer's disease.

FINDING MAY OPEN WINDOW

The discovery won't translate into practical help anytime soon, but Thies says, "it might give us a window on a mechanism that could be useful."

The next step might be to find out if people with Alzheimer's had a genetic variation that caused them to produce less of Pin1.

As a footnote to this study, Lu's lab has also found that Pin1 is overexpressed in many human cancers and plays an important role in the development of cancer. "It would appear that certain cancers share common genetic elements with Alzheimer's disease, suggesting that Pin1 may prove to be the missing link between these two seemingly distinct areas of disease, both of which grow much more common with age," Lu says.

info For more information about Alzheimer's disease, visit the National Institute of Neurological Disorders and Stroke at *www.ninds.nih.gov.*

Uncovered: A Real Cause of Alzheimer's

Neuroscience.
Saint Louis University news release.

Many researchers believe Alzheimer's disease results from the buildup of toxic, tangled proteins in the brain. A recent study offers a twist on that theory, suggesting that the brains of Alzheimer's patients aren't able to expel the harmful molecules.

At the heart of the finding is a harmful protein called amyloid beta. Restoring the brain's natural ability to shed it could provide scientists with a new approach for treating Alzheimer's, experts say.

"It's going to be a big piece toward solving the Alzheimer's disease puzzle," says lead author Dr. William A. Banks, a professor of geriatrics and pharmacological science.

In healthy people, the dangerous protein can leave the brain by crossing through the blood-brain barrier, a semi-permeable defensive wall that usually stops harmful molecules from entering the brain. In people with Alzheimer's disease, amyloid beta protein can't pass through that barrier to leave the brain. As more amyloid beta protein accumulates in a person's brain, he/she becomes more and more mentally disabled.

Banks says that finding ways to repair the system that transports amyloid beta protein across the blood-brain barrier could lead to treatments for Alzheimer's disease.

"We need to find therapies to bring the transportation system back on line to pump the amyloid beta protein out of the brain," Banks says.

Discovery of Alzheimer's 'Protein' Could Mean Better Drugs

Proceedings of the National Academy of Sciences.
Northwestern University.

A protein that may be responsible for the memory loss suffered by people with Alzheimer's disease has been identified by researchers at Northwestern University.

This protein could provide scientists with information about the progression of Alzheimer's and help develop new drugs capable of reversing memory loss in those diagnosed and treated at an early stage of the disease.

The Northwestern University researchers found that the brain tissue of people who had Alzheimer's contained up to 70 times more small, soluble aggregated proteins, called ADDLs (amyloid b-derived diffusible ligands), than normal brain tissue.

HOW THEY WORK

Their study supports a recent theory which suggests that ADDLs accumulate at the beginning of Alzheimer's disease and block the memory function by a process that scientists believe is reversible.

ADDLs attack the memory-building activity of synapses, which are communication points in the brain where neurons exchange information. ADDLs affect the synapses, but do so without killing neurons.

"For more than a decade, researchers thought it was big molecules, the 'amyloid fibrils,' that caused memory problems, but we think the real culprits are extremely small molecules—what we call ADDLs," explains research team leader William L. Klein, a professor of neurobiology and physiology.

"Now we've shown that ADDLs are present in humans and are a clinically valid part of Alzheimer's pathology. If we can develop drugs that target and neutralize these neurotoxins, it might be possible to not only slow down memory loss, but to actually reverse it, to bring memory function back to normal," Klein adds.

Penny for Your Thoughts? Copper May Shield Brain From Alzheimer's

David Westaway, associate professor, University of Toronto, Ontario, Canada.

Thomas Bayer, PhD, associate professor, Saarland University Medical Center, Homburg/Saar, Germany.

Proceedings of the National Academy of Sciences.

In the past, the element copper was thought to play a role in the development of Alzheimer's disease, but two recent studies turn that theory on its head.

New research indicates that mice with more copper in their brain cells are less likely to develop the toxic protein fragments called amyloid beta that are associated with Alzheimer's.

TWO STUDIES

In one study, German scientists found mice with a genetic predisposition to the brain disease lived longer and had less amyloid beta when they drank copper-laced water than did those that didn't get the supplements.

In a second study, scientists in Canada and the United States showed that mice with high amounts of copper in their brain cells had approximately half as much amyloid beta buildup as mice with lower amounts of copper in their brains.

"There has been the suggestion that elevations of copper can help drive Alzheimer's disease, but we don't get that," says study leader David Westaway, a brain researcher at the University of Toronto. "When we drove up levels of copper in the brain, some of the hallmarks of Alzheimer's disease improved."

Thomas Bayer, a neuroscientist at Saarland University Medical Center, in Homburg/Saar, Germany, and leader of the first study, says, "If you give mice copper, either in water or by genetic manipulation, you reduce amyloid beta" and prolong their life.

How copper and amyloid beta are related isn't yet understood. Bayer's group thinks the link involves an enzyme in the brain called *amyloid beta precursor protein,* or APP.

Copper normally controls this molecule. But as people age, the copper levels in their brains fall. As a result, Bayer speculates, APP can generate the amyloid beta proteins that destroy neurons.

"If copper is bound to APP, you don't get amyloid beta. If APP is copper-free, amyloid beta is produced directly," he says.

Bayer is not recommending that people take copper supplements at this point. Much more study is needed.

info For more information on Alzheimer's disease, visit the National Library of Medicine's MedlinePlus Web site at *www.nlm. nih.gov/medlineplus/alzheimersdisease.html.*

MRI May Predict Dementia Before Symptoms Appear

Henry Rusinek, PhD, associate professor, radiology, New York University School of Medicine, New York City.

Mony J. de Leon, EdD, professor, psychiatry, and director, Center for Brain Health, New York University School of Medicine, New York City.

Radiology.

L osing brain mass is a natural part of getting older, but people who lose it quickly are at increased risk for Alzheimer's disease, a study says.

"With the help of MRI imaging over time, we are capable of detecting cognitive impairment, which may lead to Alzheimer's disease, before the patient shows clinical symptoms," says lead researcher Henry Rusinek, an associate professor of radiology at New York University School of Medicine.

Symptoms of Alzheimer's disease include memory loss, language deterioration, poor judgment, confusion, restlessness and mood swings. Eventually the disease destroys cognition, personality and the ability to function.

THE STUDY

Rusinek and his team of researchers studied 45 healthy patients, 60 years and older. These patients underwent six years of MRI imaging of their medial temporal lobe at two-year intervals. The medial temporal lobe is near the middle of the brain, which includes areas critical to forming new memories.

The researchers compared the images from year to year. "The normal brain shrinks at a very slow rate," Rusinek explains. "However, we can pick up the surge in brain shrinkage in patients who were found later on to be impaired," he adds.

Rusinek notes that, over a period of time, there is an increased accumulation of cerebrospinal fluid, which indicates a loss of brain cells. By comparing the increases in fluid over time, the researchers can establish the rate of cell loss.

Over the six years of the study, 13 of the patients showed cognitive decline. The researchers noted that the rate of loss of mass in the medial temporal lobe was the most significant predictor of decline. The overall accuracy of this measure was 89%.

Rusinek believes that measuring brain shrinkage can be used to test the effectiveness of drugs to delay or prevent Alzheimer's and to diagnose other types of dementia.

FUTURE USES

In the future, this method may be used as a screening technique to identify those at risk for Alzheimer's and other forms of dementia, Rusinek says. "But right now it's too expensive and, of course, even if we know that Alzheimer's is likely, there is no cure," he says.

"This is the beginning of an era of diagnosing future Alzheimer's disease in people who are within the normal limits of cognition and will put us in a position to start preventive therapy," says co-researcher Mony J. de Leon, a professor of psychiatry and director of the Center for Brain Health at New York University School of Medicine.

However, he cautions that in addition to MRIs, other tests are still necessary to make a definitive diagnosis of Alzheimer's.

info To learn more about dementia and Alzheimer's disease, visit the American Academy of Family Physicians at *http://family doctor.org.*

Amazing: Teaching Alzheimer's Patients Boosts Memory

Howard Hughes Medical Institute news release.

S ome forms of memory may remain intact in people with Alzheimer's disease, a study says. This finding may help improve rehabilitation programs aimed at boosting cognitive function in healthy older people and in those with Alzheimer's.

Researchers from the Howard Hughes Medical Institute found that people in the early stages of Alzheimer's disease still possess a form of memory used for rote learning of skills, even when they have lost the memories of loved ones and previous life events.

THE STUDY

The study looked at 24 older adults in the early stages of the disease, 33 healthy older adults and 34 young adults. The researchers compared the groups' memory capabilities. Each person was shown a series of words and asked to decide whether these words represented living or nonliving objects.

"We discovered that, with practice, all three groups showed a significant reduction in the time required to decide on a word, which is the hallmark of implicit learning," says researcher Randy L. Buckner.

The people were then asked to repeat the task while their brains were scanned using magnetic resonance imaging (MRI).

"What was surprising and novel in this study is that the brain region with the greatest activity during the task was the high-level region of the frontal cortex," Buckner says.

"We didn't expect this because high-level cognition is affected in Alzheimer's disease. From this and other studies we have done, it appears that a number of brain systems are more intact in Alzheimer's than we had anticipated," Buckner says. "These findings suggest that if we can help people use these brain systems optimally by providing the right kinds of cues or task instructions, we may be able to improve their function," he adds.

Alzheimer's Risk Higher In Diabetics

Sam Gandy, MD, PhD, vice president, Medical and Scientific Advisory Council, Alzheimer's Association and director, Farber Institute for Neurosciences, Thomas Jefferson University, Philadelphia.

Zoe Arvanitakis, MD, neurologist, Alzheimer's Disease Center, Rush University Medical Center, Chicago.

Archives of Neurology.

Having diabetes appears to be linked to a 65% higher risk of developing Alzheimer's disease, according to a study that is the first to look at how cognitive systems might be affected differently in people with diabetes.

The issue of a link between diabetes and Alzheimer's is an increasingly important one as the prevalence of type 2 diabetes grows in this country and around the world. Approximately 20% of Americans older than 65 years have the disease, and if left unchecked it can lead to heart and kidney problems, cognitive impairment and more.

Although previous research has looked at the association between dementia and diabetes, results were inconclusive.

"This [study] strengthens the evidence that tight control of diabetes may be important, not only to manage vascular complications but to lower your risk for Alzheimer's," says Dr. Sam Gandy, vice president of the Medical and Scientific Advisory Council of the Alzheimer's Association. "It's now possible with oral agents and insulin and relatively painless glucometers to monitor and maintain your blood sugar in a very tight range."

THE STUDY

This study made use of data from the Religious Orders Study, an ongoing study of Catholic nuns, priests and brothers, to analyze the relationship between Alzheimer's and diabetes. Approximately 824 participants were followed up for more than five years, undergoing periodic neuropsychological testing of several cognitive systems, including general knowledge, working memory, perceptual speed (the speed with which simple comparisons can be made) and the ability to recognize spatial patterns.

During the study period, 151 participants developed Alzheimer's, including 31 who had diabetes. This represents a 65% higher risk of developing Alzheimer's for the people who had diabetes compared with the subjects who did not.

UNCERTAIN HYPOTHESES

"One of the first thoughts that comes to mind is that [the connection] would be through a vascular process, because we know that diabetes is associated with vascular diseases that affect the brain and thinking ability," says study author Dr. Zoe Arvanitakis, a neurologist with the Alzheimer's Disease Center at Rush University Medical Center in Chicago.

It's also not certain whether this is a cause-and-effect relationship or simply an association. Gandy believes that a cause-and-effect scenario would make a certain amount of sense. "We know that diabetes increases atherosclerosis and high cholesterol, and high cholesterol can aggravate Alzheimer's," Gandy said.

info The National Diabetes Information Clearinghouse has more information on the blood-sugar disorder at *http://diabetes. niddk.nih.gov.*

Higher Testosterone Levels Lower Alzheimer's Risk by 26%

Susan Resnick, PhD, investigator, National Institute on Aging, National Institutes of Health, Baltimore.

Eva Hogervorst, PhD, associate professor, University of Arkansas for Medical Sciences, Little Rock, and research scientist, University of Oxford, England.

Neurology.

M en who have low testosterone levels may have a higher risk of developing Alzheimer's disease, a study says.

THE STUDY

In the study, 574 men were followed up for an average of 19 years as part of the Baltimore Longitudinal Study of Aging. Their testosterone levels were checked periodically, and none of the men had Alzheimer's at the beginning of the study. During the follow-up period, 54 of the men developed Alzheimer's disease.

Men who developed Alzheimer's had approximately half the amount of testosterone compared with men who didn't get the disease. And for some men, this drop in testosterone was found 10 years before Alzheimer's was diagnosed, the report says. The results showed a 26% decrease in the risk of Alzheimer's for every 50% increase in the amount of free testosterone in the blood.

Although testosterone levels normally decline with age, they dropped significantly more in men who developed Alzheimer's.

"This is one more piece that we need to understand—whether testosterone will protect men from developing Alzheimer's disease," says study author Susan Resnick, an investigator with the National Institute on Aging. "The logical next step would be to see if men should be raising their levels of testosterone. We don't know the answer to that yet."

SUPPLEMENTATION NOT ENCOURAGED

The connection between testosterone and Alzheimer's disease is complicated. Simply raising testosterone levels might not do the trick. "There may be some optimal level of testosterone that is beneficial, but levels that are too high or too low may not be beneficial," Resnick explains.

Resnick says more men are taking testosterone supplements, but she warns that little is known about the side effects, which may include an increased risk of prostate cancer and stroke.

"This is certainly an area that is worth exploring, but," Resnick cautions, "we certainly do not encourage anyone to use testosterone supplements to improve memory or prevent Alzheimer's disease."

Alternative Therapies Help Ease Alzheimer's Symptoms

E. Jane Byrne, MD, FRC Psych, senior lecturer, Manchester Royal Infirmary, Manchester, UK.

Elaine Perry, PhD, professor, neurochemical pathology, Newcastle General Hospital, Newcastle upon Tyne, UK.

Presentation, International Psychogeriatric Association, Chicago.

A romatherapy and bright-light therapy appear to help Alzheimer's patients sleep better and get less agitated, according to the findings of two British studies presented at the 11th Congress of the International Psychogeriatric Association in Chicago. The Association includes health professionals and scientists who are devoted to geriatric mental health.

The practical applications of the preliminary research might be as simple as suggesting that Alzheimer's patients sit facing a sunny window or that caregivers massage them with aromatherapy skin cream.

BRIGHT-LIGHT STUDY

In the bright-light study, researchers from the Manchester Royal Infirmary in Manchester, England, evaluated 47 nursing home residents who had been diagnosed with Alzheimer's or other problems that lead to mental confusion, memory loss and dementia.

About half were assigned to the bright-light group and they sat in front of a light box for two hours daily for two weeks.

The other patients sat in front of a light box that gave off much dimmer light.

The treatment with the bright light made a difference during the shorter days of winter, says Dr. E. Jayne Byrne, a senior lecturer at the Infirmary and the study's coauthor. "On short days, the treatment group slept longer," she says.

The study was done over the course of one year and was conducted on the short days of winter and the longer days during the other seasons. On short days, those in the bright light group also were less agitated.

"We think the bright light is affecting the circadian rhythm" in a good way, Byrne says, perhaps resetting the rhythm to normal. The circadian rhythm is defined as the 24-hour biological timer that regulates numerous bodily functions.

More research is needed, Byrne adds, and perhaps a more practical approach than sitting in front of a light for two hours. Perhaps light visors could give the same result, she says, without the need to sit in one place.

CALMING LEMON BALM

The aromatherapy study, done by a team at the University of Newcastle in Newcastle upon Tyne, evaluated lemon balm. The researchers applied it daily with a short massage to 36 agitated nursing home residents and applied sunflower oil to another 36 residents who made up the control group.

During the four weeks of treatment, 35% of those in the lemon balm group showed improvement in agitation scores, compared with only 11% of the placebo group, says Elaine Perry, a neurochemical pathology professor at the university.

How does aromatherapy—the use of natural extracted essences from plants to promote health—work to reduce agitation? "There are lots of theories," Perry says, noting that one says the essences may act on body systems and substances, such as serotonin, involved in agitation and mood.

info For information on aromatherapy, visit the National Association for Holistic Aromatherapy at *http://naha.org*.

■ ■ ■ ■

Aromatherapy...For Much More Than Pleasant Smells

When you hear the word "aromatherapy," you probably think of a scented bath or a fragrant candle.

But medical practitioners in America and around the world are using distilled oils of aromatic plants medicinally. According to Jane Buckle, RN, PhD, president of RJ Buckle Associates LLC, which teaches aromatherapy to health care professionals, essential oils activate the *parasympathetic nervous system,* causing relaxation, which speeds healing.

AROMATHERAPY IN ACTION

Plant oils can be used in a warm bath...a "carrier oil"—such as almond or sesame oil —for massage...or a lotion.

The oil aromas can also be sniffed from a bottle...a cotton ball...or a *diffuser*—a machine that emits the aroma into the air.

Clinical and scientific studies support the use of aromatherapy as an adjunct to medical care for treating...

•**Anxiety.** Essential oils that were inhaled for three minutes relieved anxiety in men and women, according to research published in the *International Journal of Neuroscience.* Use rosemary, Roman chamomile or patchouli.

Typical treatment: Sniff one to three drops when anxious.

Caution: Avoid using rosemary if you have high blood pressure.

•**Bronchitis.** Use spike lavender.

Typical treatment: One drop of spike lavender in a bowl of three cups of boiling water. Drape a towel over your head, close your eyes and inhale the steam. Do this for five minutes, four times a day.

•**Hair loss.** In people with patchy hair loss due to *alopecia areata,* essential oils helped restore hair growth, notes an *Archives of Dermatology* study that used a carrier oil containing a mixture of thyme (two drops), rosemary (three drops), lavender (three drops) and cedarwood (two drops).

Typical treatment: Massage the mixture into scalp for two minutes daily.

•**Headache.** Use peppermint. If pain isn't gone in five minutes, try Roman chamomile or true lavender.

Typical treatment: Five drops in one teaspoon of carrier oil. Apply to temples or sniff.

•**Hot flashes.** Use clary sage, fennel, geranium or rose.

Typical treatment: Ten drops in two cups of water in a spray bottle. Spray on face during hot flash.

•**Insomnia.** Use ylang ylang, neroli or rose.

Typical treatment: Five drops in a diffuser placed in the bedroom.

•**Low back pain.** Use lemongrass. If you feel no relief in 20 minutes, try rosemary or spike lavender.

Typical treatment: Five drops in one teaspoon of carrier oil. Apply to the painful area every three hours.

•**Menstrual cramps.** Use geranium.

Typical treatment: Five drops added to one teaspoon of carrier oil. Rub on the lower abdomen and lower back every three hours.

•**Muscle spasms.** Use clary sage, sage or lavender.

Typical treatment: Five drops added to one teaspoon of carrier oil. Apply to the affected muscles at least every three hours.

•**Osteoarthritis.** Use frankincense, rosemary or true lavender.

Typical treatment: Five drops added to one teaspoon of carrier oil. Apply to the painful area every three hours.

WHAT TO BUY

Aromatherapy is most effective when the essential oils are prepared with no extraneous ingredients.

Good brands include Northwest Essence (*www.pacificmassage.com*) and Scents & Scentsibility (*www.scentsibility.com*). They are also available in health-food stores.

USING AROMATHERAPY SAFELY

Some essential oils can irritate or burn skin if applied undiluted. Always dilute oils before using topically. If skin stings or becomes red, dilute with a plain carrier oil and wash with unperfumed soap.

Essential oils are flammable. Store them away from candles, fires, cigarettes and stoves. Don't pour oil on lightbulbs to scent a room.

Caution: Essential oils can be lethal if they are ingested—even in tiny doses. Keep away from children and pets. People with asthma or epilepsy and pregnant women should consult their doctor before using aromatherapy.

■ ■ ■ ■

Inexpensive Aromatherapy

The scent of hair conditioner relieves anxiety just as well as scents of essential oils, according to Ellen Wiebe, MD, an assistant professor at the University of British Columbia in Vancouver.

Study: Researchers gave 66 women awaiting a surgical procedure either a mixture of expensive essential oils—vetivert, geranium and bergamot—or pleasant-smelling hair conditioner to sniff, without the patients or the experimenter knowing which was which.

Result: They found that both groups reported less anxiety, with each experiencing an equal reduction in anxiety. Researchers suggest that while pleasant smells may make patients feel better, it does not matter what pleasant smells are used.

Alzheimer's Reduces Life Span

Eric Larson, MD, MPH, director, Center for Health Studies, Group Health Cooperative, Seattle.

Katie Maslow, MSW, associate director for Quality Care Advocacy, Alzheimer's Association.

Barry Reisberg, MD, psychiatrist, New York University Medical Center, and clinical director of the Silberstein Aging and Dementia Research Center, New York University School of Medicine, New York City.

Annals of Internal Medicine.

Although it is known that Alzheimer's disease greatly reduces the quality of life, a study says the disease also decreases life expectancy.

Researchers found that the average survival after a diagnosis of Alzheimer's disease was 5.7 years for women and 4.2 years for men.

The study also found that symptoms of the disease, such as problems walking and urinary incontinence, were associated with a shorter life expectancy.

"People often wonder what the future will portend and make plans based on how long they think they'll live," says Dr. Eric Larson, author of the study and director of the Center for Health Studies at Group Health Cooperative in Seattle.

This information, he said, may help people make plans for the long-term care of a loved one with Alzheimer's. The data may also be useful for refining public health policies and allocating limited health-care resources.

THE STUDY

Larson and his colleagues gathered data on 521 people diagnosed with Alzheimer's disease between 1987 and 1996. All were from the Seattle area, and their ages ranged from approximately 65 years to almost 90 years.

The researchers collected information on other existing diseases (heart disease, high blood pressure, diabetes, stroke and depression), education and Alzheimer's symptoms, including falls, wandering, paranoia and urinary incontinence. They also performed a Mini-Mental State Examination on each person.

They found that people with Alzheimer's have approximately half the average life expectancy at the time they're diagnosed with the disease than people without the disease.

Example: A healthy American woman who lives to be 70 years old can expect to live another 15.7 years. But the study found a 70-year-old woman with Alzheimer's only will live another eight years.

A healthy 70-year-old American man typically lives another 9.3 more years, but a 70-year-old man with Alzheimer's will only live another 4.4 years, according to the study.

The presence of other medical conditions and more severe Alzheimer's symptoms indicated a shorter life expectancy.

"Certain people with Alzheimer's disease have a worse prognosis than others," Larson says. In particular, people with heart disease, diabetes, poor cognitive function, wandering and walking problems don't do well.

IMPLICATIONS

According to Larson, the shorter life expectancy might not be directly related to Alzheimer's, but the disease may cause indirect consequences that decrease longevity. For example, people with Alzheimer's are less active, which may predispose them to heart disease or pneumonia. And they're less adaptable, which may make them more prone to falls and injuries, Larson said.

Katie Maslow, associate director for Quality Care Advocacy for the Alzheimer's Association, added, "For a family, while it's difficult to hear, it's good to understand what the likelihood of survival is when planning for the care of a person. And this information is particularly valuable for letting physicians know what factors influence how long a person might live."

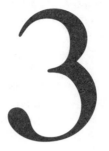

3

Asthma & Allergies

Inhaled Steroids May Trigger Cataracts

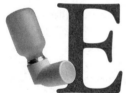

Evidence continues to indicate that long-term use of inhaled steroids to treat asthma may contribute to the formation of cataracts. Inhaled steroids are widely prescribed for asthma and other respiratory problems, including allergies. Cataracts are the number one cause of impaired vision and blindness in the world.

But experts are divided over the amount of risk posed by the steroids.

"Steroids administered systematically are well known to cause cataracts," says Dr. Richard Bensinger, a spokesman for the American Academy of Ophthalmology.

A contrary opinion is offered by Dr. Robert Cykiert, a clinical associate professor at New York University School of Medicine. Cykiert says, the association is "very rare. I've seen thousands of patients who have taken inhaled steroids for asthma and, of those I've had maybe two that have mild cataracts."

THE STUDY

The authors of the study on cataracts used data from the United Kingdom's General Practice Research Database, which contains complete prescribing and diagnostic information for almost 1.5 million patients in England and Wales.

Researchers looked at 15,479 people with cataracts and 15,479 people without this condition. The average age of the participants was 75 years old and approximately two thirds were women.

In the group with cataracts, 11.4% had been using inhaled steroids, compared with 7.6% of the group without cataracts.

Richard Bensinger, MD, spokesman, American Academy of Ophthalmology, Seattle.
Robert Cykiert, MD, clinical associate professor, New York University School of Medicine, New York City.
Robert Giusti, MD, director, Cystic Fibrosis Center, Long Island College Hospital, Brooklyn, NY.
Rajiv Luthra, MD, MPH, ophthalmologist and epidemiologist, Ochsner Clinic Foundation, New Orleans.
British Journal of Ophthalmology.

The risk apparently increased with higher dosages and long-term use. People who took up to 400 micrograms (mcg) of an inhaled steroid every day apparently had no increased risk. However, people who received doses higher than 1,600 mcg per day had a 70% increased risk.

ARE STEROIDS A NECESSARY EVIL FOR ASTHMATICS?

For many individuals who need to use inhaled steroids, this may come down to a choice between two illnesses.

"Doctors describe steroids as a wonderful awful drug," Bensinger says. "The effects are wonderful. They're absolutely critical to the practice of medicine, but they have a lot of undesirable effects."

Cataracts are one of those effects, but it is also a very treatable condition. "Treatments are extraordinarily successful," Bensinger says. "It's not a big deal to go through. [The anesthesia for cataract surgery is] almost always local anesthetic, so it's not to be feared."

Without steroids, some asthmatics may not live long enough to develop cataracts, he adds.

A PRECAUTION

There are also ways to limit the absorption of steroids in the body.

"We have patients wash out their mouth or brush their teeth after using steroids to limit systemic absorption," says Dr. Robert Giusti, director of the Cystic Fibrosis Center at Long Island College Hospital located in Brooklyn, New York. There are also second-generation inhaled steroids that the liver metabolizes and removes from the body.

The cataract study seems to be an argument for taking the lowest dose possible for the shortest time possible.

"I have no doubt in my mind [that the inhaled steroids lead to cataracts]," says Dr. Rajiv Luthra, an ophthalmologist and epidemiologist at the Ochsner Clinic Foundation located in New Orleans.

"If they're taken on a constant basis, which is every day or every other day for months to years, they will cause a problem," he adds.

info The National Eye Institute at *www.nei. nih.gov* has additional information on cataracts and other eye disorders.

It Can't Be True! These Asthma Inhalers Make It Harder to Breathe

Tom Stibolt, MD, senior physician, Department of Pulmonary and Critical Care Medicine, Kaiser Permanente, Portland, OR.

Stephanie Shore, PhD, senior physiology lecturer, Harvard School of Public Health, Boston.

Journal of Clinical Investigation.

US Food and Drug Administration release.

Scientists say that they finally understand why asthma patients who use the most common types of inhalers often suffer from a rebound effect that makes their condition worse.

Airway-opening inhalers—including *albuterol, ventolin* and *salbutamol*—appear to cause a biochemical reaction that exacerbates swelling in the body's airway. The swelling, in turn, can block airflow and make breathing more difficult.

According to Dr. Tom Stibolt, a pulmonologist with the Kaiser Permanente health plan located in Portland, Oregon, "Everyone knew that effect was there, but no one knew why. Now we know."

INHALERS EFFECTIVE

Over the past two decades, a new generation of medications known as beta2-agonists, commonly found in bronchodilating (airway-opening) inhalers, has let asthmatics breathe more easily by opening their airways.

These "relievers" are certainly a good temporary measure "because they save lives while you do the things you need to do to reduce the inflammation," Stibolt says. But patients often are so impressed by the rapid response of the inhalers that they don't use the anti-inflammation inhalers—called "controllers"—that prevent a recurrence.

As the inflammation on the walls of the airway gets worse, the reliever inhalers become overwhelmed and fail to work properly, Stibolt explains. "It actually worsens the problem in the long term."

The airway constriction can last for weeks after a patient stops using the relievers, says Stephanie Shore, a senior physiology lecturer at the Harvard School of Public Health located in Boston.

However, she adds, the number of affected patients appears to be small. Some of these patients may have inherited a propensity to develop the problem.

THE STUDY

In the study, researchers at the University of Cincinnati examined genetically altered mice that were designed to have different levels of a receptor that works to keep the airway open and unblocked by swelling.

The research team reports that through the study they discovered an interaction between chemicals that contributes to the growth of inflammation.

Shore believes researchers will need to test humans to see if the findings translate.

IF YOU HAVE ASTHMA, ALWAYS USE BOTH INHALERS

For the present time, Stibolt says, people who have asthma need to understand how important it is to use both the reliever and controller inhalers.

"If you're using enough controller medication, you hardly use any reliever medication," he says, adding most people should just have to use the reliever inhalers a couple of times a week.

Some patients, however, incorrectly accept their poor breathing.

"The problem is they don't come in and say, 'I'm using a lot of reliever medication, help me.' They just figure that's the way it is," he says.

info To learn more about asthma medications, visit the American Academy of Allergy, Asthma & Immunology at *www.aaaai.org* or the American Lung Association at *www.lungusa.org*.

What a Pain! Acetaminophen May Raise Asthma Risk

R. Graham Barr, MD, DRPH, associate professor, medicine and epidemiology, Columbia University, New York City.

Susan Redline, professor, pediatrics, Rainbow Babies and Children's Hospital, Cleveland.

American Journal of Respiratory and Critical Care Medicine.

Frequent use of the popular painkiller acetaminophen may increase a person's risk for developing asthma, a study says. But experts caution that it's far too early to tell consumers to avoid it.

Women who were taking acetaminophen at least 15 days a month for six years had a 63% higher risk of developing asthma compared with women who didn't use the analgesic, according to researchers.

Individual reactions to pain relievers vary and "we are not trying to say that all asthmatics should stop using acetaminophen," says study author Dr. R. Graham Barr, associate professor of medicine and epidemiology at Columbia University.

Soaring rates of asthma across the United States have alarmed public health officials and puzzled asthma experts.

People estimate that in the past 30 years, asthma cases approximately doubled in younger children, says Susan Redline, an asthma expert at Rainbow Babies and Children's Hospital in Cleveland.

However, the exact cause of this steep climb remains unclear.

Rising rates of obesity—which can impair lung function—have been cited as a possible culprit, as have indoor pollutants, such as dust mites and mold.

But the upswing in new asthma cases also coincided with the increasing popularity of over-the-counter acetaminophen, the researchers say. According to the American Medical Association, approximately 200 over-the-counter drugs contain acetaminophen.

THE STUDY

In their study, Barr and his colleagues examined data from the Nurses Health Study, which included nearly 122,000 adult women. As part of the study, each participant kept a record of her analgesic use, as well as the development of any new medical conditions, including asthma.

Among women who used acetaminophen for more than half of the days in a given month, "there was a significant increase—63%—in the risk of a new diagnosis of asthma," Barr says.

POSSIBLE EXPLANATION

Scientists know that acetaminophen lowers blood levels of a natural compound called *glutathione.* "Glutathione has an antioxidant effect in the body, particularly in the lungs," Barr explains. When glutathione levels plummet, "that may reduce the antioxidant defenses in the body and increase the possibility of developing asthma."

However, the study only demonstrates an association between acetaminophen and increased asthma—not a cause-and-effect relationship. And Barr notes that other analgesics such as aspirin, ibuprofen and nonsteroidal anti-inflammatory drugs (NSAIDs), such as Celebrex, have also been shown to affect asthmatics in various ways.

"If individuals happen to notice that their asthma gets worse after they take aspirin or nonsteroidals or acetaminophen, it's worth reassessing that usage," Barr says. "But we're not making any blanket statements."

info For information on controlling asthma symptoms, visit the Asthma and Allergy Foundation of America at *www.aafa.org.*

■ ■ ■ ■

Asthma Cases Increasing

Asthma rates have been climbing in the United States in recent decades. This chronic condition now affects more than 20 million Americans, including more than 5 million children.

Asthma kills nearly 5,000 people every year in the US, according to the American Academy of Allergy, Asthma & Immunology. This illness leads to 1.8 million emergency room visits and 14 million missed days of school annually, the group says.

In addition to air pollution, other factors that can trigger an asthma attack include respiratory infections, cigarette smoke, vigorous crying or laughing and irritants such as pet dander, dust mites, cockroaches, pollen and mold, as well as weather and temperature extremes.

Even 'Safe' Ozone Levels Aggravate Asthma

Janneane F. Gent, PhD, associate research scientist, Yale University School of Medicine, New Haven, CT.

George D. Thurston, ScD, associate professor, environmental medicine, New York University School of Medicine, Tuxedo, NY.

Journal of the American Medical Association.

A level of air pollution considered safe by the federal government can cause breathing problems for children with asthma—and maybe for a lot of other people.

"We looked at particularly vulnerable members of society and at the effect daily levels of ozone had on their respiratory system," says Janneane F. Gent, leader of the study and an associate research scientist at Yale University School of Medicine. "But the ozone blanketing our region is affecting all of us. Not everyone has asthma, but we are all breathing the same air."

THE STUDY

Gent and her team of researchers studied 271 children younger than 12 years who had active asthma, measuring their response to two air pollutants—ozone and very small particulate matter. A one-hour exposure to air containing 50 parts per billion caused a significant increase in wheezing and chest tightness in those children, and increased their use of symptom-relieving drugs.

No ill effects of exposure were seen in a control group of children who were not taking asthma medication, the researchers say.

But that doesn't necessarily mean that normal lungs are not being hurt by that level of ozone exposure, says George D. Thurston, an associate professor of environmental medicine at the New York University School of Medicine. He notes that the asthmatic children may serve as early detectors of air problems.

Ozone is an unusually reactive form of oxygen, Thurston notes. One early test of the effects of ozone was to see how much damage it caused to a rubber band, he says.

"If it can damage the elasticity of rubber, you can imagine what it does to the lining of the lungs," he says. "It certainly has some effect on the lining of the lungs of a healthy person, but the effect is much stronger for a child with asthma."

Atmospheric ozone is produced through the burning of fossil fuels, such as coal and oil, and in chemical production.

The EPA tightened its ozone standards five years ago, and is now studying health data to see if the standards should be tightened further, Thurston says.

info An overview of ozone can be found at the Environmental Protection Agency Web site at *www.epa.gov.*

Flu Shots Make It Easier For Adults with Asthma To Breathe

Seymour Williams, MD, medical epidemiologist, US Centers for Disease Control and Prevention, Atlanta.

Stephen Wasserman, MD, professor, medicine, University of California, San Diego, and fellow, American Academy of Allergy, Asthma & Immunology.

Chest.

Adults who have asthma are advised to get flu shots every year, but only one third do so, according to a US government survey.

Younger adults who have asthma are even less likely to heed the advice, report researchers from the Centers for Disease Control and Prevention (CDC). Only 21% of all asthmatics aged 18 to 49 got the flu vaccine in 2001, the researchers say.

People with asthma are considered a high-risk group for developing bacterial infections that frequently follow flu, such as pneumonia, bronchitis and ear infections.

MISCONCEPTION BLAMED

The lack of compliance is partially due to a misconception, says Dr. Seymour Williams, a medical epidemiologist at the CDC's National Center for Environmental Health and also a co-author of the report. Many people who have asthma think a flu shot worsens their condition, he says.

In fact, the flu can trigger asthma attacks, Williams says. If you catch influenza and have asthma, you get a double whammy, he explains. Getting the vaccine annually results in one less trigger for asthma.

The flu-vaccine recommendation for those patients who have asthma is long-standing, yet people either remain unaware of it, fail to comply or both.

Williams and his team found that among respondents with asthma, only 35.1% got a flu vaccine in 1999, only 36.7% in 2000 and only 33.3% in 2001.

Williams says all doctors should make sure that their asthmatic patients are aware of the recommendation.

Dr. Stephen Wasserman, a professor of medicine at the University of California, San Diego, and also a fellow of the American Academy of Allergy, Asthma & Immunology, says that this new research underscores what doctors already know.

"We all know that flu vaccine is not as aggressively pursued as it should be by patients or their physicians," he says.

"Most people think flu vaccine is for older people. I recommend it to all my asthmatic patients," Wasserman says.

Wasserman also cautions his patients that getting a flu shot is not a cure-all for asthma. Lots of viral illnesses that trigger asthma are not influenza, he tells them. But getting vaccinated can still be a great help to staying healthy.

■ ■ ■ ■

The Facts About the Flu

The influenza virus infects 10% to 20% of the United States population every year, according to the CDC, and approximately 36,000 people die from the illness annually. Symptoms of influenza include fever, body aches, fatigue and cough. Most people recover in one to two weeks if there are no complications.

Vaccines are designed to target the flu strain expected to be prevalent during the upcoming season. Flu season generally runs from October to mid-May. October and November are the best months to get the vaccine so there's enough time to stimulate the immune system to resist the infection. Late November or early December is less ideal, but the vaccine may still be effective if people get it at that time.

Melatonin Makes Asthma Worse

Rand Sutherland, MD, MPH, assistant professor, medicine, National Jewish Medical and Research Center, University of Colorado Health Sciences Center, Denver.

Charles Irvin, PhD, professor, medicine, and director, Vermont Lung Center, University of Vermont, Burlington.

Journal of Allergy and Clinical Immunology.

Melatonin, a hormone that is found naturally in the body and that helps regulate the body's circadian rhythms, could make asthma worse at night, researchers have found.

"We found that patients who have nocturnal asthma have higher levels of melatonin than patients who do not have asthma," says study author Dr. Rand Sutherland, an assistant professor of medicine at the National Jewish Medical and Research Center in Denver. "Higher levels of melatonin were associated with a greater worsening of lung function overnight," he says.

Melatonin is produced by the pineal gland in the brain, and many people take supplemental melatonin to help them sleep and to combat jet lag.

THE STUDY

Sutherland and his colleagues at the University of Colorado Health Sciences Center looked at seven patients who had nocturnal asthma, 13 patients who had non-nocturnal asthma and 11 patients who did not have asthma.

While the patients slept, the researchers took blood samples every two hours. Sutherland's team also measured lung function before the patients went to bed and again after they woke up.

Results showed the patients with nocturnal asthma had the highest levels of melatonin and the biggest decrease in lung function. Among those with nocturnal asthma, levels of melatonin were an average of 68 picograms per milliliter (pg/mL), compared with 61 pg/mL for patients with non-nocturnal asthma and 54 pg/mL for patients without asthma.

In addition, among patients with nocturnal asthma, lung function dropped an average of 19% compared with 5% in patients with non-nocturnal asthma. Among non-asthmatic patients, lung function increased about 2%.

In other experiments, melatonin has been shown to rev up the inflammation process, Sutherland notes.

Sutherland speculates that "high melatonin levels may be one way in which the worsening of nocturnal asthma is regulated."

"These findings raise concern that high melatonin levels may play a role in making asthma worse at night, and therefore people who have asthma should avoid taking supplemental melatonin," Sutherland advises.

WARNING IS 'JUST RIGHT'

Charles Irvin, a professor of medicine and director of the Vermont Lung Center at the University of Vermont, comments that, "this is a very important paper and could be a very exciting development."

This study is the first real attempt to find out the cause of nocturnal asthma, he says: "The conclusion by Sutherland that patients with asthma should be cautious about using melatonin is just right."

Patients are desperate to find nonpharmaceutical treatments for sleep disorders, Irvin explains, but many of the alternatives are not benign. Many like melatonin are very powerful, he adds. And people need to be careful about how they use these supplements.

"Patients with mild asthma may try melatonin, but if their asthma gets worse, they should stop it right away. However, people with nocturnal asthma should avoid taking melatonin altogether," Irvin cautions.

Tired? It Could Be a Sinus Infection

Alexander C. Chester, MD, clinical professor of medicine, Georgetown University Medical Center, Washington, DC.

Philip Perlman, MD, chief of otolaryngology, St. Francis Hospital, Roslyn, NY.

Archives of Internal Medicine.

Feeling beat and don't know why? You might have sinusitis, one of the most common chronic health problems for people in the United States.

Sinusitis affects an estimated 34 million people every year, according to the National Institute of Allergies and Infectious Diseases. More women are afflicted than men.

The condition is characterized by inflammation of the nasal passages, and can be caused by any number of triggers, including colds, allergies and fungal infections. The inflammation narrows the nasal passages so that mucus can't drain properly, causing discomfort and sometimes infection.

Left untreated, sinusitis can become chronic, lasting for weeks, months or even years, according to the NIAID.

Dr. Alexander Chester, an internist at Georgetown University Medical Center, interviewed almost 300 of his patients and found that those who reported unexplained chronic fatigue were nine times more likely to have sinusitis symptoms than those who felt well.

Also, patients who said they had unexplained body pain were six times more likely than the pain-free patients to have such symptoms of sinusitis as facial pressure, heavy-headedness or frontal headache, Chester says.

Doctors who specialize in sinusitis—otolaryngologists—know that almost one third of sufferers experience severe fatigue and pain, Chester says, but the news hasn't gotten to the general practitioner.

As a result, he adds, many patients may not be getting treatment for sinusitis that could alleviate their fatigue or pain.

THE STUDY

Chester surveyed 297 of his patients. Sixty-five (22%) of the patients reported unexplained chronic fatigue, described as a sleepiness unrelieved by rest. And 33 (11%) of the patients reported unexplained body pain.

Although there were more men than women in the study (54% versus 46%), more women than men reported unexplained chronic fatigue (60% versus 42%).

"People are not aware of how global the effects can be from sinusitis," Chester says. "Sufferers can feel a general sense of malaise even without direct sinus symptoms. My hope is to raise awareness among internists as to the fact that unexplained chronic fatigue can be caused by sinusitis."

SYMPTOMS

Fatigue is one of the "top five" symptoms of sinusitis, says Dr. Philip Perlman, a New York otolaryngologist. The others are pain, facial pressure, nasal congestion and fever.

"To say that everyone who has unexplained chronic fatigue should be worked up for sinusitis is pushing it a bit," Perlman says.

"But a few easy questions—like, 'Do you have a history of sinusitis?' or 'Do you feel facial pressure or have frontal headaches?'—could pick out those patients who do have sinusitis," he notes.

The good news: There are now treatments that include nasal sprays, as well as intranasal nebulized antibiotics, certain antihistamines, topical antifungals and antibiotics that target the fungi and bacteria that often plague sinusitis sufferers.

info An explanation of sinusitis and its symptoms can be found at the National Institute of Allergy and Infectious Diseases Web site, *www.niaid.nih.gov.*

■ ■ ■ ■

Symptoms and Treatment For Sinusitis

The National Institute of Allergy and Infectious Diseases (NIAID) offers the following information on the symptoms of sinusitis and some treatments that might be effective…

SYMPTOMS

- **Headache when you wake up.**
- **Pain in your forehead** when it is touched.
- **Pain in your upper jaw and in your teeth.** Cheeks tender to the touch.
- **Swelling of the eyelids and the tissues around your eyes,** and pain between your eyes. Tenderness when the sides of your nose are touched, as well as a loss of smell and a stuffy nose.
- **Earaches, neck pain** and deep aching at the top of your head.

In addition, the drainage of mucus, called postnasal drip, can cause a sore throat. Mucus drainage also can irritate the membranes lining your larynx (upper windpipe). Not everyone with these symptoms, however, has sinusitis.

TREATMENT

After diagnosing sinusitis and identifying a possible cause, your doctor can suggest treatments that will reduce the inflammation and relieve your symptoms.

- **Decongestants** to reduce congestion.
- **Antibiotics** to control a bacterial infection, if present.
- **Pain relievers** to reduce any pain.

You should, however, use over-the-counter or prescription decongestant nose drops and sprays for only a few days. If you use these medicines for longer periods, they can lead to even more congestion and swelling of your nasal passages.

If bacteria is present, antibiotics used along with a nasal or oral decongestant will usually help. Your doctor can prescribe an antibiotic to fight the type of bacteria most commonly associated with sinusitis.

Many instances of acute sinusitis will end without antibiotics. If you have an allergic disease along with infectious sinusitis, however, you may need medicine to relieve your allergy symptoms.

In addition, your doctor may prescribe a steroid nasal spray to reduce your sinus congestion, swelling and inflammation.

America's Autumn Allergy Capitals

Derek K. Johnson, MD, Temple University Children's Medical Center, Philadelphia, and spokesman, Asthma and Allergy Foundation of America.

Planning a visit to Harrisburg, Pennsylvania, this fall? Or Raleigh, North Carolina? How about Louisville, Kentucky? If so, bring plenty of tissues and a cache of eye drops.

Based on autumn pollen levels, the length of peak seasons for the worst allergens, and the number of antihistamine prescriptions written in recent years, these cities top the list of places where fall allergies are most severe.

"We broadly classify allergies as seasonal, but seasonal can be spring, summer and fall. We want people to realize that, even in the fall, their itchy throat and runny nose may be allergy symptoms," says Dr. Derek K. Johnson, an allergist at Temple University Children's Medical Center in Philadelphia.

Weed pollens are the most common and irritating of the fall allergens, Johnson says, and they often remain in the air until the first freeze. In the Midwest, these irritants include English plantain and lambsquarter. Ragweed is the main culprit in the Northeast.

The list of the top 50 cities [see next article] for fall allergens was compiled by the Asthma and Allergy Foundation of America (AAFA), as part of its Allergy Action Plan education program.

Johnson, a spokesman for the AAFA, says allergy symptoms often mimic cold symptoms —runny nose, watery eyes, itchy throat. But colds run their course in seven to 10 days.

"If your symptoms last longer than that, you may be having an allergic reaction" and you should see a doctor, he says.

REDUCE YOUR EXPOSURE TO ALLERGENS

Prevention is key, says Johnson, who recommends the following steps to reduce your chances of pollen exposure...

•**Spend more time indoors** when pollen and mold counts are high.

•**Decrease allergens in your home** by keeping windows closed and using an air filter that's cleaned regularly.

•**Reduce the number of dust mites** in the home by washing bedding often and in hot water.

Johnson says that even if your city isn't high on the list, you should be alert to possible allergies.

An estimated 40 to 50 million Americans have allergies, according to the American Academy of Allergy, Asthma & Immunology. Of those, some 36 million have seasonal allergic rhinitis, otherwise known as hay fever.

Asthma is quite common as well. It affects more than 15 million adults and children in the United States, according to the National Heart, Lung and Blood Institute (NHLBI).

Each year asthma leads to 1.5 million trips to the emergency room, roughly half a million hospitalizations, and more than 5,500 deaths. Asthma is more common in children and in African-Americans.

■ ■ ■ ■

Ah-choo! Where the Allergen Hot Spots Are

These are the places the Asthma and Allergy Foundation of America says cause the most problems for allergy sufferers...

1. Harrisburg-Lancaster-Lebanon-York, PA.
2. Raleigh-Durham-Fayetteville, NC.
3. Louisville, KY.
4. Austin, TX.
5. Grand Rapids-Kalamazoo-Battle Creek, MI.
6. Memphis, TN.
7. Oklahoma City, OK.
8. Dallas-Ft. Worth, TX.
9. Kansas City, MO.
10. St. Louis, MO.
11. Indianapolis, IN.
12. Columbus, OH.
13. Minneapolis-St. Paul, MN.
14. Charlotte, NC.
15. San Antonio, TX.
16. Birmingham-Tuscaloosa, AL.
17. Cincinnati, OH.
18. Milwaukee, WI.
19. Houston, TX.
20. Detroit, MI.
21. New Orleans, LA.
22. Nashville, TN.
23. Phoenix, AZ.
24. Greenville-Spartanburg-Anderson, SC.
25. Pittsburgh, PA.
26. Denver, CO.
27. Hartford-New Haven, CT.
28. Albuquerque-Santa Fe, NM.
29. Atlanta, GA.
30. Chicago, IL.
31. Greensboro-High Point-Winston-Salem, NC.
32. Las Vegas, NV.
33. Cleveland-Akron-Canton, OH.
34. Jacksonville-Brunswick, FL.
35. Salt Lake City, UT.
36. Orlando-Daytona-Melbourne, FL.
37. Albany-Schenectady-Troy, NY.
38. Philadelphia, PA.
39. Boston, MA.
40. Sacramento-Stockton-Modesto, CA.
41. Tampa-St. Petersburg-Sarasota, FL.
42. Baltimore, MD.
43. Washington, DC.
44. Providence, RI.
45. Norfolk-Portsmouth-Newport News, VA.
46. Seattle-Tacoma, WA.
47. New York, NY.
48. Los Angeles, CA.
49. Portland, OR.
50. San Francisco-Oakland-San Jose, CA.

Now You Can Stop Suffering from Annoying Allergies

Gillian Shepherd, MD, clinical associate professor of medicine, Weill Medical College of Cornell University and an attending physician at New York Presbyterian Hospital, both in New York City.

Bottom Line/Health.

If you have seasonal or chronic allergies, identifying and limiting exposure to your triggers is the first step to minimizing your misery. Unfortunately, many people with allergies suffer unnecessarily because they are misinformed about their condition.

Common misconceptions about allergies…

Misconception #1: Spring is the peak allergy season.

Fact: The time of year that you have nasal and/or eye allergies (allergic rhinitis or conjunctivitis) depends on what triggers your attacks. Although tree allergies typically flare in the spring and grass allergies peak in late spring and summer, weed allergies are most likely to strike in the fall. Late September through December can also be high season for mold allergies, since damp, rotting piles of leaves are a breeding ground for spores.

Caution: Fall allergies may often linger into cold and flu season, which leaves you more vulnerable to upper-respiratory infections. That's because inflamed, mucous-filled nasal passages act like magnets to viruses.

To reduce your cold and flu risks, treat fall allergy symptoms promptly.

Decongestants…over-the-counter (OTC) antihistamines, such as *loratadine* (Claritin)…or prescription antihistamines, such as *fexofenadine* (Allegra) or *cetirizine* (Zyrtec), relieve mild symptoms, including congestion and sneezing.

For more severe or chronic symptoms, consult an allergist, who may recommend a prescription nasal steroid spray.

Misconception #2: Smoke from cigarettes, household cleaners and perfumes are common allergens.

Fact: Although such strong-smelling irritants can aggravate the nerves that are located in the nose and cause allergy-like symptoms (stuffiness, sneezing, etc.), they are not actually allergens. That's because they don't trigger an immune response.

When an allergic person encounters a true allergen (for example, mold or pollen) his/her immune system overreacts, launching a massive defense against the foreign invader.

However, in people who have a "hyperactive" nose, strong odors may cause nerve endings in the nose to overreact. And this results in congestion and sneezing. But this is not an immune reaction.

Nearly half of all people who think they have airborne allergies may instead suffer from a hyperactive nose.

Misconception #3: Indoor molds are a trigger for allergies.

Fact: Bathroom mold rarely causes allergies. Because mold sticks to surfaces and must be scrubbed off, it is unlikely that this type of mold will become airborne. Even toxic molds, such as *stachybotrys,* may cause health problems, but not allergies.

The overwhelming majority of mold allergies are triggered by outdoor molds that are found growing in damp, shady areas, on rotting wood or vegetation, in fields, pastures and on freshly cut lawns. This outdoor mold can be tracked inside on shoes or clothing, triggering symptoms indoors.

That's why testing and cleaning for household molds won't necessarily ease your symptoms. Your best defense to ease your allergy symptoms is to avoid outdoor areas where molds thrive.

If symptoms persist, consult an allergist about appropriate drug treatments.

Misconception #4: Pollen counts that are broadcast locally can prepare you for high-allergy days.

Fact: Pollen counts are typically 24 to 36 hours old by the time they're reported. Pollen must be collected on slides for as long as 24 hours, then identified and tallied under a microscope. These pollen counts can confirm the cause of yesterday's misery and can give you the approximate amount of pollen present in a given week. However, the specific amount of pollen in the air fluctuates daily, so counts may not accurately predict the severity of on-coming symptoms.

Misconception #5: People with pet allergies won't suffer symptoms when they're exposed to "hypoallergenic" breeds.

Fact: There is no such thing as a hypoallergenic dog or cat. Scientists once believed that animal allergies were triggered by dander, skin particles that stick to and are shed along with the hair of the animal. This led to the theory that non-shedding breeds—poodles, bichons frises and terriers—would not trigger allergy symptoms.

We now know that dog and cat allergies are caused by chemicals that are in the animal's saliva, skin secretions and urine. These fluids dry on the pet's hair, then flake off and become airborne. All cats and dogs produce these allergens to varying degrees and have the potential to trigger allergies.

Cats cause more allergies than dogs—probably because they lick themselves more and often use indoor litter boxes.

A small, non-shedding dog will typically produce less allergen than a large, shedding breed. So it may be tolerated by people who are mildly allergic.

Allergic pet owners often mistakenly believe that vacuuming will minimize symptoms. But vacuuming often exacerbates symptoms, because it sucks up allergen particles from the carpet and disperses them in the air, where they can linger for hours and trigger flare-ups.

Helpful: If you are determined to keep your pet despite allergies, invest in a vacuum cleaner with a *high-efficiency particulate-arresting* (HEPA) filter, designed to trap very small particles. If possible, delegate vacuuming duties. If you must vacuum, wear a HEPA mask and immediately change and wash clothes when finished. HEPA products are sold in appliance stores and by Allergy Control Products, 800-422-3878, *www.allergycon trol.com.*

Washing your pet may also lessen symptoms for two days following the bath. Soap isn't necessary, but you do have to dunk the animal in a tub (wiping down with a damp cloth won't do it).

Misconception #6: All nasal allergy sprays are addictive.

Fact: Over-the-counter decongestant sprays, such as Afrin and Neo-Synephrine, are a good option for immediate, short-term relief of nasal congestion. They shrink swollen nasal membranes and can safely be used twice a day for up to three consecutive days. If they are used longer or more frequently, they can produce rebound congestion, causing nasal passages to swell even more severely once the drug wears off. With repeated use, patients may become addicted to these sprays and unable to breathe without them.

Prescription nasal steroid sprays, such as *fluticasone* (Flonase), *mometasone* (Nasonex) and *budesonide* (Rhinocort), are nonhabit-forming and can safely be used daily. They work by reducing inflammation and blocking the allergic reaction.

To properly administer nose sprays: Clear the nostrils of mucus, lean your head slightly forward and spray one nostril at a time while pressing a finger against the other. Aim straight up the center of your nostril or slightly inward, toward the eye area. A common mistake is to aim toward the outside of the nostril. After spraying, lean your head back for a few seconds.

Beyond the Sniffles: Allergies Can Trigger Very Surprising Symptoms

Thomas Brunoski, MD, specialist in the treatment of medical problems and food and environmental allergies through the use of nutritional and preventive methods. *Bottom Line/Personal.*

Allergic reactions to pollen, mold, food and other substances affect the *entire* body—not just the nose or sinuses. The symptoms can be far more serious than sniffles and sneezes. Yet few people connect persistent illness to allergies.

CASE STUDY #1: SKIN RASH

A young woman had been treated successfully for allergy-triggered skin rashes as well as sinus problems. She came back with head-to-toe eczema that had appeared after she moved into a new home.

Testing showed several allergies. The strongest was to dogs, yet none of her neighbors owned a dog.

Solution: Although the new house had been professionally cleaned, urine stains from the previous owner's dog were embedded in the wood floor. After the stains were removed—part of the floor had to be replaced—her eczema vanished.

CASE STUDY #2: ASTHMA

A nine-month-old child had severe asthma and eczema, which had not improved even after the doctor had prescribed an oral steroid.

Because this medication can stunt a child's growth and damage the immune system, the mother was understandably distraught.

I uncovered a powerful allergy to oranges. Yet the baby did not eat oranges or drink orange juice.

Solution: I advised the mother to check around her home. She discovered the furniture polish she used contained orange fragrance. When she discarded the polish and removed all traces from the furniture, her son's symptoms cleared up.

CASE STUDY #3: CANKER SORES

For years, a woman suffered from unpredictable and recurring canker sores. Despite a range of treatments, from medicated mouthwash to antibiotics, the sores persisted.

Since allergies can aggravate inflammation, I advised an allergy test. The results showed a reaction to dairy products.

Solution: An analysis of her diet revealed that her on-and-off consumption of dairy products—ice cream in the summer—explained why the sores appeared sporadically. Avoiding dairy products completely has kept the sores away.

CASE STUDY #4: SINUS TROUBLE

A man had no relief from recurrent sinus infections, even after many courses of antibiotics. Allergy tests revealed that he was allergic to pollen, dust and molds.

He followed instructions to remove these allergens from his environment—but still experienced symptoms.

Solution: The environment is not the only source for molds. Diet may also be a supplier. I advised him to avoid products that are fermented, such as cheese, vinegar (he had to check salad dressings) and pickles (which might garnish a hamburger and be in tartar sauce and other dressings)...and to switch to a low-yeast bread, such as sourdough. His sinus problems cleared.

DIAGNOSING ALLERGIES

It is estimated that 17% to 21% of us suffer from allergies. Pollution is thought to be the main cause. The first step in discovering an allergy trigger is testing. Skin tests, once the sole diagnostic tool, can yield false-positive or false-negative results.

Instead, I use a blood test called the amplified ELISA. This highly accurate test identifies a broad range of allergens. No one is ever allergic to just one substance. This blood test also measures the intensity of the individual's reaction to each trigger.

Once the trigger is discovered, the source might still be unclear. Additional detective work generally uncovers the source, as the four case studies illustrate.

OVERCOMING ALLERGIES

Identifying an allergen—and avoiding heavy exposure to it—are only the first two steps.

Because it's impossible to avoid many common allergens, I also recommend *desensitization*. During this process, a person is exposed gradually to increasing amounts of an allergen. Allergy shots—an injectable "cocktail" composed of multiple allergens—are typically prescribed. However, they sometimes have disappointing results...and can cause swelling, redness and soreness.

More effective: Allergy drops, a concentrate of a specific allergen. Patients take a weekly dose, under the tongue, for about two years.

I retest for allergies after one year. By then, most patients show great improvement.

With consistent therapy, the individual will eventually be able to withstand exposure to a once-troublesome allergen with little or no reaction.

To find a practitioner: American Academy of Environmental Medicine, 316-684-5500 ...*www.aaem.com.*

STAYING HEALTHY

Follow these basic steps to build good health and minimize your risk of allergic reactions...

•**Eat a variety of foods.** Humans evolved as hunter-gatherers who sampled many foods. We still do best with this type of diet. Even a moderate allergy may intensify with the daily consumption of trigger foods. And alternating foods makes it easier to spot possible triggers if symptoms occur.

•**Avoid processed foods.** Processing removes nutrients. Additives, preservatives and dyes are common triggers of allergic symptoms. Eat lots of fresh vegetables and fruits. Use cold-pressed, extra-virgin olive oil when cooking and in salad dressing. It contains essential fatty acids.

•**Take nutritional supplements.** With heavy processing and soil deletion, food may not always provide essential nutrients. *I recommend the following daily supplements to my patients...*

•Multivitamin/multimineral containing 50 milligrams (mg) or more of B-complex vitamins.

•Chelated calcium to keep bones strong, 1,200 mg.

•Magnesium, which aids in absorption of calcium, 600 to 750 mg.

•Folic acid, which reduces the blood level of *homocysteine,* an amino acid that is harmful to the heart, 800 micrograms (mcg). The amount that is available in over-the-counter pills is limited. Your doctor can write a prescription if you need a higher dose.

•Vitamin C, an antioxidant, 1,000 mg. Take 500 mg twice daily.

•**Exercise regularly.** Try to fit in at least a one-hour workout three times a week, preferably a combination of some kind of aerobics and strength training.

Pets May Protect Against Animal Allergies

Eva Rönmark, PhD, Obstructive Lung Disease in Northern Sweden Study Group (OLIN), department of medicine, Central Hospital of Norrbotten, Lulea-Boden, Sweden.
Marjan Kerkhof, PhD, medical researcher, University of Groningen, Netherlands.
Journal of Allergy and Clinical Immunology.

A recent study has found that although an allergy to cats was the most common airborne childhood allergy, owning a cat didn't necessarily increase the risk of developing allergies in children.

In fact, the study found that persistently high exposure to cat and dog allergens appeared to protect both boys and girls equally from developing allergies.

Children who had continuously owned cats or dogs developed fewer allergies to them than new pet owners and those who had only been exposed earlier in life. Among children who were allergic to cats, 80% had never kept a cat at home.

"Our research has found no increased risk of sensitization in children due to exposure to pets in the home," says Eva Rönmark, an allergy expert at the department of medicine at the Central Hospital of Norrbotten in Lulea-Boden, Sweden.

"Sensitization is genetic. The big risk factor for [developing an allergy is] if you already have it in your family," she adds.

THE STUDY

Rönmark and colleagues from the University of Virginia at Charlottesville gave 2,454 7- and 8-year-olds in northern Sweden skin sensitization tests every four years. Parents also completed annual questionnaires on their children's risk factors.

"Parents also need to be aware that just because you don't have a pet [doesn't mean that] your child won't develop sensitization," adds Rönmark.

"Cat [and other] allergens can also be found where there are no cats—in schools, for example, where they can be transferred by clothes," she explains.

"At this time, though, we don't really know why these high exposure levels decrease the risks," says Rönmark.

Researchers note that when a child with an existing allergy comes into contact with a cat or dog, naturally they begin to show more symptoms. Traditional thinking had been to assume that avoiding pets altogether would prevent these allergies.

OLD VIEW UNDERMINED

The study suggests the new findings are antithetical to the traditional views that exposure causes more severe symptoms.

"Studies we have done show that exposure to microorganisms has been shown to play a role in protecting against developing allergies," says medical researcher Marjan Kerkhof of the University of Groningen in the Netherlands. "And pets certainly would carry a lot of microorganisms."

"But," she cautions, "I think there needs to be more work done on this subject."

Sunscreen and Bug Spray: A Dangerous Brew

Xiaochen Gu, PhD, University of Manitoba.
University of Manitoba, Canada, news release.
James A. Duke, PhD, past chief of the US Department of Agriculture's medicinal plant laboratory and author of *The Green Pharmacy*. Rodale Press.
Robert Norris, MD, chief, division of emergency medicine, Stanford University Medical Center, CA.

Although both serve an important purpose, slathering on sunscreen and mosquito repellent at the same time may not be a good idea, especially for children.

Recent research from Canada suggests that the combination could lead to serious side effects, including skin allergies, high blood pressure, headaches and seizures. The risk may be especially high in children.

University of Manitoba pharmaceutical researcher Dr. Xiaochen Gu says using sunscreen and mosquito repellent together increases their absorption rates.

Gu studied DEET, which is the active ingredient in many bug repellents, and oxybenzone, an agent in sunscreen. He studied them separately and then combined the two substances and measured their penetrative value.

STRONGER SIDE EFFECTS

When DEET and oxybenzone are combined, there's a marked increase in the rate of absorption through the skin. Gu says this could mean the side effects of the chemicals may be heightened when they're used together.

He is trying to modify the nonmedicinal ingredients found in bug repellents and sunscreens to reduce these high absorption rates. That would make the products more effective and smaller amounts would then be needed to achieve the desired protective effect.

Gu is especially interested in how using sunscreens and bug repellents simultaneously affect children and seniors.

SPECIAL CONCERNS

"Children have tender skin, making them more prone to cross-skin absorption. People over 65 tend to have thinner skin and have had years of exposure to sun, which also makes their skin absorb more of these chemicals," according to Gu.

■ ■ ■ ■

How to Use Bug Repellents Safely

The Environmental Protection Agency (EPA) offers the following tips for the safe use of bug repellents…

●**Apply repellents only to exposed skin and/or clothing** (as directed on the product label). Do not use under clothing.

●**Never use repellents over cuts,** wounds, or irritated skin.

●**Do not apply to the eyes and mouth,** and apply sparingly around ears. When using sprays do not spray directly onto face; spray on hands first and then apply to face.

●**Do not allow children to handle the products,** and do not apply to children's hands. When using on children, apply to your own hands and then put it on the child.

●**Do not spray in enclosed areas.** Avoid breathing a repellent spray, and do not use it near food.

●**Use just enough repellent that is necessary to cover exposed skin and/or clothing.** Heavy application and saturation is generally unnecessary for effectiveness; if biting insects do not respond to a thin film of repellent, then apply a bit more.

●**After returning indoors,** wash treated skin with soap and water or bathe. This is particularly important when repellents are used repeatedly in the same day or on consecutive days. Also, wash treated clothing before wearing it again. If you suspect that you or your child is reacting to an insect repellent, discontinue use, wash treated skin, and then call your local poison control center. If you go to a doctor, take the repellent with you.

●**Obtain specific medical information about the active ingredients** in repellents and other pesticides by calling the National Pesticide Information Center (NPIC) at 800-858-7378. NPIC operates from 9:30 AM to 7:30 PM (Eastern Time), seven days a week. The NPIC Web site is *www.npic.orst.edu.*

■ ■ ■ ■

Preventing and Relieving Mosquito Bites

Rubbing a handful of fresh basil leaves on your skin should protect you from mosquitoes for a few hours, according to James A. Duke, PhD, past chief of the US Department of Agriculture's medicinal plant laboratory. The herb does not contain hazardous chemicals and is less likely than synthetic bug sprays to cause skin irritation. It's also cheaper.

If you do get bitten, you can stop the itch by swabbing the bite with an antiseptic—alcohol or witch hazel.

Dr. Robert Norris, chief of emergency medicine at Stanford University Medical Center, suggests using caution when applying creams that contain *diphenhydramine,* such as Benadryl. If the cream is applied too heavily or used in conjunction with oral Benadryl, children can absorb toxic amounts of the chemical.

Also avoid: Iodine and Merthiolate. These substances can slow healing by killing the white blood cells that help repair wounds.

info You can learn more about insect repellents from the Centers for Disease Control and Prevention (CDC) at *www.cdc.gov.*

Allergies Driving You Nuts? These Test Kits Help

US Food and Drug Administration news release.

Three kits that test for peanut proteins in cereal, cookies, ice cream and milk chocolate have been approved by the Association of Official Analytical Chemists (AOAC). And this is good news for the nearly 7 million Americans who have various food allergies, especially the estimated 1.5 million people who have severe allergic reactions to peanuts.

RELIABLE HELP

These test kits provide the food industry with a quick, reliable method to detect the presence of peanuts in food items that are not labeled as containing peanuts. The kits will help prevent such products from making their way onto store shelves.

Research as well as industrial food operations and other packagers with limited laboratory facilities will be the most likely users of these test kits.

The tests will let these operations quickly determine whether their food-processing operations prevent the inclusion of peanuts in foods declared to be peanut-free.

The test also will reveal whether plant cleanup operations are successfully avoiding cross-contamination and whether the finished product is peanut-free.

The US Food and Drug Administration (FDA) performed a joint review and evaluation with the AOAC on the test kits. An FDA laboratory prepared and distributed coded samples to participating laboratories. Approximately 40 analyses can be done with each kit. The cost per kit ranges from $450 to $650.

A COMMON FOOD ALLERGY

Peanuts have become one of the world's most allergenic foods because they are progressively finding their way into more and more food products, according to the American Academy of Allergy, Asthma & Immunology.

Even food products that don't list peanuts as an ingredient may be dangerous for people who have an allergy to them. People with allergies should read the ingredient label, looking for specific ingredients that could indicate the presence of peanut protein. These include peanuts, mixed nuts, ground nuts, mandelonas, peanut butter, peanut oil, goober nuts, goober peas, beer nuts, peanut flour, artificial nuts or hydrolyzed peanut protein.

■ ■ ■ ■

Peanuts Can Be Deadly

Approximately 8% of children younger than three years and approximately 2% of adults are affected by food allergies.

Almost 90% of all food allergy reactions are caused by eight foods: peanuts, eggs, milk, shellfish, wheat, soy, fish or tree nuts.

If you mistakenly eat peanuts and are allergic to them, you run the risk of going into anaphylactic shock. This reaction can begin and proceed rapidly, occasionally proving fatal within minutes.

Anaphylactic shock must be treated with epinephrine immediately at the first signs of reaction. Epinephrine is a synthetic form of adrenaline, a hormone that boosts the body's reaction to a threat.

People who have a history of anaphylactic shock may carry an EpiPen, a form of self-injectable epinephrine. You can slip back into shock even after receiving treatment, so ongoing observation and care are required.

Other possible reactions people may have to peanuts include...

• **Foreboding,** fear or apprehension.

• **Flushed face,** hives, swollen or itchy lips, mouth, eyes or tongue.

• **Tightness in mouth,** chest or throat.

• **Difficulty breathing or swallowing,** drooling, wheezing, choking, coughing.

• **Running nose,** voice change.

• **Vomiting,** nausea, diarrhea, stomach pains.

• **Dizziness,** unsteadiness, sudden fatigue, rapid heartbeat, chills.

• **Pallor,** loss of consciousness, coma, death.

Every year, thousands of people are rushed to emergency departments because of shock that is caused by peanut allergies, and approximately 50 to 100 people die after accidentally eating peanuts.

info The Mayo Clinic's Web site has more information about food allergies at *www.mayoclinic.com.* Click on "Diseases & Conditions."

4

Breast Cancer Treatments

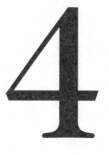

Encouraging News! Breast Cancer Procedure May Save More Lives

For a large part of the last century, women with aggressive breast cancer have been advised to have their armpit tissue removed—a clean-sweep operation intended to prevent the disease from spreading. But now doctors are rethinking that strategy.

A far less invasive procedure called *sentinel node biopsy* looks for signs of cancer in the sentinel lymph nodes, which are the first to collect fluid and cells draining from breast tumors. If these nodes are positive for cancer, the armpit, or axillary, tissue is removed. If not, the tissue is left intact.

THE STUDY

A study suggests this procedure may be a safe and accurate alternative to the one-size-fits-all surgery. The study followed 516 women with small breast tumors (less than an inch in diameter). Half of the women had the sentinel node biopsy procedure and half had the conventional operation.

After five years, the two groups had about the same odds of their cancer recurring, the researchers say. Yet women who underwent sentinel node biopsy reported less pain and nerve problems, and better arm mobility.

FALSE-NEGATIVE READINGS

Unfortunately, previous research has shown sentinel node samples have a false-negative reading between 5% and 15% of the time, a relatively high figure. A false-negative reading means that although the test results come back as normal, there really is an abnormality.

Still, Dr. Umberto Veronesi, director of the European Institute of Oncology in Milan and leader of the research, believes that in the long

Umberto Veronesi, MD, professor, surgery, University of Milan, and director, European Institute of Oncology, Milan, Italy.

David Krag, MD, professor, surgery, University of Vermont, Burlington.

New England Journal of Medicine.

run the procedure may save more lives than removing all the lymph nodes. "We believe that leaving normal lymphatic tissue [in the armpit] will help protect women and help patients do better," Veronesi says.

QUESTIONS REMAIN

Dr. David Krag, a University of Vermont cancer surgeon who helped develop the sentinel node biopsy, says two major questions about the surgery remain. Do the reduced side effects and discomfort over conventional surgery come at the price of an increased risk of death? And does sentinel node biopsy offer inferior control of cancer in the breast itself?

Two studies now under way should answer those questions, says Krag. Each is a head-to-head comparison of sentinel node surgery with immediate axillary tissue removal.

info For more information on sentinel node biopsy, visit the M.D. Anderson Cancer Center at *www2.mdanderson.org.*

■ ■ ■ ■

Warning Signs

Breast cancer is the second most common form of cancer in women in the United States, after skin cancer.

Approximately 212,000 women were diagnosed with the disease in 2003, according to the National Cancer Institute. Another 1,300 men were found to have the illness, too.

Although breast cancer can be deadly, if caught early the disease responds well to treatment. As a result, health officials recommend that women get screened regularly for breast tumors.

NCI advises that…

• **Women in their 40s and older** should have mammograms every one to two years.

• **Women who are at higher than average risk of breast cancer** because of family history should talk with their health care providers about whether to have mammograms before age 40 and how often to have them.

Many women also perform self-examinations of their breasts. Those that do should be aware of changes that might signal the presence of a tumor. *These include…*

• **A lump or thickening** in or near the breast or in the underarm area.

• **Nipple tenderness.**

• **A change in breast size or shape.**

• **A nipple that is turned inward** into the breast itself.

• **The skin of the breast,** areola or nipple may be scaly, red or swollen. The skin may also have ridges or pitting so that it looks like the skin of an orange.

• **Fluid discharge** from the nipple.

If a woman is found to have breast cancer, she may undergo a combination of treatments —chemotherapy, surgery to remove the mass, radiation to kill off any cancer cells left behind and medication to prevent the growth of additional tumors.

Some women choose to undergo complete removal of the affected breast (or even both breasts), a procedure called mastectomy.

Too Many Biopsies Bias Study Results

Stephen B. Edge, MD, medical director, breast and soft tissue surgery, Roswell Park Cancer Institute, Buffalo, NY.
Journal of the National Cancer Institute.

An investigational procedure is now routinely performed on women who have early-stage breast cancer, but some experts say this may be premature.

Although a sentinel node biopsy involves less surgery than the standard procedure to detect the spread of cancer, adopting this investigational method too soon may compromise ongoing clinical trials, experts say.

In the standard procedure, called *axillary node dissection,* the lymph nodes under the arm of the patient are removed so the doctor can evaluate if there has been any spread of the disease. If it has spread, more treatment, such as chemotherapy, is ordered.

However, the standard procedure results in approximately 25% of women developing pain or chronic swelling of the arm, called lymphedema, according to the American Cancer Society.

The newer procedure, called sentinel node biopsy, involves identifying the first—or sentinel—node under the arm, and testing it. The theory is that if the breast cancer is going to spread, it will first travel to the sentinel node. If the cancer is not in that node, additional surgery can be avoided. If it has spread there, the surgeon can follow-up with the axillary node dissection.

"This is a complex issue," says study author Dr. Stephen B. Edge, medical director of breast and soft tissue surgery at Roswell Park Cancer Institute in Buffalo, New York.

"On the one hand, there is an enormous body of literature showing the technique of sentinel node biopsy is accurate. On the other hand, there is not [yet] a head-to-head comparison with full lymph node dissection."

Edge and his colleagues examined the pattern of how the sentinel node technique was used, evaluating 3,003 women with stage I or II breast cancer.

Overall, the sentinel node biopsy alone was used in 13% of the women, sentinel node and axillary node dissection in 22%, axillary node dissection was used in 59% and no axillary surgery in 6%.

The use of the new technique in the 1,763 women with stage I cancers treated with breast-conserving surgery increased over the study period from 8% to 58%.

"It appears that the surgical teams at these centers, reviewing the available evidence, felt they could accept [the new procedure] as the standard of care," Edge says.

Edge questions whether that might bias the results of the ongoing clinical trials comparing the techniques.

But the counterargument, he acknowledges, is that putting off the use of sentinel node biopsy while awaiting the results of ongoing clinical trials—expected in 2007—means more women would experience side effects such as lymphedema.

■ ■ ■ ■

Facts About Surgery

Many myths exist about the dangers of breast cancer surgery. *A not-for-profit organization, Breastcancer.org, debunks the following two myths...*

Myth #1: Surgery opens up the cancer to the air and makes it spread.

You're feeling just fine, and then something suspicious is discovered in your breast. Surgery is performed and the diagnosis is cancer. When later tests show cancer elsewhere, you may think that it was the surgery that released the cancer cells, allowing them to spread all over the body. "After all, I couldn't feel them before," you might say. But metastatic breast cancer (cancer that has spread outside of the breast to other areas of the body) can be silent for a long time before surgery. Surgery does not cause cancer to spread.

Myth #2: Mastectomy is safer than lumpectomy with radiation therapy.

Not necessarily true. For women who have one site of breast cancer, with a tumor (less than four centimeters) that is removed with clear margins, lumpectomy with radiation is likely to be equally as effective as mastectomy.

New Drug Lowers Breast Cancer Recurrence by 50%

Teleconference with Paul Goss, MD, PhD, Princess Margaret Hospital, Toronto, Ontario, Canada.
New England Journal of Medicine online release.

The results of a major international trial of the cancer drug *letrozole* were so promising that investigators decided to stop the trial early.

Breast cancer patients taking letrozole, one of a new class of drugs called aromatase inhibitors, had about half the rate of cancer recurrences as women taking a placebo.

"The results are absolute, confirmed and credible," says study investigator Dr. Paul Goss. "An independent monitoring committee recommended that we stop the study by preset statistical boundaries, which we exceeded by at least tenfold."

TAMOXIFEN BENEFITS AND RISKS

An older drug called *tamoxifen* has helped women who have estrogen-receptor-positive breast cancer; that is, cancer fueled by the hormone estrogen.

Tamoxifen reduces the risk of recurrence by 47% and the risk of death by 26% for five years after surgery.

Unfortunately, when tamoxifen is used for longer than five years, it may actually promote the growth of cancer cells. Women who are more than five years past surgery represent the largest subgroup of women with breast cancer, Goss says.

"What is unrecognized is that over 50% of recurrences unfortunately occur beyond five years after diagnosis," Goss says. "Because it continues to relapse almost indefinitely, there is no limit to the disease."

Doctors have lacked any appropriate tools for the hundreds of thousands of women who enter that post-five-year period every year. Until now.

THE STUDY

The letrozole trial started enrolling participants in 1998 and ended up with 5,187 women in Canada, the United States and Europe who were postmenopausal, had hormone-receptor-positive tumors and had been taking tamoxifen for approximately five years. All of the women had to be within three months of stopping tamoxifen and all were disease-free when enrolled. The trial was coordinated by the National Cancer Institute of Canada.

The participants in Goss's study received either 2.5 milligrams (mg) of letrozole or a matching placebo daily for five years. Letrozole reduced the risk of recurrence by 43%.

SIDE EFFECTS

The median follow-up was only 2.4 years when the trial was stopped. There are some drawbacks to stopping a trial early, including questions about side effects and the effectiveness of the drug over time.

At the time of the study's early closure, the number of women who were experiencing side effects in the placebo and the letrozole groups was approximately the same, except in the rate of bone thinning, which was slightly higher in the letrozole group.

Tamoxifen provides protection against bone fractures, but it contributes to endometrial cancer and blood clots. Women considering letrozole therapy need to discuss with their doctor ways to mitigate the risk of osteoporosis.

Letrozole has been approved by the Food and Drug Administration (FDA) for the treatment of some forms of breast cancer.

Current and future studies of aromatase inhibitors will look at whether letrozole could be used instead of tamoxifen, whether this drug could be used for women who have been off tamoxifen therapy for longer than three months and whether the success of letrozole will continue over longer time frames.

info The American Cancer Society has more information on cancer drugs at *www. cancer.org.*

Limited Radiation Shows Promise for Breast Cancer Treatment

Frank A. Vicini, MD, chief of oncology, William Beaumont Hospital, Royal Oak, MI.
Paul Wallner, DO, chief of radiation oncology, National Cancer Institute, Bethesda, MD.
Journal of the National Cancer Institute.

A woman who undergoes limited-field radiation after breast cancer surgery has similar survival and recurrence rates as a woman who receives whole-breast radiation, researchers report.

"For about 10 years, we have been looking at whether limited-field radiation, which limits radiation to the tumor site and a small surrounding area, is as effective as treating the whole breast in patients with early-stage breast cancer," says Dr. Frank A. Vicini, the chief of oncology at William Beaumont Hospital in Royal Oak, Michigan.

THE STUDY

The report compares five-year results of 199 women with early-stage breast cancer who were treated with limited-field radiation after breast-conserving surgery with 199 similar women who were treated with whole-breast radiation therapy.

The researchers found that there was no difference in the median time until the recurrence of cancer at the same location. They also found that there was no difference in the spread of the cancer beyond the breast, or in overall survival rates.

Vicini says he thinks limited-field radiation is appropriate therapy in women with an early-stage cancer that has not spread to the lymph nodes and with a clearly defined tumor.

The advantages of limited-field radiation therapy include a shorter treatment cycle—five days compared with six—and fewer side effects, he says.

FUTURE TRIALS

Although randomized trials that compare both treatments are being conducted in Europe, Vicini would like to see a randomized study done in the United States. The advantage of such a study is that it would identify the kind of patients most likely to benefit from limited-field radiation therapy. The disadvantage is that it will take many years to complete.

Meanwhile, many physicians are offering limited-field radiation therapy. Vicini cautions that this type of therapy may become the standard of care without proper study.

Dr. Paul Wallner, chief of radiation oncology at the National Cancer Institute, and his colleagues also recommend randomized trials before limited-field radiation therapy is widely used.

"But we recognize that physicians will use this therapy now and trials will take a long time," Wallner says. "We are raising a note of caution. One of our concerns is that people will think this therapy is applicable to a different group of patients than it was tested on.

Physicians should be sure to tell their patients that the results are based on small studies among highly selected patients."

(info) To learn more about breast cancer treatments, visit the National Cancer Institute at *www.cancer.gov.*

Stop Hormone Therapy Immediately if You Have Breast Cancer

Nigel Bundred, MD, professor, surgical oncology, South Manchester University Hospital, Manchester, England.
David Decker, MD, chief, hematology/oncology, William Beaumont Hospital, Royal Oak, MI.
Cancer.

By now it's well known that hormone therapy, and estrogen in particular, slightly increases the risk of breast cancer. Less clear is what women taking estrogen should do if they develop a breast tumor.

A recent study has found that women who develop breast cancer while taking hormone therapy should stop taking the drugs.

The reason: Tumors that grow more rapidly in the presence of estrogen become less aggressive when the hormone is withdrawn.

When hormone replacement therapy (HRT) is stopped, the tumors "stop growing," says study leader Dr. Nigel Bundred, a breast cancer expert at South Manchester University Hospital in England.

HRT AND BREAST CANCER

The majority of breast cancers in women taking HRT are sensitive to estrogen, meaning they grow more quickly when supplied with the hormone. Indeed, the hormone stimulates tumors that might otherwise remain hidden, Bundred says.

In the United States, halting estrogen therapy is the common course for women newly diagnosed with breast cancer. But, occasionally, doctors may continue to prescribe HRT for these patients because suddenly stopping the drugs can lead to an uncomfortable rush of hot flashes, vaginal dryness and various other symptoms of menopause. The latest study indicates that practice might be harmful.

THE STUDY

Bundred and his colleagues looked at 140 women treated for breast cancer in England during a four-year period. All had been taking HRT at the time of their diagnosis, but 125 immediately stopped taking the hormones when they learned that they had cancer.

The remaining 15 women continued taking HRT until they had surgery to remove the cancer, a period lasting up to one month. The researchers also studied 55 other women with breast cancer who weren't taking HRT, and used them as a control group.

Of the 125 women who stopped HRT, 106 (approximately 85%) had breast tumors that were sensitive to estrogen. Twelve of the 15 women who continued taking hormones had such cancers.

Cancer growth that was sensitive to estrogen slowed down markedly in the women who stopped taking HRT between diagnosis and surgery.

Cancers that were not estrogen-sensitive didn't slow down, and for women with these cancers HRT is not harmful, Bundred says.

OTHER RESEARCH CONTRADICTS STUDY

However, at least one recent study found that women who continued taking HRT after a diagnosis of breast cancer did not fare any worse than those who stopped taking hormones. "We didn't have any adverse outcomes in terms of breast cancer," says Dr. David Decker, chief of hematology/oncology at William Beaumont Hospital in Royal Oak, Michigan, who led that study.

Decker is willing to let women continue treatment with HRT after breast cancer turns up, but admits he's in the minority in this country and that most doctors cease the hormones immediately.

info Visit the Women's Health Initiative at *www.nhlbi.nih.gov/whi* for more information on HRT's risks and benefits.

Genetics Determine Best Breast Cancer Treatment

William D. Foulkes, MB, PhD, director, program in cancer genetics, and associate professor in the departments of medicine, human genetics and oncology, McGill University, Montreal.
Julia Smith, MD, oncologist, clinical assistant professor, New York University School of Medicine, New York City.
Cancer.

Not all breast cancer tumors are the same, according to a study, and this finding may dramatically affect the course of the disease and the choice of treatment.

In the past, the medical community thought that most breast tumors were predictable, with a correlation between tumor size, the spread of the cancer cells to the nearby lymph nodes and the severity of the disease, says William D. Foulkes, study author who is also director of the program in cancer genetics at McGill University in Montreal.

But the new study found that even when tumors are small or the cancer does not invade lymph nodes, women with the BRCA1 gene mutation—an inherited genetic defect —still frequently experience a virulent form of this disease.

"We may need to apply a different set of rules when investigating the benefits of screening, early detection and treatment, in carriers of BRCA1," according to Foulkes. "Now research shows not all tumors play by the same rules."

THE STUDY

The study gathered data from 10 medical centers in the United States, Canada and Switzerland. The research group, led by Foulkes, looked at 1,555 women with invasive breast cancer. Of that group, 276 women carried the BRCA1 gene, 136 had the BRCA2 gene (a slightly less aggressive gene mutation) and 1,143 women had no known genetic link to breast cancer.

THE RESULTS

The disease of each patient was categorized according to the size of her tumor. The researchers then used a mathematical calculation to estimate the chance of lymph node involvement for each tumor size. Lymph node involvement indicates a more aggressive form of the disease and the need for more dramatic treatment, including chemotherapy.

Foulkes' team found a significant correlation between tumor size and lymph node involvement in the women who did not carry any gene mutations, as well as for women who carried the BRCA2 gene. Specifically, the larger the tumor, the greater the chance that the cancer would invade the lymph nodes.

THEORY DOESN'T HOLD

But the calculations did not apply to the cancer patients who carried the BRCA1 genetic mutation.

For these women, Foulkes says, the tumor size did not appear to predict the course of the disease. He says this may indicate an entirely new and different disease progression when gene mutations are a part of the diagnostic picture.

Breast cancer expert Dr. Julia Smith agrees that the study represents an important new direction in breast cancer diagnosis and ultimately may affect the treatment of many different types of cancers.

"More and more, we are realizing that not all tumors behave or act the same way, and that, in many instances, you cannot apply general rules of treatment simply based on a diagnosis of breast cancer," Smith says.

All New Test— Nomogram—Tells if Breast Tumors Will Spread

Annals of Surgical Oncology.
Memorial Sloan-Kettering Cancer Center news release.

A new tool called the *nomogram* may give doctors a better sense of how likely breast tumors are to spread.

The nomogram was developed by researchers at Memorial Sloan-Kettering Cancer Center in New York City. It helps doctors calculate the likelihood that breast cancer will spread beyond the sentinel lymph nodes under the arms. This information is a key factor in determining whether a breast cancer patient is likely to benefit from additional surgery to remove all of the nodes.

THE STUDY

In a study, researchers assessed the pathological features of the primary breast tumor and the sentinel lymph node metastasis of 702 breast cancer patients.

The researchers then used that information to develop nomogram calculations to predict the presence of additional cancer in the axillary lymph nodes. They concluded the nomogram predictions were accurate to within a few percentage points.

"This easy-to-use nomogram will allow patients and their physicians to obtain accurate estimates of a patient's risk for additional disease in the axillary lymph nodes, and can assist greatly in individualized decision-making regarding further treatment," says lead author and breast cancer surgeon Dr. Kimberly Van Zee.

Ugly News: Cosmetics Linked to Breast Tumors

Philippa D. Darbre, PhD, senior lecturer, oncology, University of Reading, England.

Bert Petersen, MD, breast surgeon and director, Family Risk Program, Beth Israel Medical Center, New York City.

Cosmetic, Toiletry and Fragrance Association.

Journal of Applied Toxicology.

The most common group of chemical preservatives in cosmetics and deodorants has been found in human breast cancer tissue.

Although the discovery links breast tumors and this group of chemicals, called *parabens,* it is not clear what the relationship is and whether the use of these products might be hazardous.

A BETTER SCREENING METHOD

In a study, Colorado scientists showed how adding a contrast dye to digital mammography can reveal tumors not otherwise visible with conventional screening, particularly in certain high-risk women.

"We expect [that this method] will become an alternative to breast magnetic resonance imaging [MRI] in evaluating difficult-to-interpret mammograms or for screening women who have an elevated risk for breast cancer," says John Lewin, a radiologist and an author of the study.

The technique may also be useful for identifying potentially malignant breast abnormalities in women who have already been diagnosed with one breast cancer, according to Lewin.

Current studies show conventional mammography, which uses X-ray film to image the breast, misses up to 20% of all breast cancers. Nine percent of these missed tumors could actually be felt in the breast.

THE TECHNIQUE

The new technique—called *dual-energy contrast-enhanced digital subtraction mammography*—is filmless. Instead, it uses two ultra-sharp computerized images of the breast.

One image is taken much like a regular mammogram, but displayed as a digital picture on a computer screen.

The second image is taken in conjunction with a contrast dye that tries to "light up" areas of new blood vessel growth commonly associated with tumor development.

The two images are laid on top of each other and the matching areas of both are subtracted or removed. What's left is very often the image of a tumor—one that might otherwise be too small to be seen or one that is hidden in dense breast tissue.

For breast imaging specialist Dr. Michael Cohen, the technique represents a step toward much more accurate diagnoses of breast cancer, particularly in women who may be at very high risk for the disease.

"This is good science, and we need pioneers like Dr. Lewin to push the envelope and that's exactly what he's doing. He's laying the groundwork for what may be an exciting diagnostic option for certain women in the future," says Cohen, who is director of the Memorial Sloan-Kettering Guttman Diagnostic Center in New York City.

THE STUDY

Lewin and his research team looked at 26 women who had traditional mammograms. These breast exams had found lumps or other types of abnormalities, indicating that there was a need for a biopsy, but without verification of a malignancy.

All 26 received the dual-energy contrast-enhanced digital subtraction mammogram. Of this group, 14 of the women were ultimately shown to have a cancerous tumor.

Eleven of those tumors appeared as "strongly enhanced" images on the high-contrast mammogram, one appeared moderately enhanced and two were weakly enhanced.

For the 12 women who were found to be free of cancer, the high-contrast mammogram that was used showed either a weak enhancement or no enhancement at all.

Lewin points out that the contrast dye mammograms actually "lit up" every single malignancy and let the doctors see the breast cancer tumors that had been virtually invisible on traditional mammograms.

NOT FOR EVERYONE

Currently, there is no commercial machine that is available to perform this particular type of mammogram.

In addition, Lewin has not yet determined the precise level of radiation needed to obtain the clearest pictures.

And Cohen added that even if the system should become commercially available, it would not be necessary for all women.

"However, for those women who could benefit—someone who has dense breasts, for example, or when we can feel a lump, but it does not appear on a traditional mammogram—this technique could one day be an excellent diagnostic tool that is fast and easy and may yield important, even lifesaving answers," Cohen says.

info For more information on high-contrast X rays, visit the University of North Carolina at Chapel Hill at *www.rad.unc.edu* and click on "Research."

Mammograms Can Save Lives—Even in Those Over 65

Jeanne Mandelblatt, MD, MPH, professor of medicine, Georgetown University Medical Center, and director, Cancer and Aging and Cancer Outcomes Research, Lombardi Cancer Center, Washington, DC.

Cheryl Kidd, MPH, director of education, Susan G. Komen Breast Cancer Foundation.

Annals of Internal Medicine.

A study finds that the benefits of screening women who are older than age 65 for breast cancer every two years outweigh the costs and possible side effects. That conclusion is drawn from a review of 10 published cost-effectiveness studies.

Based on current medical spending, it costs an additional $34,000 to $88,000 per year-of-life saved to perform those biennial tests, the study found.

"It's very comparable with other spending," says Dr. Jeanne Mandelblatt, a cancer outcomes researcher at Georgetown University's Lombardi Cancer Center and the lead author of the study.

Treating adults who have mild to moderate hypertension with a medication that lowers blood pressure, for example, costs approximately the same—$16,000 to $72,000 per year-of-life saved, the researchers note.

However, a lot of older women are being screened every year, rather than every other year, "especially because Medicare covers that," according to Cheryl Kidd, director of education at the Susan G. Komen Breast Cancer Foundation in Dallas.

The cost-benefit question looms, in part, because of a lack of data on the issue. Few older women were included in the original trials of mammography screening, according to the report.

WHEN MAMMOGRAPHY MAY NOT BE BENEFICIAL

Most women are urged to have an annual mammogram beginning at age 40 to detect breast cancer before symptoms arise.

But some women older than 65 years who have other health problems, such as diabetes, heart disease, hypertension or other cancers, may not find any benefit in early breast cancer detection. A woman might die of a heart attack, for instance, before breast cancer would kill her, Mandelblatt says.

The authors of the study also note that diagnosing and treating breast cancer in a woman who is dying of another disease can reduce her quality of life, especially if treatment fails to extend her life.

Individual health status also makes a difference. A vigorous 80-year-old may get more out of a mammography screening than a frail 70-year-old, Mandelblatt says.

Screening "becomes more costly and harms begin to outweigh the benefits in the sickest women, such as those who have dementia" or other conditions that limit life expectancy, the authors note.

WOMEN STILL NEED TO MAKE THEIR OWN DECISION

Mandelblatt says the report is intended to guide future research and policymaking, not a woman's decision to get screened. Women need to make those decisions in consultation with their health-care providers, she says.

The report's findings are consistent with recommendations from the American Cancer Society, which says further research is needed on the risks and benefits of mammography for women with serious chronic health problems or short life expectancy.

Although many Americans remain squeamish about rationing health care, studies like this one help to put a fine point on the costs, benefits and risks of investing in certain services and tests, the researchers say.

info To learn more about mammography, visit the National Library of Medicine at *www.nlm.nih.gov/medlineplus.*

More Men Stricken with Breast Cancer

Sharon Giordano, MD, assistant professor, breast medical oncology, M.D. Anderson Cancer Center, Houston.

Kathleen Wilson, MD, senior internal medicine specialist, Ochsner Clinic Foundation, New Orleans.

Alison Estabrook, MD, breast surgeon, Comprehensive Breast Center, St. Lukes–Roosevelt Hospital, New York City.

Cancer, online edition.

Although it is still rare, the incidence of breast cancer in men has increased significantly over the past 25 years, a study says. Researchers found that the number of cases rose from 0.86 to 1.08 cases per 100,000 men.

They also found that men typically were diagnosed at a later age and at a later stage of the disease than women.

The study was led by Dr. Sharon Giordano, an assistant professor of breast medical oncology at the M.D. Anderson Cancer Center in Houston, Texas.

"Because it is very rare, we have not had good information about male breast cancer epidemiology, treatment or prognosis," Giordano says.

"We had not even been able to determine whether the disease presents the same way in both sexes. Our examination and analysis of the National Cancer Institute's data has helped fill in some of those gaps in our knowledge," he adds.

SOME THEORIES

The study did not provide any clue about why male breast tumors are on the rise. But other medical experts have some ideas.

"There are at least three factors that could be associated with the increase observed," says Dr. Alison Estabrook, a breast surgeon at the Comprehensive Breast Center at St. Luke's–Roosevelt Hospital in New York City.

"The first is an increase in carcinogens in the environment; the second is more awareness that males can have this type of cancer leading to more such diagnoses; and the third is the current epidemic of obesity."

Estabrook explains that increases in body fat are associated with increases in circulating estrogen, a factor that is associated with the development of breast cancer in both men and women.

TREATMENT

"Men whose families carry the breast cancer gene and have a strong family history of female breast cancer have a higher risk," says Dr. Kathleen Wilson, senior internal medicine specialist at the Ochsner Clinic Foundation in New Orleans.

The treatment that is usually recommended for male breast cancer is modified radical mastectomy surgery.

"The lumpectomy that is performed in women is not practical because there is so little breast tissue in men. Lymph nodes that are under the arm are sampled or a PET scan can show if there is cancer outside of the breast," she adds.

STATISTICS

Approximately 1,300 men are diagnosed with breast cancer and nearly 400 die from it in the United States each year, according to Wilson. There is one man diagnosed with breast cancer for every 150 women with the diagnosis, she says.

info To learn more about men and breast cancer, visit the University of Maryland Medicine Web site at *www.umm.edu/men/brstcan.htm.*

Tamoxifen Cuts Breast Cancer Risk by 50%

Henry M. Kuerer, MD, PhD, director, Breast Surgical Oncology Training Program, University of Texas M.D. Anderson Cancer Center, Houston.

Cancer, online edition.

Tamoxifen has been shown to cut breast cancer risk by nearly 50%, yet many women at high risk of the disease are not taking the drug.

A study found that although 63% of women were offered the drug, only 26% accepted it.

The researchers believe that physician practices are responsible for the low rates of tamoxifen use.

TAMOXIFEN HISTORY

Tamoxifen, a drug that doctors have been using to treat breast cancer since 1978, was approved in 1998 for use in women who are at high risk of developing the disease.

The Food and Drug Administration (FDA) based its approval on a National Cancer Institute (NCI) study of more than 13,000 women who were believed to be at an increased risk of breast cancer. The trial was halted 14 months early when interim results showed tamoxifen slashed the incidence of breast cancer nearly in half.

Tamoxifen works by blocking cancer cell multiplication, but it can cause a range of side effects, including hot flashes, irregular periods, vaginal dryness and the need to use a barrier form of birth control. It is also linked to an increased risk of blood clots, endometrial cancer and eye problems.

THE STUDY

Researchers at Northwestern University reviewed the records of 219 women who were seen at the Lynn Sage Breast Center for risk evaluation in the wake of the pivotal NCI study. Their hope was to identify markers that would predict which women would be offered and accept tamoxifen.

Two risk factors stood out as significant predictors. Women with a history of *atypical hyperplasia*—a noncancerous condition that indicates higher risk for breast cancer—or *lobular carcinoma in situ*—a precancerous condition—were twice as likely to be offered and accept tamoxifen therapy as women without those risk factors.

In general, if a woman is being offered tamoxifen, she is at an increased risk of breast cancer, the authors report.

TREATMENT CHOICES ARE PERSONAL

Dr. Henry M. Kuerer, director of the Breast Surgical Oncology Training Program at the University of Texas M.D. Anderson Cancer Center, says that patients need to hear the potential benefits and risks of tamoxifen, but the decision to take tamoxifen is ultimately a personal one.

"They're not universally taking a pill just because on the surface it sounds like they are going to decrease their chance of developing breast cancer," he insists.

If you are at an increased risk of breast cancer, talk to your doctor about the risks and benefits of tamoxifen so you can make your own informed decision.

Bone-Up on This Amazing New Breast Cancer Drug

Study report, European Cancer Conference, Copenhagen, Denmark, at the European Cancer Conference. Cancer Conference news release.

Concerns that a promising breast cancer drug might not be given to patients because of its propensity to increase the risk of broken bones seem to be easing, due to the results of a recent study.

Anastrozole has shown somewhat better disease-free survival rates than tamoxifen, the current standard treatment for women who have breast cancer.

Anastrozole also has proven better at reducing the recurrence of cancer, according to results from an international study known as the ATAC[1] trial.

THE STUDY

The study, involving more than 9,000 postmenopausal women in 21 countries, compared anastrozole, tamoxifen and a combination of the two drugs.

Women in the study who were taking anastrozole had nearly 60% more bone fractures after two years than those who were taking tamoxifen, reports Professor Anthony Howell, a medical oncologist at the Christie Hospital in Manchester, England, and chairman of the study's steering committee.

The bright side, Howell says, is that after four years the fracture risk with anastrozole was only 30% higher than the risk with tamoxifen.

"It is now important to see what happens when patients stop their treatment after five years," he says.

■ ■ ■ ■

Prevention and Early Detection

With many other forms of cancer, such as lung cancer, experts know at least some ways of preventing the tumors—such as quitting smoking. But with breast cancer, scientists haven't identified any simple and powerful way of preventing the disease.

However, women with a strong family history of breast cancer, those who've already had cancer in one breast, and those who inherit genes that put them at particularly high risk of breast cancer can take steps to reduce their chances of developing the disease.

Taking tamoxifen as a preventive measure is one way. Studies show that women who take tamoxifen for five years reduce their risk of breast cancer by nearly 50% compared with those not taking the drug.

Breast removal surgery is another option. Some women who are at high risk of breast cancer choose to have their breasts removed. This approach is highly effective, but because some breast tissue remains after the operation cancer may still occur.

The most important thing any woman can do to reduce her chances of dying from breast cancer is to be vigilant about screening for the disease.

The American Cancer Society suggests that all women aged 40 and older have a routine screening mammogram every year.

Women who are in their 20s and 30s should have a clinical breast exam at least once every three years.

All women who are older than 20 should also perform regular breast self-examinations and report any changes that they notice in their breasts to their doctor.

Block Breast Cancer Risk In Hodgkin's Treatment

Flora van Leeuwen, PhD, professor, epidemiology, Netherlands Cancer Institute, Amsterdam.

Journal of the National Cancer Institute.

In young women with Hodgkin's disease, the threat of breast cancer is a particular concern following radiation therapy. But research suggests that this risk can largely be avoided by blocking the effects of estrogen with drugs like tamoxifen.

"Tamoxifen has not been used in this [group of women], but it might be something that we should consider," says lead researcher Flora van Leeuwen, an epidemiologist at the Netherlands Cancer Institute in Amsterdam.

HODGKIN'S DISEASE

Hodgkin's disease, which is also known as Hodgkin's lymphoma, is a blood-related cancer that affects 7,000 people every year in the United States, according to The Leukemia & Lymphoma Society.

Advances in treatment since World War II, including radiation and a variety of drug combinations, have greatly improved the odds for patients with the disease, and five-year survival rates now hover around 90%.

However, secondary cancers that are brought on by treatment have bedeviled many Hodgkin's patients.

Although many of these secondary malignancies aren't especially serious, some can be life-threatening.

RESEARCH REVEALS TWO KEY FINDINGS

The study made two key findings: First, it showed that a woman's risk of breast cancer after radiation treatments for Hodgkin's disease rose based on the dose she received. Women who got the most radiation had a 4.5 times greater risk of developing breast cancer than those who got the smallest dose.

"In Hodgkin's disease treatment, the mediastinal lymph nodes are irradiated and various portions of the breast receive different doses" in the process, van Leeuwen says.

"Calculating this dose was a labor-intensive part of the study, but crucial," he adds.

The second finding was that the chances that radiation for Hodgkin's disease would promote breast cancer was 60% lower in women whose treatment also called for chemotherapy, van Leeuwen says.

The likely reason: Chemotherapy can hasten the onset of menopause, van Leeuwen says. Since menopause is a hormone-suppressed state, and many cases of breast cancer are sparked by the female sex hormone estrogen, inducing menopause may blunt the ability of radiation to trigger breast tumors.

"We now know that with higher [doses of radiation], the risk of breast cancer is higher. But we now see that there may be a way to substantially reduce the risk of these cancers," says van Leeuwen.

info For more on Hodgkin's disease, visit the National Institutes of Health Web site at *www.nih.gov* or The Leukemia & Lymphoma Society Web site at *www.leukemia.org*.

Breast Cancer Survivors Have Lower Heart Attack Risk

Elizabeth B. Lamont, MD, assistant professor of hematology and oncology, Massachusetts General Hospital Cancer Center, Boston.

A recent study has found that men age 67 or older who survived Stage 1 or Stage 2 breast cancer were 34% less likely to have a heart attack than women of the same age without a history of breast cancer.

Theory: Estrogens that cause breast cancer may protect the heart.

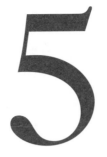

5

Cancer Breakthroughs

Prostate Cancer Test That's Wrong 80% of The Time

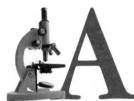

A leading screening tool misses more than 80% of prostate cancers, according to a researcher in Chicago. This test, called *prostate-specific antigen* (PSA), detects blood levels of a protein produced by the prostate gland, a chestnut-sized gland surrounding the urethra, at the base of the bladder.

Men with prostate cancer have a high PSA level, but not all men with a high PSA level have cancer.

Therefore, there is an ongoing debate about what numbers should actually be considered "high" by medical professionals.

THE STUDY

Dr. William J. Catalona and his colleagues evaluated 6,691 men who had PSA screening between 1995 and 2001. Of the men studied, 11%, or 705, then had a biopsy of the prostate.

STUDY RAISES QUESTIONS ABOUT WHEN BIOPSY IS NECESSARY

Many doctors order a biopsy for PSA levels of more than 4 nanograms of protein per milliliter of blood.

But Catalona found that up to 82% of cancers in men younger than 60 years, and 65% of cancers in men 60 and older, may be missed using that threshold.

A biopsy should be done when the PSA reading reaches 2.5, says Catalona, director of the clinical prostate cancer program at Northwestern Memorial Hospital and professor of urology at Northwestern University's Robert H. Lurie Comprehensive Cancer Center in Chicago.

William J. Catalona, MD, director, clinical prostate cancer program, Northwestern Memorial Hospital and professor of urology, Robert H. Lurie Comprehensive Cancer Center, Northwestern University, Chicago.

Herman Kattlove, MD, medical editor and spokesman, American Cancer Society, Los Angeles.

New England Journal of Medicine.

"Even using the 2.5 [as a cutoff], there will be some cancers that have spread," Catalona says.

In his own practice, Catalona has been following the 2.5 cutoff for eight years and is confident it makes a difference.

"If your PSA is 2.5, get a biopsy, no matter what your age," he says. There's one exception, he adds. "There are a lot of men whose PSA will jump up because of inflammation in the prostate. Try a course of antibiotics first. If it doesn't come down, then ask for a biopsy."

Not everyone agrees, including Dr. Fritz H. Schroder of the Erasmus Medical Center in Rotterdam, The Netherlands, who says, "This recommendation is not ready for routine clinical practice" and calls for ongoing, randomized studies.

Dr. Herman Kattlove, a medical editor and spokesman for the American Cancer Society, says, "I think you would find a lot more prostate cancer if you biopsy at 2.5. But I am not sure it would be necessary to treat all of them." The cancer may be small, slow-growing, or both, he says. And the side effects of treatment, including incontinence and impotence, must be weighed against the benefits, he says.

If a man's PSA reaches 2.5, Kattlove recommends that the doctor keep an eye on it to see if it rises.

info To learn more about prostate cancer, visit the National Prostate Cancer Coalition at *www.4npcc.org*.

■ ■ ■ ■

What the PSA Test May Show

The US Food and Drug Administration has approved the *prostate-specific antigen* (PSA) test for use in conjunction with a *digital rectal exam* (DRE) to help detect prostate cancer in men age 50 and older. Doctors often use these as prostate cancer screening tests in men who have no symptoms of the disease.

PSA is a protein produced by the cells of the prostate gland. The test measures the level of PSA in the blood. Normal levels of PSA range from 0 to 4 nanograms per milliliter (ng/mL). When the prostate gland enlarges, PSA levels tend to rise. The higher a man's PSA level, the more likely it is that cancer is present. But PSA levels can also rise due to benign conditions.

The most common benign prostate conditions are *prostatitis* (inflammation of the prostate) and *benign prostatic hyperplasia* (BPH, enlargement of the prostate).

Although PSA levels alone do not give doctors enough information to distinguish between benign prostate conditions and cancer, the doctor will take the result of this test into account in deciding whether to check further for signs of prostate cancer.

Age is the most common risk factor, with more than 96% of prostate cancer cases occurring in men age 55 years and older. Other risk factors for prostate cancer include family history and race.

Hair-Raising Drug May Block Prostate Cancer

Peter Greenwald, MD, DrPH, director, division of cancer prevention and control, Early Detection Program and Community Oncology Program, National Cancer Institute, National Institutes of Health, Bethesda, MD.

Leslie Ford, MD, associate director, Early Detection Program and Community Oncology Program, National Cancer Institute, National Institutes of Health, Bethesda, MD.

Ian M. Thompson, MD, professor and chairman, division of urology, University of Texas Health Science Center, San Antonio.

New England Journal of Medicine.

A drug used to combat male baldness and shrink benign prostate glands may also prevent prostate cancer, according to a government-sponsored study.

Men who took the drug *finasteride* for a period of seven years had a 25% lower chance of developing prostate cancer. In fact, the trial was halted 15 months early because of these promising results.

"This trial proves that prostate cancer, at least in part, is preventable," says Dr. Peter Greenwald, director of the National Cancer Institute's division of cancer prevention and control and also a participant in the trial. "It is a huge step forward for cancer research."

STUDY LIMITATIONS

Finasteride is the first drug shown to prevent prostate cancer, but a few problems exist. Although the men who took the medication had fewer prostate tumors, the tumors that did develop seemed more likely to be aggressive. Also, the drug was linked to an increase in sexual side effects, such as impotence, which may deter some men from taking it.

The results of the study suggest that finasteride could prevent or delay as many as 15 cases of prostate cancer in every 1,000 men who take it. However, it may also lead to an additional four cases of aggressive tumors in the men who do develop the disease.

Finally, the researchers say, there's no evidence yet that taking finasteride over time can reduce the death rate from prostate cancer. That question "is impossible to answer at this time," says study co-author Dr. Leslie Ford, a researcher at the National Cancer Institute, which funded the trial.

African-American men and men with a strong family history of prostate cancer may be inclined to embark on the therapy, says Dr. Ian M. Thompson, a urologist at the University of Texas Health Science Center and leader of the research. Any man considering finasteride to reduce his risk of prostate cancer should talk with his doctor.

info The National Cancer Institute has more information on prostate cancer at *www. cancer.gov*.

The Cancer–Hereditary Connection

International Journal of Cancer.
John Wiley & Sons, Inc., news release.

Men with brothers who have already had prostate cancer may face the greatest hereditary risk for the same disease, according to a study led by the Fox Chase Cancer Center in Philadelphia.

The study found a much greater risk of prostate cancer for men who have a brother with prostate cancer than for men who have a father, or any other combination of relatives with the disease.

THE STUDY

The researchers reviewed nearly two dozen studies and found the increased risk was 1.8 times greater if a man had a grandfather or uncle who had prostate cancer, 2.1 times greater if a man had a father who had prostate cancer and 2.9 times greater if a man had a brother who had prostate cancer.

"This study is the first to report a statistically higher risk associated with having a brother with prostate cancer than having an affected father," the study authors write.

The researchers suggest this strong link between brothers may be related to environmental or occupational factors, dietary exposures or age of onset.

■ ■ ■ ■

Prostate Cancer Warning Signs

The prostate gland is the part of a man's reproductive system that makes and stores seminal fluid. Seminal fluid is a milky substance that nourishes sperm and is released during ejaculation.

Prostate cancer is classified as the second most common form of cancer in American men, after skin cancer.

According to statistics from the American Cancer Society, an estimated 230,000 men in the United States are diagnosed with the disease every year, and approximately 30,000 men in this country will die from it.

In the United States, prostate cancer is primarily found in men older than 55 years. The average age of patients at the time of diagnosis is 70 years.

Risk factors include family history, race and diet. Prostate cancer is much more common in African-American men than in white men, and less common in men of Asian and American Indian descent.

Some evidence suggests that a diet high in animal fat may increase the risk of prostate cancer and a diet high in fruits and vegetables may decrease the risk.

Although prostate cancer is quite common, it's not especially lethal and the death rate has been falling.

Early detection and treatment of prostate cancer could reduce the chances of dying from the disease.

The National Cancer Institute lists the following warning signs of prostate cancer…

• **Frequent urination,** especially at night.

• **Difficulty starting urination** or holding back urine.

• **Inability to urinate.**

• **Weak or interrupted flow of urine.**

• **Painful or burning urination.**

• **Difficulty having an erection.**

• **Painful ejaculation.**

• **Blood in urine or semen.**

• **Frequent pain or stiffness in the lower back,** hips or upper thighs.

info See your doctor if you have any of these symptoms. You can learn more about prostate cancer from the American Cancer Society at *www.cancer.org.*

Zinc May Double Risk of Prostate Cancer

Michael F. Leitzmann, MD, epidemiological investigator, National Cancer Institute, Bethesda, MD.

Janet Stanford, MD, research professor, epidemiology, Fred Hutchinson Cancer Research Center, Seattle.

Journal of the National Cancer Institute.

Men who overdo it with zinc supplements may double their risk of developing prostate cancer.

Zinc has been a target of prostate cancer research for a long time because it is found in high concentrations in the prostate gland, but studies of its effects on cancerous tumors have yielded mixed results.

THE STUDY

In this study, researchers looked at 46,974 men and found an increased risk of prostate cancer in men who took the most zinc for the longest amount of time.

According to study author Dr. Michael F. Leitzmann, an epidemiological investigator at the National Cancer Institute, no increased risk was found in men who took up to 100 milligrams (mg) of zinc per day.

However, men who took more than that amount daily were 2.29 times more likely to develop prostate cancer than those who took less. And the risk was 2.37 times greater for men who took zinc supplements for 10 or more years.

Zinc is known to increase blood levels of an insulin-like growth factor and testosterone, both of which are directly related to prostate cancer, Leitzmann says.

Its possible malignancy occurs because high levels of zinc increase the growth rate of slow-growing prostate cancers, he says.

PREVIOUS STUDY RESULTS DO NOT PRESENT CONFLICT

One study that was released four years ago found an association between daily doses of zinc and a reduced risk of prostate cancer.

But this doesn't necessarily present a conflict between the two trials, according to Dr. Janet Stanford, a research professor of epidemiology at the Fred Hutchinson Cancer Research Center located in Seattle and a leader of the earlier study.

"Our study was not designed to assess supplement use," Stanford says.

The new study "does raise a question about the role of zinc [supplements] in prostate cancer. But it is not the basis for making decisions," she says.

info For more information on the risk factors for prostate cancer, go to the Fred Hutchinson Cancer Research Center Web site at *www.fhcrc.org.*

Doctors See Prostate Cancer Treatment Results In Just Three Months

University of Texas Health Science Center at San Antonio news release.

Presentation, American Society for Therapeutic Radiology and Oncology, Salt Lake City.

Men who have had radiation treatment for prostate cancer must endure an equally grueling waiting game to see if their disease will return.

For many people, the success or failure of the therapy isn't clear until one year—and sometimes two—has passed without a return of their tumor.

But a study by researchers at the University of Texas Health Science Center at San Antonio suggests that the effectiveness of radiation therapy for men with prostate cancer can be predicted as early as three months after they complete treatment.

THE STUDY

Lead author, Dr. Sean Cavanaugh, a fourth-year radiation oncology resident, studied blood samples of 855 men treated with external beam radiotherapy. Cavanaugh and his colleagues compared the early prostate-specific antigen (PSA) levels of the men with their clinical outcome.

"At the three-month mark in this study, we established that if a patient's PSA level was lower than 3.0 ng/mL [nanograms per milliliter], his chance of long-term, relapse-free survival was 87.8%, compared with patients whose levels were above 3.0 at three months and who had only a 57.2% chance of relapse-free survival," Cavanaugh says.

"Patients generally have their PSA tested soon after therapy, but unless there is a dramatic increase, many physicians wait a year or two [before they] analyze the trend and interpret the information. My colleagues and I disagree with that approach," says Cavanaugh.

"We found that PSA levels at three or six months after radiotherapy were significantly prognostic for long-term outcome. Analysis of

early PSA response enables us to accurately identify those patients who have an 80% or better chance of being cured of prostate cancer. Once confirmed by follow-up studies, this method may help us identify men who will benefit most from the addition of hormone therapy, which has some serious side effects and should not be started in all men," Cavanaugh says.

How Often Do You Really Need a Colon Cancer Test?

Robert E. Schoen, MD, associate professor, medicine and epidemiology, University of Pittsburgh Cancer Center.

Polly Newcomb, PhD, director of prevention, Fred Hutchinson Cancer Research Institute, Seattle.

Journal of the American Medical Association.
Journal of the National Cancer Institute.

How frequently your doctor thinks you should be tested for colon cancer may depend on which of two studies has the most impact.

Health officials in the United States currently recommend that healthy people have a *sigmoidoscopy* every five years.

Sigmoidoscopy is a procedure in which a flexible tube is used to inspect the lower portion of the colon, where 60% of all colon cancers occur. The tube allows doctors to look for *polyps*—growths that can become cancerous. There is a slight risk the intestine may be damaged during this procedure.

THE FIRST STUDY

A study that was conducted by Dr. Robert E. Schoen and colleagues at the University of Pittsburgh Cancer Institute, included 11,583 people who had an initial sigmoidoscopy and 9,317 who had a second examination conducted three years later.

Schoen found that there is approximately a 1-in-100 chance that someone who tested negative on the sigmoidoscopy will develop a cancer, or an intestinal growth that leads to cancer, within three years of the last exam.

THE SECOND STUDY

The second study, which was led by Polly A. Newcomb, director of prevention at the Fred Hutchinson Cancer Research Institute in Seattle, collected information on the screening history and colon cancer risk factors of 1,668 cancer patients and 1,294 healthy people.

This study found that a single sigmoidoscopy reduced the risk of undetected cancer for as long as 15 years, suggesting that the length of time between tests could be extended.

There was a four-fold reduction in the incidence of colon cancer among people who recalled having at least one sigmoidoscopy, compared with people who said they never had one. The reduction in cancer lasted for at least 15 years, the report says.

When researchers rely on a person's memory of a procedure, it's not as reliable as a written record. But, Newcomb says, "We have found that people can accurately report if they have had a sigmoidoscopy."

IMPLICATIONS

Newcomb says her study supports lengthening the recommended period between sigmoidoscopies. It takes a long time for most polyps to become cancerous, she says.

"The five-year period recommended by organizations such as the American Cancer Society doesn't appear to be data-based, unlike other recommendations," she contends.

Schoen's group says the five-year recommendation should stay—for now.

"We need more data," Schoen says, adding he'd like to see what the cancer rate was five years after the first screening. "Maybe it's not that different."

"I do not think the results of [my] paper should be interpreted as saying that everyone has to come back in three years," Schoen says. But "it does look like the more screening, the less chance there is of missing something," he adds.

info To learn more about colorectal cancer and sigmoidoscopy, visit the National Library of Medicine Web site at *www.nlm. nih.gov.*

■ ■ ■ ■

Colon Cancer Symptoms

If it's diagnosed early enough, colon cancer is almost always curable. According to the American Society of Colon and Rectal Surgeons, the most common symptoms are rectal bleeding and changes in bowel habits, such as constipation or diarrhea. (These symptoms are also common in other diseases so it is very important you receive a thorough examination should you experience them.) Abdominal pain and weight loss are usually late symptoms possibly indicating extensive disease.

Unfortunately, many polyps and early cancers fail to produce symptoms. Therefore, it is important that your routine physical includes colon cancer detection procedures when you reach age 40. Those detection methods are a digital rectal exam (DRE) and a chemical test of stool for blood. A sigmoidoscopy—the inspection of the lower bowel with a lighted tubular instrument—should be part of routine physical check-ups.

info For more on colorectal cancer, visit the American Society of Colon and Rectal Surgeons Web site at *www.fascrs.org.*

Virtual Colonoscopy Results Disappointing

Peter B. Cotton, MD, director, Digestive Disease Center, Medical University of South Carolina, Charleston. *Journal of the American Medical Association.*

A computer-assisted test for colon cancer is gaining popularity because it is less intrusive than the conventional screening method, but a recent study suggests that it's not ready for widespread use.

Virtual colonoscopy is the examination of computer-generated images made from data received through an abdominal CT scan.

Researchers have found that the accuracy of virtual colonoscopy in detecting cancers is substantially lower than that of conventional colonoscopy. And they also advise that the use of this technique should be limited until the technology and training are improved.

"The accuracy of this technique was surprising and disappointing," says lead researcher Dr. Peter B. Cotton, director of the Digestive Disease Center at the Medical University of South Carolina.

The goal of this study was to see if regular radiologists could reproduce the results of the other studies, done at expert centers, which found that virtual colonoscopy was reasonably accurate. "And the answer was that they couldn't," Cotton says.

THE STUDY

Cotton and his team had 615 participants undergo both a virtual colonoscopy and a standard colonoscopy. The researchers compared the accuracy of both methods in detecting colon polyps.

The virtual colonoscopy found only 39% of the polyps that were at least 6 millimeters (mm) in size and only 55% of the polyps that were at least 10 mm in size.

The standard colonoscopy detected 99% of the polyps at least 6 mm in size and 100% of the polyps that were at least 10 mm in size, according to the report.

INSURANCE COSTS

Based on the findings of this study, Cotton says, "People should think hard before they spend money on a procedure that is not yet proven to be accurate."

Virtual colonoscopy is not covered by most health insurance, Cotton adds. "If you read some of the hype, it sounds very attractive, but it's only valuable if it does the job, and our study shows that in the real world, it may not do so."

Cotton also explains that even with a virtual colonoscopy, patients must perform the same bowel preparation as done for a standard colonoscopy. This preparation involves not eating solid foods and using laxatives to clean out the bowel.

Moreover, with a standard colonoscopy any polyps that are found can be removed during the procedure. If any polyps are found during a virtual colonoscopy, the patient will then have to undergo a standard colonoscopy and the bowel preparation again.

The virtual colonoscopy technique shows promise, however. With continuing improvements in scanners and the software that runs them, coupled with better and more specific training of radiologists, Cotton says virtual colonoscopy will be a valuable addition to the arsenal of tools used to detect colon cancer.

Cotton stresses that people who are experiencing colon cancer symptoms should have a colonoscopy, as should anyone over 50 years of age and all people who have a family history of colon cancer.

info The National Digestive Diseases Information Clearinghouse can tell you more about virtual colonoscopy at *http://digestive. niddk.nih.gov.*

DNA Test Identifies Colon Cancer

Martin Widschwendter, MD, professor, Department of Obstetrics and Gynecology, Medical University Innsbruck, Austria.

Douglas K. Rex, MD, professor of medicine, Indiana University School of Medicine, Indianapolis, and president, American College of Gastroenterology.

The Lancet.

A new test that identifies changes in cell DNA could lead to a noninvasive way of screening for cancer of the colon, researchers have found.

Scientists in Austria say that by testing stool samples for changes in DNA methylation—a genetic alteration that is common in colon cancer cells—they were able to identify colon cancer in approximately 90% of the cases that were studied.

"There are certain types of changes in DNA that are specific to certain tumors," says lead researcher Dr. Martin Widschwendter, a professor of obstetrics and gynecology at the Medical University of Innsbruck.

According to Widschwendter, earlier fecal DNA tests for colon cancer that have looked at gene mutations were not nearly as accurate as this new one.

THE STUDY

Widschwendter and his team tried to find the most promising markers for colon cancer by looking for DNA changes in the stools of cancer patients and healthy controls.

To confirm their finding, they then tested for these potential markers in stool samples from 49 subjects—some cancer patients and some healthy controls, according to their report. They found a gene that could be used to predict colon cancer.

Although other DNA markers have been identified in stool that predict colon cancer, this gene is the most accurate predictor found so far, Widschwendter said.

"What we are aiming for is to combine all these markers with gene mutation markers to develop a simple test that will be 100% accurate," he says. Patients who have a positive test would then go on to have a colonoscopy, Widschwendter adds.

Widschwendter believes this method can also be used to identify cervical cancer and other types of cancer by getting samples of blood and other body fluids and looking for specific DNA changes.

"This approach will open up a new and exciting way to screen for cancers," he says.

FINDINGS ENCOURAGING BUT PRELIMINARY

Dr. Douglas K. Rex, a professor of medicine at Indiana University School of Medicine and president of the American College of Gastroenterology, called the Austrian work "encouraging" with the potential to make a big advance in colon screening.

Using this marker along with other markers may be an effective way of diagnosing colon cancer, Rex says.

But he cautions that until a large screening test is done to see how well this test detects cancers in a large population, it remains only an interesting preliminary finding.

info The Colon Cancer Alliance has more information about screening for the disease at *www.ccalliance.org*.

Hard Alcohol May Increase Risk of Colon Cancer

Gurvinder Sethi, MD, assistant instructor, medicine, and Joseph Anderson, MD, assistant professor, medicine, Stony Brook University, NY.

Ann Silverman, MD, gastroenterologist, William Beaumont Hospital, Royal Oak, MI.

Presentation, American College of Gastroenterology annual meeting, Baltimore.

Toast to good health with wine, not a martini. Research has found that study subjects who consumed more than nine drinks per week that contained distilled spirits, such as vodka and whiskey, were three times more likely to have colon cancer. However, wine consumption appeared to reduce that risk.

THE STUDY

The study group included almost 2,000 volunteers, approximately 90% Caucasian. The equal number of men and women (*average age:* 57 years) had colonoscopies, a procedure in which doctors examine the colon using a thin, flexible tube equipped with a light and a camera.

In addition, information was gathered from each volunteer about their drinking habits, weight, family medical history, diet, smoking habits, education and exercise.

The researchers found that those participants who drank more than nine beverages containing hard alcohol per week had three times the risk of having cancer or a suspicious lesion on the colon compared with people who didn't drink at all. Heavy beer drinkers appeared to face a higher risk, but Anderson says the difference wasn't statistically significant. Drinking wine appeared to have a protective effect, and reduced the risk of having cancer or a suspicious lesion.

There was a strong association between spirits and the presence of a lesion on the colon that may be cancerous, according to one of the study's authors, Dr. Gurvinder Sethi, an assistant instructor in medicine at Stony Brook University in Stony Brook, New York. "The risk was 3.3 times higher than for people who didn't drink at all."

Dr. Joseph Anderson, an assistant professor of medicine at Stony Brook University, who was also involved in the research, says he's not sure why spirits would be associated with more suspicious lesions.

Dr. Ann Silverman, a gastroenterologist at William Beaumont Hospital in Royal Oak, Michigan, says it's possible there may be chemicals involved in the processing of these products that lead to the lesions, or they could be caused by another factor altogether, such as a history of aspirin use, that the volunteers had in common.

Because only 66 people in the study group drank more than nine glasses of spirits per week, Silverman says, the sample is too small to really draw any conclusions.

Anderson says the most important thing people need to remember is that "lifestyle, including alcohol consumption, has an impact on your risk of getting colorectal [cancer]."

'Keyhole' Surgery Recovery Time Faster For Colon Cancer Patients

The Lancet news release.

Minimally invasive, or laparoscopic, surgery for colorectal cancer offers quicker patient recovery times and has a similar five-year survival rate compared with conventional surgery, according to a study by researchers at the University of Hong Kong.

In laparoscopic surgery, doctors make tiny "keyhole" incisions to enter the body.

THE STUDY

Over a 10-year period, researchers compared the survival rates of approximately 400 patients with colorectal cancer, some of whom had conventional and some laparoscopic surgery. They found the five-year survival rate was 76% for those who had laparoscopy and 73% for patients who had conventional surgery.

Although operating time was much longer for laparoscopic surgery than for conventional surgery, recovery time was much shorter for patients who had laparoscopy. The study also found that laparoscopy was more expensive than conventional surgery.

According to the Society of Laparoendoscopic Surgeons, which represents practitioners of laparoscopy, nearly every organ is a candidate for for this type of surgery. The procedure is now routine for operations on the gallbladder, stomach, intestines, pancreas, spleen, kidneys, bladder and female reproductive organs, as well as the prostate in men.

The less invasive nature of laparoscopy returns the greatest benefits in its ability to reduce post-operative pain and infections associated with conventional surgery, experts say. On the downside, the technique requires expensive equipment and surgical expertise that smaller hospitals might lack.

Colorectal cancer is the second leading cancer killer in the United States, after lung tumors. Each year, more than 130,000 Americans are diagnosed with the disease and 50,000 die from it, according to the National Institutes of Health.

info Visit the Colorectal Cancer Network for more information on this disease at *www.colorectal-cancer.net.*

Some Colon Cancer Patients Don't Need Chemotherapy

Manish A. Shah, MD, assistant attending physician, gastrointestinal oncology, Memorial Sloan-Kettering Cancer Center, New York City.

Michael Spencer, MD, assistant clinical professor, surgery, University of Minnesota, Minneapolis.

New England Journal of Medicine.

Individuals who have colon cancer with a specific genetic characteristic may not benefit from chemotherapy, which is often a standard practice after surgery, a study says.

Colorectal cancer is the second most fatal cancer in the United States. Tumors are surgically removed, but some patients, especially those whose cancer has spread, are advised to get chemotherapy.

"In patients with a certain stage of the disease, the chance of recurrence is 50% to 60%," says Dr. Manish A. Shah, an assistant attending physician and gastrointestinal oncology specialist at Memorial Sloan-Kettering Cancer Center in New York City. "Chemotherapy reduces the chance of recurrence."

Or so doctors thought.

THE STUDY

The authors of this multicenter study, which was led by researchers at Mount Sinai Hospital in Toronto, wanted to see if microsatellite areas could predict how a patient responded to chemotherapy. A microsatellite area describes that part of a tumor cell that has an abnormally repeated sequence of DNA. Cells with many sections of abnormal repeats are said to have *high-frequency instability*. Cells with just a few such areas have *low-frequency instability,* and those that have no such abnormalities are considered stable.

The researchers analyzed tissue specimens from 570 colon cancer patients who had participated in previous studies of chemotherapy.

Interestingly, the patients with high-frequency instability had a better five-year survival rate when they did *not* receive chemotherapy than patients with low-frequency instability who did not receive chemotherapy.

Chemotherapy after surgery improved overall survival among patients who had stable tumors or tumors displaying low-frequency instability.

FINE-TUNING TREATMENT

No one knows for sure why the results turned out the way they did.

Although the findings form part of a larger movement to fine-tune cancer treatment to the individual, the study authors and others caution that therapies should not be changed until there is more confirmation of the findings.

"What we're looking for are specific aspects of tumors and genetic markers to see if they may be more amenable to more chemotherapy regimens," says Dr. Michael Spencer, an assistant clinical professor of surgery at the University of Minnesota in Minneapolis.

■ ■ ■ ■

What to Ask Your Doctor About Chemotherapy

Chemotherapy is usually given in cycles, with a treatment period followed by a recovery period, and then another treatment period. Usually, a patient has chemotherapy as an outpatient, but a short hospital stay may be needed depending on which drugs are given and the patient's general health.

Questions patients may want to ask their doctor before starting chemotherapy include…

● **What is the goal of this treatment?**

● **What drugs will I be taking?**

● **Will the drugs cause side effects?** What can I do about them?

● **What side effects should I report?**

● **How long will I need this treatment?**

● **What should I do to take care of myself during treatment?**

● **How will we know if the drugs I'm being given are working?**

When You Should Hold Off on Chemo

News release, *The Lancet.*

Delaying chemotherapy until symptoms develop could be the best option for patients with asymptomatic, advanced, low-grade non-Hodgkin's lymphoma.

THE STUDY

That opinion comes from a British study of 309 participants in which half were given immediate chemotherapy using oral medication. The other half of the participants were treated with "watchful waiting"—chemotherapy was delayed to see if the disease progressed. Local radiotherapy was given to people in both groups if their lymph nodes showed evidence of the disease.

People in the watchful waiting group had about a 20% chance of not requiring chemotherapy after 10 years. In patients older than 70 years, that rate doubled to 40%.

"An initial policy of watchful waiting in patients with asymptomatic, advanced stage, low-grade non-Hodgkin's lymphoma is appropriate, especially in patients over 70 years of age," says researcher Dr. Kirit M. Ardeshna.

The average follow-up of patients in both groups was 16 years. The study found no difference in overall survival (about six years) between the two groups.

■ ■ ■ ■

Non-Hodgkin's Lymphoma Symptoms

The symptom that is most common in non-Hodgkin's lymphoma is a painless swelling of the lymph nodes in the neck, underarm, or groin, according the National Cancer Institute. *Other symptoms may include the following...*

- **Unexplained fever.**
- **Night sweats.**
- **Constant fatigue.**
- **Unexplained weight loss.**
- **Itchy skin.**
- **Reddened patches on the skin.**

These symptoms are not sure signs of non-Hodgkin's lymphoma, and could be caused by other, less serious conditions, such as the flu or other infections.

If you experience any of these symptoms, it is important to see a doctor so that any illness can be diagnosed and treated as early as possible. Don't wait to feel pain—early non-Hodgkin's lymphoma may not cause pain.

info You can learn more about non-Hodgkin's lymphoma from the National Institutes of Health's Medline Plus at *www.nlm. nih.gov/medlineplus/ency/article/000581.htm.*

Mono Virus May Cause Hodgkin's Disease

Alan Kinniburgh, PhD, vice president, research, The Leukemia & Lymphoma Society, White Plains, NY.

Jay Brooks, MD, chief, hematology/oncology, Ochsner Clinic Foundation, New Orleans.

Mads Melbye, MD, PhD, professor and head, department of epidemiology research, Statens Serum Institute, Copenhagen, Denmark.

New England Journal of Medicine.

Scientists have discovered a link between the virus that causes mononucleosis and Hodgkin's disease.

Researchers from Denmark and Sweden report that the Epstein-Barr virus (EBV), the microbe that causes mono, is associated with an increased risk of certain types of Hodgkin's lymphoma in young adults.

Hodgkin's lymphoma is a type of cancer that affects the body's lymphatic system.

The finding from this study could be a milestone in understanding the possible causes of Hodgkin's disease.

"It confirms what we believed about Hodgkin's lymphoma—that as many as one third or more of the patients have EBV, the causative agent of mononucleosis," says Alan Kinniburgh, vice president of research at The Leukemia & Lymphoma Society. "That's important, because there's a possibility that something can be done for those patients."

Scientists have long suspected an association between Hodgkin's disease and EBV because people who have had mononucleosis caused by EBV also have an increased risk of developing Hodgkin's.

"This is probably one of the largest studies ever done," adds Jay Brooks, chief of hematology and oncology at the Ochsner Clinic Foundation in New Orleans.

"We've had hints, but this [study] is the most conclusive," he says.

THE STUDY

This study involved one group of 38,555 people who had had symptoms of mononucleosis and whose blood tested positive for

EBV. A second group included 24,614 people who showed symptoms of mono but had no evidence of the viral infection in the blood. The researchers then tested biopsy specimens of those who had cancer for the presence of EBV in cancer cells.

Overall, 29 tumors were traced to patients who had had mononucleosis. Of those, 16 (55%) had evidence of EBV. Those patients whose blood tested positive for EBV had a two to three times greater risk of developing Hodgkin's disease.

CANCER RISK STILL LOW FOR INFECTED

The authors stress that the chances of developing Hodgkin's even after a bout of mononucleosis is slim: Approximately one in 1,000 (versus one in 2,000 for the general population).

According to Dr. Richard Ambinder of Johns Hopkins University, more than 90% of adults are infected with EBV and, quite clearly, 90% of adults do not develop Hodgkin's.

"Most of us will be infected with EBV at some point during our lifetime, but very few of us will get mononucleosis," says study author Dr. Mads Melbye, head of the department of epidemiology research at the Statens Serum Institute in Copenhagen, Denmark. Even fewer will develop Hodgkin's.

However, knowing who is susceptible may help develop ways to head off the disease. "You can't avoid getting mono, but if we could identify certain individuals who are highly susceptible to [cancer] activity, then perhaps we could find strategies to prevent the disease in them," Brooks says.

"I certainly think this investigation has put us closer to that fact that EBV appears to play a causal role," Melbye says.

"It's not the only cause and other factors must be involved as well, but EBV is involved in the causal pathway of the development of some cases of Hodgkin's, though surely not all of them," he adds.

info For more on Hodgkin's lymphoma, visit The Leukemia & Lymphoma Society Web site at *www.leukemia.org*.

Psoriasis Linked to Lymphoma Risk

Archives of Dermatology.
American Medical Association news release.

People who have the skin condition psoriasis appear to have an increased risk of developing lymphoma, a group of cancers that affect tissues in the lymph nodes and spleen.

A study by scientists at the University of Pennsylvania found people who had psoriasis had three times more lymphoma than people who did not have the skin condition.

THE STUDY

The researchers studied a random sample of patients 65 years or older (2,718 who had psoriasis and 105,203 who did not) from the General Practice Research Database in the United Kingdom.

People who had psoriasis developed an additional 122 lymphomas per 100,000 patients each year compared with those without the skin disorder.

"Additional studies are necessary to determine if the increased rate of lymphoma is related to psoriasis severity, psoriasis treatment or an interaction between these risk factors," the study authors say.

Combo Scans Speed Cancer Treatment

Gerald Antoch, MD, resident, diagnostic and interventional radiation, University Hospital Essen, Germany. *Journal of the American Medical Association.*

Using two body imaging tests may be a promising tool for cancer diagnosis and prognosis, German researchers report.

THE STUDY

A combination of *positron emission tomography* and *computed tomography* (PET/CT) was more effective than *magnetic resonance imaging* (MRI) in determining the spread of cancer in a study of 98 patients.

All the patients, who had a variety of cancers, had both imaging tests.

According to the researchers at the University Hospital Essen, "PET/CT had a direct impact on patient management in 12 patients. Results from MRI changed the therapy regimen in two patients."

THE TECHNIQUES

A PET scan is done by injecting a radioactive tracer into a patient. The tracer can give information about cells. CT imaging generates a three-dimensional picture by computer manipulation of X-ray plates. MRI puts patients in a magnetic field to generate a three-dimensional image.

It's too early to tell whether the combined PET/CT technique will improve the ultimate outcome for patients, says Dr. Gerald Antoch, study author and a resident in diagnostic and interventional radiology at Essen.

"PET/CT has only been available for a limited time," Antoch says. "Thus, data on the effect of increased diagnostic accuracy on patient survival are not yet available. Studies addressing this issue will be required in the future."

The combined technique does give doctors more information faster, he says. A basic requirement of cancer treatment is knowledge about the stage of the disease, he notes.

"In most centers, tumor staging is still performed by more than one imaging procedure, thus increasing the time between tumor diagnosis and complete tumor staging, as well as the overall cost," Antoch says.

STUDY HERALDS CHANGE IN CANCER DIAGNOSIS AND CARE

The Essen report is greeted enthusiastically by cancer specialists at the Karolinska Hospital in Stockholm, Sweden.

"The day in which futuristic movies show a patient lying on a table, entering a tunnel-like device with blinking lights, only to return a few moments later with a rapid diagnosis and a specific treatment plan, does not seem as far away as once thought," says Dr. Lennart Blomqvist and Dr. Michael R. Torkzad.

If the combined technique lives up to its early promise, changes will be needed at cancer centers, Antoch says. There are currently only approximately 400 PET/CT units available worldwide, he says. MRI units are much more common.

Skin Cancer Raises Risk of Other Cancers In Women

Cancer.
John Wiley & Sons, Inc., news release.

Women who have a history of the most common forms of skin cancer have a greater risk of getting other cancers, according to a study by researchers in the United States.

AFRICAN-AMERICAN WOMEN FACE GREATEST RISK

The study found that women who had been diagnosed with nonmelanoma skin cancers—such as *basal cell* or *squamous cell* carcinomas—were more than twice as likely to develop other cancers, regardless of age, socioeconomic background, smoking status or other lifestyle factors.

African-American women who had some type of nonmelanoma skin cancer faced a much greater risk of developing other cancers than Caucasian women who had a history of nonmelanoma skin cancer.

In addition to these results, researchers discovered that African-American women with a history of nonmelanoma skin cancer were approximately seven times more likely to develop a second cancer than African-American women who never had skin cancer.

"This cross-sectional study, undertaken in a large, ethnically diverse and clinically well-characterized sample, supports an association between a history of nonmelanoma skin cancer and a history of other cancers in women," according to the study authors.

Roughly 1 million Americans per year are diagnosed with skin cancer, according to the US National Cancer Institute (NCI). Of these people, the vast majority will have basal cell or squamous cell tumors, which can almost always be cured.

■ ■ ■ ■

Sun Protection

The leading risk factor for skin cancer is exposure to sunlight. Sunlight can sometimes cause damage to the DNA that is found in skin cells.

The Skin Cancer Foundation offers the following seven tips for sun safety…

1. Don't sunbathe. A tan might seem glamorous, but it's not worth the risk.

2. Avoid unnecessary exposure to the sun, especially between the hours of 10 am and 4 pm, the peak period of time for harmful ultraviolet (UV) radiation.

3. Use sunscreens rated SPF 15 or higher. Apply them liberally and frequently.

4. Wear clothing that is protective, such as long pants, long-sleeved shirts, broad-brimmed hats and UV-protective sunglasses.

5. Avoid artificial tanning devices.

6. Teach your children good sun protection habits at an early age. The skin damage that leads to skin cancers in adults often starts in early childhood.

7. Examine your skin head-to-toe at least once every three months.

In addition to exposure to the sun, scientists have identified several other risk factors for nonmelanoma skin tumors. These include exposure to certain types of chemicals, such as arsenic, industrial tar, coal and paraffin, as well as exposure to radiation.

People with severe bone infections and inflammatory diseases, smokers and those people who have weakened immune systems—transplant patients, for example—also are at greater risk of the tumors.

Worried About Skin Cancer? Check Your Feet and Ankles First

Foot and Ankle Surgery.
American College of Foot & Ankle Surgery news release.

Melanoma, the deadliest form of skin cancer, is always a concern. But when the disease strikes the feet and ankles, it's particularly lethal.

THE STUDY

A study by Rhode Island podiatric foot and ankle surgeon Susan M. Walsh found that the overall five-year survival rate for people who had primary melanoma of the foot or ankle was 52%, compared with 84% for those people who had melanoma on the thigh or calf.

"The results of this study should serve as a strong reminder for physicians and patients to be vigilant in checking the feet carefully for evidence of skin cancer," Walsh says.

"A malignant melanoma on the foot, especially if it isn't painful and if it's on the bottom of the foot, won't be as readily noticed as a lesion on the face or arm. Foot melanomas, therefore, are more advanced and more dangerous," Walsh says.

RISK FACTORS AND HOW TO PROTECT YOURSELF

Melanomas can be found anywhere on the foot—even under a toenail. Risk factors for foot and ankle melanomas are similar to other skin cancers, and include excessive sun exposure, family history of skin cancer, numerous moles on the body and having fair skin, blue eyes or red hair.

Doctors should be highly suspicious when a patient has a pigmented or unusual lesion on the foot, Walsh advises. Anyone with moles on their feet should have the moles removed and biopsied if they change color or shape.

According to the National Cancer Institute, more than 53,000 Americans are diagnosed with melanoma each year, accounting for only 4% of the total number of skin cancers, but causing the vast majority of skin cancer deaths.

Formaldehyde Linked to Leukemia, Lung Cancer

Samuel S. Epstein, MD, professor emeritus, environmental and occupational medicine, University of Illinois School of Public Health, Chicago.

Michael Hauptmann, biostatistics researcher, National Cancer Institute, Bethesda, MD.

Journal of the National Cancer Institute.

Formaldehyde, the chemical that is used in everything from insect preservation to film manufacturing, is at the center of a debate over the danger it poses to workers who are exposed to the chemical.

A major United States federal analysis discovered that workers exposed to the chemical may have higher rates of leukemia. In addition, a study conducted in the United Kingdom suggests these workers also face a greater lung cancer risk.

Federal regulations have limited exposure to formaldehyde in the US since the 1980s, but some experts are calling for less research and more restrictions.

"We need more science like we need a hole in the head," says Dr. Samuel S. Epstein, professor emeritus of environmental and occupational medicine at the University of Illinois School of Public Health.

THE STUDY

For the US study, Michael Hauptmann, a biostatistics researcher at the National Cancer Institute, and his colleagues launched the largest-ever analysis of formaldehyde exposure. They examined the medical records of 25,619 employees at 10 industrial plants who began working with formaldehyde before 1966. Researchers followed up the workers through 1994.

The workers who were exposed to high levels of formaldehyde were up to 3.5 times more likely to develop leukemia than those who were exposed to the lowest levels. In total, 69 workers died of leukemia.

"The study definitely suggests that exposure should be kept to a minimum in the workplace and the environment," Hauptmann says.

Although it is not exactly clear how formaldehyde may lead to leukemia and lung cancer, Epstein says that both studies are "more than enough to warrant the toughest regulatory proposals."

■ ■ ■ ■

Where Formaldehyde Is Used

Most workers are exposed to formaldehyde during the manufacturing of certain products, including particleboard, plywood, plastic, photographic film and permanent press clothing. Scientists and pathologists also work with formaldehyde, which acts as a preservative and gives some laboratories their very distinctive smell.

Formaldehyde usually comes in liquid form, from which solutions are prepared. During this process, a colorless, pungent-smelling gas is released.

Exposure to high levels of the chemical can cause nausea, watery eyes, burning sensations in the eyes and throat and difficulty in breathing in some people, according to the US Environmental Protection Agency (EPA).

info To learn more about the use of formaldehyde in industry, visit the US Department of Labor's Occupational Safety & Health Administration at *www.osha.gov/SLTC/formaldehyde.*

Test that Helps Lung Cancer Patients Choose The Best Treatment

Vanderbilt University Medical Center, Nashville, news release.

The Lancet.

Doctors can now accurately predict the course of lung cancer with a new protein profile that has been identified by Tennessee researchers.

Scientists at Vanderbilt University Medical Center in Nashville found that a distinct pattern of 15 proteins in lung tumors can predict whether a person who has lung cancer has a good or poor prognosis.

The ability to assess an individual's prognosis may help doctors determine the most appropriate form of treatment.

Based on the information that is provided by the protein profile, the doctor may opt for more aggressive therapy if a patient has a good prognosis.

Patients who have a poor prognosis, however, may decide to avoid cancer therapies that may extend their lives slightly but at great physical and emotional cost.

PROTEIN PROFILE IDENTIFIES SAMPLES WITH 100% ACCURACY

The team of researchers at Vanderbilt analyzed 79 cell samples from lung tumors and 14 samples from normal lung tissue. *Based on patterns of protein expression that they found, the researchers were able to distinguish with 100% accuracy...*

- **Normal lung tissue** from tumor tissue.

- **Primary nonsmall cell lung cancer** from normal lung cells.

- **Primary nonsmall cell lung cancer** from cancer that had spread to the lungs from other organs.

- **Adenocarcinomas** from squamous cell carcinomas, and squamous cell carcinomas from large cell carcinomas.

Every patient who received a poor prognosis from the protein profile died within a year of diagnosis, while all the patients who got a good prognosis were still alive one year after the diagnosis was made.

MORE STUDY IS NECESSARY

"If this pattern is confirmed in large studies, its prognostic power exceeds that of virtually any previously published standard molecular marker," the study authors wrote.

The researchers also discovered that this protein profile can accurately determine the risk that the cancer has already spread to nearby lymph nodes.

Lung Tumor Patients In Clinical Trials Live 30% Longer

Cancer.
John Wiley & Sons Inc., news release.

Lung cancer patients who volunteer for clinical trials live longer than those patients who receive standard cancer treatment, at only a modest increase in medical costs, researchers have discovered. The study provides the first evidence that clinical trials offer cost-effective treatment for people with nonsmall cell lung cancer.

THE STUDY

Researchers at the Center for Cancer Economics, Technology Assessment, Innovation and Development in Detroit compared the outcomes for people with nonsmall cell lung cancer taking part in clinical trials with the outcomes of those receiving standard therapy. They also evaluated the cost-effectiveness of each treatment.

Clinical trials were 22% more expensive than standard treatment ($41,734 versus $34,191), but there was a major difference in overall survival, according to the study. People in the clinical trials lived approximately 30% longer than those who received standard care (1.3 years versus 0.9 years).

"The increase in costs associated with clinical trials may, in part, reflect increased costs associated with these new agents, but these effects appear to be offset by the improved survival," the study authors say.

■ ■ ■ ■

About Lung Cancer

Lung cancer is the nation's leading cancer killer, claiming more lives each year than cancers of the breast, prostate, colon and pancreas combined.

There are two forms of lung cancer—small cell and nonsmall cell tumors. Although many patients can have an excellent prognosis if lung cancers are detected early, the outlook becomes much less encouraging in more advanced cases.

Smoking is the chief cause of lung cancer in the United States, attributed to nearly 90% of all cases, according to the American Cancer Society (ACS). Men who smoke raise their risk of death from lung cancer more than 22-fold, and women who smoke face a 12 times greater risk of death from the disease, the US Centers for Disease Control and Prevention (CDC) says.

However, you don't have to be a smoker to be at an increased risk of smoking-related lung cancer. People exposed to secondhand smoke —such as those who live with smokers—have much higher odds of developing the disease than those who aren't exposed to smoke. Secondhand smoke is blamed for some 3,000 lung cancer deaths annually, the ACS says.

Another cause of lung cancer is exposure to radon gas. This toxic element is linked to between 15,000 and 22,000 of the nation's lung cancer deaths every year.

The good news is that quitting smoking significantly cuts your chances of dying from lung cancer—even if you've smoked for years. After 10 tobacco-free years, your risk of dying from lung cancer falls to about half that of a smoker's, according to the government's National Women's Health Information Center.

Because smoking is also a major cause of heart and vessel disease, quitting can lead to quick and dramatic improvements in cardiovascular health.

Cancer Virus Linked to Deadly Lung Disease

Norbert F. Voelkel, MD, professor of medicine, University of Colorado, Denver.

Ethel Cesarman, MD, PhD, associate professor, pathology, Weill Medical College, Cornell University, New York City.

Pulmonary Hypertension Association.

New England Journal of Medicine.

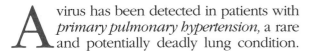virus has been detected in patients with *primary pulmonary hypertension,* a rare and potentially deadly lung condition.

If the finding is confirmed, it will be the first clue to discovering the cause of the illness.

Pulmonary hypertension is abnormally high blood pressure in the lung arteries, which can ultimately cause heart failure.

Most cases of pulmonary hypertension are labeled "secondary," meaning they are caused by another breathing disorder, such as chronic bronchitis.

Primary pulmonary hypertension, for which the cause is unknown, occurs in approximately two out of every 1 million Americans.

THE STUDY

A group led by Dr. Norbert F. Voelkel, professor of medicine at the University of Colorado Health Sciences Center, reports that evidence of infection with *human herpesvirus-8* (HHV-8) has been detected in 10 of 16 patients with primary pulmonary hypertension.

Tests were done on cells from patients who have either primary or secondary pulmonary hypertension. Immune system antibodies generated by exposure to HHV-8 were found in 10 of the patients with primary hypertension, but none were found in the patients with the secondary form of the disorder.

FINDING OFFERS HOPE

The finding offers hope for patients who have primary pulmonary hypertension. If HHV-8 does cause the lung condition, "that would help us find treatments for the disease," says Dr. Ethel Cesarman, an associate professor of pathology at Cornell University's Weill Medical College. "And you can have other defenses, such as vaccinations."

Until now, with no apparent cause evident, treatment has consisted of a continuous infusion of artery-widening medication.

"The current treatment is expensive and has not generated a cure," Voelkel says. At best, it has lengthened survival time to four or five years. Now that the condition can be regarded as "a form of malignancy," new approaches are possible, he says.

"The paper suggests that the virus causes it, but it requires confirmation," Cesarman says. The researchers acknowledge that "we cannot conclude that infection alone causes this condition." One possibility is that having pulmonary hypertension increases the risk of HHV-8 infection, they say.

info You can learn about primary pulmonary hypertension from the Pulmonary Hypertension Association Web site at *www.ph association.org*.

New Discovery: Common Gene Flaw Raises Cancer Risk

Virginia G. Kaklamani, MD, oncologist, Northwestern Memorial Hospital, Chicago, IL.
Loren S. Michel, MD, research fellow, Memorial Sloan-Kettering Cancer Center, New York, NY.
Journal of Clinical Oncology.

In the past, researchers who were interested in the genetic causes of cancer have focused on relatively rare mutations.

Now, scientists report that they have found that a common gene error appears to raise the risk of many types of cancer when combined with environmental carcinogens such as cigarette smoke or other toxins.

This research reflects an important shift in emphasis in cancer genetics research. Until recently, scientists have concentrated on *high-penetrance genes,* relatively rare mutations that run in families and greatly increase the risk of specific cancers. These include mutations in the *BRCA1* and *BRCA2* genes that sharply raise a woman's risk of developing breast and ovarian tumors.

Now researchers are looking at more common *low-penetrance genes.* Mutations in these genes are less likely to lead to specific inherited tumors, but they somehow interact with environmental factors to increase the risk of many different cancers.

THE STUDY

The new study by researchers at Northwestern Memorial Hospital in Chicago, used data from seven studies that included more than 2,000 patients with various types of cancer. They found that a mutation in a gene for a protein called *transforming growth factor beta* (TGF-beta) increases the risk of all cancers by 26%.

The TGF-beta mutation may increase the risk of breast cancer by 48%, ovarian cancer by 53%, and colon cancer by 38%, according to the researchers.

Now the Northwestern researchers are doing studies in which carriers of the mutation are being identified and followed up to determine their risk of cancer. "In the future, we hope that we can identify individuals at high risk because they carry the mutation," says Dr. Virginia G. Kaklamani, author of the study and an oncologist at Northwestern Memorial.

STILL A LONG WAY TO GO

The ultimate goal is to develop a model that includes a large number of low-penetrance mutations and that would assess overall cancer risk with a single genetic test, Kaklamani says.

The effort is being pushed in a number of laboratories because "finding these genes is going to be the frontier in cancer biology, giving us a new understanding of how cancer develops," says Dr. Loren S. Michel, a research fellow at Memorial Sloan-Kettering and a member of the research team.

info Get an overview of cancer genetics from the Medical College of Wisconsin at *http://healthlink.mcw.edu.*

New Drug Approach Offers Hope for Brain Cancer

Jeremy Rich, MD, assistant professor, medicine, Brain Tumor Center, Duke University, Durham, NC.
Mitchel Berger, MD, professor, neurosurgery, and chairman, department of neurological surgery, University of California, San Francisco.
Presentation, Molecular Targets and Cancer Therapeutics meeting, Boston.

Drugs that target small proteins in malignant brain tumors may be the weapons that will be used in the future to combat this disease.

Initial tests of some experimental versions of these drugs appeared to be very successful in both mice and human cancer cells when studied in a laboratory, according to a presentation at a conference about cutting-edge cancer research.

"We have targeted ways cancer cells stimulate tumor growth, promote their survival and create new blood vessels," says lead researcher Dr. Jeremy Rich, an assistant professor of medicine in the Brain Tumor Center at Duke University.

THREE TREATMENTS

In his presentation at the Molecular Targets and Cancer Therapeutics Meeting, Rich discussed three treatments. One is a drug called ZD6474, which blocks vascular endothelial growth factor (VEGF), and epidermal growth factor (EGF), both of which are involved in blood vessel growth, Rich says.

What is unusual about ZD6474 is that it blocks both VEGF and EGF, whereas most drugs block only one or the other.

"In clinical trials, single blockers have not worked great," Rich says. "But the combination has worked fantastically well."

"This combination has worked against gliomas, the most common type of brain tumor, but also other types of tumors. That's a pretty exciting finding," he adds.

SB431542, the second new compound, was tested with some success in fighting human malignant glioma cell lines.

The third compound, a combination of AEE788 and RAD001, blocked tumor growth more effectively than either drug alone.

HOPE FOR THE FUTURE

In the future, Rich sees treating brain cancer and other cancers with a combination of these drugs, customized for each patient, in addition to chemotherapy and radiation. He believes that eventually drug therapy alone may prove effective, eliminating the serious side effects associated with chemotherapy and radiation.

"These developments will enable us to design a cocktail approach to treating each patient," Rich says. "We can tailor [treatment to] the particular needs of each patient, based on the type of tumor."

"There is hope for the future, because treatments are changing rapidly. There are a lot of new treatments that are showing promise and that we hope will lessen side effects and increase our ability to control cancers," Rich says.

Dr. Mitchel Berger, professor of neurosurgery and chairman of the department of neurological surgery at the University of California at San Francisco (UCSF), comments, "We are all optimistic, but must remain cautious, since it is a long reach from animal models to humans. Notwithstanding, many of us committed to brain tumor research and new treatment therapies believe that we are making significant progress."

info To learn more about brain tumors, visit the National Brain Tumor Foundation at *www.braintumor.org.*

Drug Cuts Clot Risk In Half

Steven R. Deitcher, MD, head, section of hematology and coagulation medicine, Cleveland Clinic, OH.

Mark N. Levine, MD, professor, medicine, clinical epidemiology and biostatistics, McMaster University, Hamilton, Ontario.

New England Journal of Medicine.

Potentially lethal blood clots that plague many cancer patients are better treated with an injection than with a pill, according to a major international study.

Despite the clear benefit, however, financial considerations could interfere with the application of this scientific finding—the more effective treatment costs at least 10 times more per dose than the oral alternative.

THE STUDY

In the study, only 27 of 336 patients who used self-injected *dalteparin,* a sophisticated low-molecular-weight version of the clot-blocking drug *heparin,* had recurring clots. Of 336 patients who were given *coumarin,* a standard oral drug, 53 had clots.

Other studies have shown similar results, says Dr. Steven R. Deitcher, head of the section of hematology and coagulation medicine at the Cleveland Clinic. In fact, he performed one of those studies, which used another injectable low-molecular-weight heparin called *enoxaparin.*

BENEFIT VS. COST

Yet doctors continue to use coumarin, in large part for financial reasons, he says. Dose for dose, a low-molecular-weight version of heparin costs at least 10 times more than coumarin, and Medicare does not pay for it.

It's an important issue, Deitcher says. "Cancer patients are in a very high-risk group in regard to the development of blood clots, because of the underlying disease, as well as many treatments," he says.

For example, the catheters that are implanted to administer the cancer treatment drugs increase the risk of clots.

Because it is a difficult drug to manage, patients taking coumarin must have frequent blood tests, and they are often hospitalized.

But low-molecular-weight heparin doesn't have the same problems as coumarin, so it is "comparable in terms of cost-effectiveness," according to study author Dr. Mark N. Levine, professor of medicine and clinical epidemiology and biostatistics at McMaster University in Ontario, Canada.

"When you consider not only the cost of the drug, but also the cost of downstream events avoided, it's a wash," he says.

Levine says he believes doctors who treat cancer patients for blood clots will "undoubtedly" switch to injections of low-molecular-weight heparin, now that they can cite the results of this study. The switch will not come quickly, but it is already under way, he says.

info You can learn more about the danger of blood clots from the American Heart Association at *www.americanheart.org.*

One Radioisotope Injection Stops Bone Cancer Progress

Journal of Clinical Oncology.
University of Bonn news release.

A new way to more effectively treat certain kinds of cancer may have been discovered by scientists from the United States and Germany.

WHAT ARE RADIOISOTOPES?

These scientists have developed a radioisotope that emits more high-energy radioactivity than radioisotopes that are currently being used to treat bone metastases, which form when tumor cells invade bone marrow.

For many years, doctors have used radioisotopes to control the pain experienced by people with bone metastases—the end result of a multistep process in which cancer cells travel from the original organ through the bloodstream or lymphatic system to reach other parts of the body.

Metastases can occur in bones anywhere in the body, but they are mostly found in bones near the center of the body—the spine, ribs, pelvis, hip and shoulder bones.

The radioisotopes ease pain by accumulating in the area of the tumors. But the radioactivity of the standard radioisotopes that are currently being used isn't strong enough to slow or destroy those tumors.

In this study, the researchers say they've developed a radioisotope that emits higher-energy radioactivity. Although it emits high-energy beta radiation in its vicinity, its energy drops to near harmless levels in areas just a few millimeters away.

Bone metastases act like a magnet to this kind of radioactive phosphorous compound, which collects near the cancer cells and damages or destroys them.

THE STUDY

This study looked at 64 patients who had prostate cancer and bone metastases that no longer responded to the standard hormone therapy treatment.

The patients were divided into two groups. Some received one injection of the new radio-isotope medication, and others received two injections at an interval of eight weeks.

The study found that after one injection, the cancer stopped progressing for an average of 2.3 months. After more than one injection, this increased to seven months.

The survival rate of patients who received more than one injection increased from seven to 13 months.

A follow-up study is planned to investigate whether three or four injections yield even better results.

Bone metastases are not the same as primary bone cancers (cancers that begin in the bone). Primary bone cancer is much less common than bone metastasis.

■ ■ ■ ■

Bone Metastasis: Symptoms And Treatments

Bone metastasis is one of the most frequent causes of pain in people who have cancer. It can also cause fractures, dangerously high blood calcium levels and other complications.

Breast, prostate, lung, kidney and thyroid cancers are the most likely types of cancer to spread to the bones.

The first symptom of bone metastasis is almost always pain. If a cancer sufferer begins to experience pain in a bone, he or she should report it to a doctor immediately. Sometimes, if the cancer isn't promptly treated, the bone may break.

Researchers are trying to find ways to keep metastasis from occurring. They are studying drugs that might block the enzymes that help cancer cells break through blood vessel walls.

They are also studying a class of drugs known as *bisphosphonates*. Because these drugs may slow the growth of bone metastases, researchers are trying to determine if bisphosphonates can prevent bone metastases from developing in the first place.

Best Way to Treat Laryngeal Cancer

Herman Kattlove, MD, medical editor and spokesman, American Cancer Society, Los Angeles.
Arlene Forastiere, MD, professor of oncology, The Sidney Kimmel Comprehensive Cancer Center at Johns Hopkins, Baltimore.
New England Journal of Medicine.

Simultaneously administering chemotherapy and radiation to people who have laryngeal cancer offers the best chance of saving the larynx or voice box, a study says.

Researchers found the combination proved superior to chemotherapy followed by radiation and to radiation alone.

This powerful therapy is accompanied by serious side effects, such as difficulty swallowing and mouth sores.

"If you want to keep your larynx, this is the best way. But, on the other hand, you're going to suffer," says Dr. Herman Kattlove, medical editor at the American Cancer Society. But patients facing the ravages of this cancer seem to think it's worth it, experts say.

"I think there's no question that the patients view it as worthwhile, mainly because [the side effects of the treatment are] by-and-large reversible," says Dr. Arlene Forastiere, the lead author of the study as well as an oncology professor at the Sidney Kimmel Comprehensive Cancer Center at Johns Hopkins, located in Baltimore.

THE STUDY

The study compared three different therapies head-to-head—chemotherapy followed by radiation, chemotherapy concurrent with radiation and radiation alone. In all, 547 patients were randomized to one of the three groups and were followed up for an average of approximately four years to see if the larynx could be saved.

After two years, 88% of patients who had received radiation and chemotherapy concurrently still had an intact larynx, compared with 75% in the group that received chemotherapy followed by radiation and 70% in the group that received radiation alone.

Overall survival rates were similar in all three groups—approximately 75% at one year and 55% at two years.

Many patients with laryngeal cancer have other risk factors, however, such as smoking and drinking, which could affect their survival.

UNCOMFORTABLE SIDE EFFECTS

Patients in the group that received chemotherapy and radiation at the same time had more difficulty swallowing one year after the treatment.

Individuals receiving the concurrent treatment also had twice the frequency of mouth sores as the other two groups. "Think of your worst oral sore and double it. That's what they had," Kattlove says.

The patients in the study were supported with pain medication and most of them had a tube in their stomachs to provide nutrition, Forastiere says.

"There was definitely more toxicity, mouth sores, redness to the throat and mouth, and skin reaction," she adds. "These are things that are uncomfortable, but reversible."

info The University of Maryland Greenebaum Cancer Center has more information on cancer of the larynx at *www.umm.edu/cancer/overview/laryn.html.*

■ ■ ■ ■

Treating Laryngeal Cancer

Each year, 9,500 Americans are diagnosed with laryngeal cancer and 3,800 people die of it.

Small tumors can be treated with radiation or surgery without the loss of the voice.

More advanced tumors, which extend beyond the vocal cords, had been treated by removing the larynx (and thus, the voice) and administering radiation.

However, there was a breakthrough in 1991, when a clinical trial by the US Department of Veterans Affairs found that chemotherapy followed by radiation was just as effective, and in fact, preserved the larynx in approximately two thirds of the cases. This then became the standard therapy.

Surprising Strategies For Coping with Cancer

Joanna Bull, psychotherapist and founder of Gilda's Club Worldwide, a support community for people with cancer and their families.
Bottom Line/Health.

Living with cancer takes an emotional as well as physical toll. For more than 23,000 people with cancer and their families, Gilda's Club Worldwide has been the place to find—in each other—the emotional and social support they need.

Gilda's Club was founded more than a decade ago by Joanna Bull, cancer psychotherapist to the comedian Gilda Radner, who died of ovarian cancer in 1989. Gilda's Club has grown to 17 clubhouses in the US and Canada.

Ms. Bull, who has been counseling people with cancer for 25 years, offers some advice about the things that make a difference in living well with this feared disease. *Here are her suggestions...*

DISPEL MYTHS

You are the expert. It's your life and your disease. Your way is the right way, even if books, articles and well-meaning friends and relatives have different ideas. *Unfortunately, myths have developed that may make you question yourself...*

Myth #1: A positive outlook will increase your chances of survival. According to common wisdom, an optimistic, upbeat attitude will strengthen your immune system and enhance your body's ability to fight cancer. The truth is that there is no hard scientific evidence that your outlook has a significant impact on recovery.

If you can maintain an attitude of hope and a conviction that everything will turn out well, that's great—and that works for some people.

But if you ordinarily see the world through a darker lens and tend to worry rather than stride ahead with confidence, it's unrealistic to expect that having cancer will turn you into an optimist. Don't be tyrannized by the mistaken belief that being yourself puts your recovery in jeopardy.

Myth #2: You must face the facts. There's a widespread belief that it's necessary to accept the seriousness of the disease, and that anyone who doesn't achieve this level of absolute honesty with themselves is "in denial."

For some people who have cancer, minimizing the threat and even the imminence of death allows them to truly enjoy every day to the fullest.

Because cancer is full of surprises, no one really knows the facts, so the refusal to face them may be the wisest move of all for some.

Myth #3: You must be a full partner in your health-care team. Many people insist that it's crucial to take an active role in your own medical care. They say patients are obligated to educate themselves thoroughly about their disease, come to doctor visits with lists of questions and seek other medical opinions.

This approach isn't for everyone. If you feel more comfortable simply putting yourself in the hands of a health-care team you trust and doing what they think is best, go ahead.

Myth #4: This is not the time to make big changes. People living with cancer often are told not to make any significant decisions until they have the disease under control. But a look at your personal values and mortality may convince you to take steps that are difficult for others to accept.

Example: One woman came to the full realization that her marriage, which everyone thought was so wonderful, was actually stifling and even abusive. Face to face with the finitude of life, she left her husband. It made no sense to her friends who argued that now more than ever she needed caring support—but the decision was right for her.

Myth #5: Depression is normal and doesn't need to be treated. If your distress or anxiety about your disease makes it hard for you to function in everyday life, don't just assume that this is a normal, inevitable reaction to the seriousness of your illness.

Counseling or medication can help you get back on your feet, particularly if you become severely depressed. It's absolutely essential if you have thoughts of suicide. Cancer is not a death sentence.

GET EMOTIONAL SUPPORT

Emotional support is a tremendous source of strength. Plan for it. This may mean gathering your close friends and telling them what you need from them or leaning more on your spouse who also will need support.

What's been helpful for many patients is getting together with other people who are going through the same thing. These support groups relieve the tremendous sense of isolation that serious illness can bring. Also, getting to know people who are willing to share the wisdom of their experience is the best antidote to the myths that surround cancer.

Even though you've found your own way of living with cancer, hearing about what works for others can give you fresh ideas and make you more confident in your own choices.

Example: You get anxious when you undergo medical tests, such as MRIs. A fellow support-group member describes relaxation techniques he found helpful. Following his example makes the experience much less of an ordeal.

To find a group in your area, check with hospitals or social service agencies. Internet chat rooms, including those offered by the American Cancer Society, provide alternatives for people who live in isolated areas or who are more comfortable communicating on-line than face-to-face.

info For more information on how to get support for cancer patients and their families, visit Gilda's Club online at *www. gildasclub.org*.

America's Best Cancer Centers

John Connolly, EdD, editor and publisher, *America's Top Doctors*. Castle Connolly.
Bottom Line/Health.

W hen it comes to treating cancer, the top cancer centers offer the very best in high-tech diagnosis, treatment, research and prevention—a comprehensive approach that less-specialized medical centers simply can't match.

Castle Connolly Medical Ltd., publishers of *America's Top Doctors,* selected the following top cancer centers based on a variety of criteria, including status as a National Cancer Institute (NCI)–designated cancer center and the number of top-ranked physicians on its staff.*

The centers are listed here alphabetically, according to geographic region. Each offers the most advanced methods of diagnosis and cutting-edge treatments.

NORTHEAST

•**Abramson Cancer Center of the University of Pennsylvania** (Philadelphia). One of the first NCI-designated comprehensive cancer centers. Noted for programs in breast, hematologic and gastrointestinal cancers. 800-789-7366, *www.pennhealth.com/cancer.*

•**Columbia Weill Cornell Cancer Centers of New York-Presbyterian Hospital** (New York City). Noted for programs in urologic, breast and brain cancers. 877-697-9355, *www.nypcancer.org.*

•**Dana-Farber Cancer Institute** (Boston). Offers 12 specialized cancer centers and is a leading institution for cancer research. 800-320-0022, *www.dana-farber.org.*

•**Fox Chase Cancer Center** (Philadelphia). Fourth-largest hospital in the US devoted entirely to cancer. Noted for radiation oncology and noninvasive surgical approaches. 888-369-2427, *www.fccc.edu.*

•**Memorial Sloan-Kettering Cancer Center** (New York City). World leader in prevention, diagnosis and treatment of all types of cancer. Known for close collaboration between clinicians and researchers. 800-525-2225, *www.mskcc.org.*

•**Roswell Park Cancer Institute** (Buffalo, New York). Teams of specialists use a multidisciplinary approach in treating all types of cancer. 877-275-7724, *www.roswellpark.org.*

*NCI-designated cancer centers have undergone a competitive peer review process overseen by the NCI to ensure the highest standards of care. Physician rankings are based on Castle Connolly's nationwide survey of thousands of doctors who rate their peers.

•**The Sidney Kimmel Comprehensive Cancer Center at Johns Hopkins** (Baltimore). Close collaboration between clinicians and researchers allows access to innovative drugs and treatments, including bone-marrow transplantation and immunotherapy for virus-associated cancers, such as Kaposi's sarcoma as well as various types of lymphoma. 410-955-8964, *www.hopkinskimmelcancercenter.org.*

•**University of Pittsburgh Cancer Institute** (Pittsburgh). The Hillman Cancer Center has the region's largest inpatient stem-cell transplant unit. 800-533-8762, *www.upci.upmc.edu.*

•**Yale Cancer Center/Yale-New Haven Hospital and Yale School of Medicine** (New Haven, Connecticut). Noted for programs in dermatologic cancers. Also the first US center to offer transimmunization therapy for cutaneous T cell lymphoma (a form of non-Hodgkin's lymphoma). 203-785-4095, *www.yalecancercenter.org.*

SOUTHEAST

•**Duke Comprehensive Cancer Center/Duke University Medical Center** (Durham, North Carolina). Known for breast cancer research. Currently pioneering the use of random fine needle aspiration to detect precancerous breast cells in high-risk women. 888-275-3853, *www.cancer.duke.edu.*

•**H. Lee Moffitt Cancer Center & Research Institute** (Tampa, Florida). Gets more than 135,000 outpatient visits yearly for treatment of all forms of cancer. Also has largest inpatient blood and marrow transplant program in the Southeast. 888-663-3488, *www.moffitt.usf.edu.*

•**UNC Lineberger Comprehensive Cancer Center/University of North Carolina Health System** (Chapel Hill, North Carolina). Recognized for programs in breast, gastrointestinal and lung cancers. 866-828-0270, *http://cancer.med.unc.edu.*

•**University of Alabama at Birmingham Comprehensive Cancer Center.** Noted for programs in breast, lung and ovarian cancers. 800-822-0933, *www.ccc.uab.edu.*

•**University of Virginia Cancer Center** (Charlottesville, Virginia). Combines cutting-edge cancer treatments with a unique, illness-specific team approach to patient and family care. 800-251-3627, *www.healthsystem.virginia.edu/internet/cancer.*

•**Vanderbilt-Ingram Cancer Center/Vanderbilt University Medical Center** (Nashville). Known for its comprehensive programs in lung, gastrointestinal and breast cancers. 800-811-8480, *www.vicc.org.*

•**Wake Forest University Baptist Medical Center** (Winston-Salem, North Carolina). State-of-the-art care includes radiosurgery—using a Gamma Knife machine to deliver a high dose of radiation that destroys brain tumor cells noninvasively. Noted for programs in breast, prostate and brain cancer. 800-446-2255, *www.wfubmc.edu/cancer.*

MIDWEST

•**Alvin J. Siteman Cancer Center at Barnes-Jewish Hospital/Washington University School of Medicine** (St. Louis). Offers one dozen different specialty centers, covering all major types of cancer. 800-600-3606, *www.siteman.wustl.edu.*

•**Arthur G. James Cancer Hospital and Richard J. Solove Research Institute/Ohio State University Medical Center** (Columbus). Only freestanding cancer hospital in the Midwest. Noted for programs in lung and breast cancers and leukemia. Has a 24-bed bone-marrow transplant unit. 800-293-5066, *www.jamesline.com.*

•**Clarian Health Partners/Indiana University Cancer Center** (Indianapolis). Interdisciplinary programs let patients see a variety of specialists in a single visit. Known for programs in testicular, breast and lung cancers. 888-600-4822, *http://iucc.iu.edu.*

•**Eppley Cancer Center/University of Nebraska Medical Center** (Omaha, Nebraska). Noted for programs in breast and pancreatic cancers and lymphoma. 800-999-5465, *www.unmc.edu/cancercenter.*

•**Ireland Cancer Center/University Hospitals of Cleveland and Case Western Reserve University** (Cleveland). Recognized for programs in colon and blood system cancers. Has performed more than 1,000 bone-marrow transplants. 800-641-2422, *www.irelandcancercenter.org.*

•**Mayo Clinic** (Rochester, Minnesota). Known for programs in breast and colon cancer, multiple myeloma, non-Hodgkin's lymphoma and other hematologic cancers. 507-266-9288, *www.mayoclinic.org/cancercenter.*

•**Robert H. Lurie Comprehensive Cancer Center/Northwestern University** (Chicago). Noted for programs in non-Hodgkin's lymphoma, chronic lymphocytic leukemia as well as breast cancer. 312-908-5250, *www.cancer.northwestern.edu.*

•**University of Chicago Hospitals** (Chicago). Recognized for programs in prostate and colon cancer and for treating rare cancers, including hairy-cell leukemia and mesothelioma. 888-824-0200, *www.uchospitals.edu/cancer.html.*

•**University of Michigan Medical Center** (Ann Arbor, Michigan). Doctors in its 25 area clinics see more patients than any other cancer center in Michigan. Known for programs in breast and urologic cancers and melanoma. 800-865-1125, *www.cancer.med.umich.edu.*

•**University of Wisconsin Hospital and Clinics** (Madison, Wisconsin). Only NCI-designated comprehensive cancer center in Wisconsin. Noted for programs in breast, colon, lung and prostate cancers. 800-622-8922, *www.cancer.wisc.edu.*

SOUTHWEST

•**Huntsman Cancer Institute/University of Utah Hospitals** (Salt Lake City, Utah). Recognized for genetic research and for its programs in colon cancer, sarcoma, melanoma and pediatric oncology. 888-424-2100, *www.hci.utah.edu.*

•**University of Texas M.D. Anderson Cancer Center** (Houston). World leader in cancer research and multidisciplinary approach to treating and preventing common and rare cancers. 800-392-1611, *www.mdanderson.org.*

WEST

•**City of Hope National Medical Center** (Duarte, California). Has 50 beds devoted to bone-marrow transplants. Known for research on genetics, which may provide future treatment for breast and ovarian cancers. 800-826-4673, *www.cityofhope.org.*

●**Jonsson Comprehensive Cancer Center/University of California–Los Angeles Medical Center** (Los Angeles). Noted for its gene therapy program, which holds promise for treating prostate and breast cancers. 888-798-0719, *www.cancer.mednet.ucla.edu.*

●**Seattle Cancer Care Alliance** (Seattle). Alliance includes Fred Hutchinson Cancer Research Center, University of Washington and Children's Hospital and Regional Medical Center. Known for programs in bone-marrow transplantation and immunotherapy for leukemia, melanoma and breast cancers. 800-804-8824, *www.fhcrc.org.*

●**Stanford Hospital & Clinics** (Stanford, California). Noted for programs in genitourinary, prostate and gastrointestinal cancers and lymphoma. 800-756-9000, *www.cancer.stanfordhospital.com.*

●**University of California–San Francisco Comprehensive Cancer Center** (San Francisco). Offers access to a wide variety of adult and pediatric trials, including AIDS-related cancer. Clinicians are based in four Bay Area hospitals. 800-888-8664, *www.cc.ucsf.edu.*

■ ■ ■ ■

When to Travel for Cancer Care

Most US residents have a top-rated cancer center within driving distance. Although going to a nearby center makes the most sense financially and logistically, traveling to a more distant cancer center should be considered if that institution has better resources to deal with your particular type of cancer.

Travel is also warranted if your treatment is not working…to confirm a diagnosis (although, in many cases, simply sending your slides to the other institution will suffice)…or to get a second opinion on treatment options. If you do travel for therapy, follow-up care—which can last up to a year—will typically be administered at a hospital closer to your home.

CLINICAL TRIALS

You also may want to travel to a top-rated cancer center that is involved in a clinical trial for your type of cancer. Such trials, designed for patients with advanced malignancies that aren't responding to standard treatments, provide access to the newest medications and therapies, which may be more—or less—effective that current approaches.

However, only some patients enrolled in clinical trails receive the new treatment. Others are randomly assigned to a control group that gets standard care or, in some cases, a placebo.

A patient should enroll in a trial only after careful consultation with his/her oncologist. Advantages include especially close monitoring of your health throughout the treatment period and a first shot at the benefits of a new treatment—if there are any.

Potential drawbacks include side effects and other health dangers from the new treatment that may not yet be fully understood—and the risk that the new treatment may not be effective or that, even if it does have benefits, it may not work in your case.

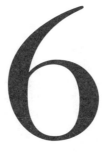

6

Diabetes Update

Coffee Cure? 5 Cups a Day Lowers Diabetes Risk

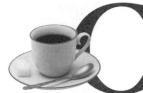

Can't do without the morning pot of coffee? This might be one addiction that actually has an upside. People who choose to drink caffeinated coffee may lower their risk of type 2 diabetes, new research suggests.

THE STUDY

The study of more than 126,000 American men and women found that people who drank more caffeinated coffee had a lower risk of type 2 diabetes than those who drank less or no coffee.

The effect was greatest for men whose regular coffee intake was more than five cups a day. This group had about half the odds of developing type 2 diabetes as men who didn't drink any coffee.

Women who drank caffeinated coffee also gained protection from type 2 diabetes, though not quite as much as men. For both the men and women in the study, the effects of coffee drinking on diabetes risk didn't become pronounced until people consumed at least four cups a day.

Although the study didn't find a statistically significant link between caffeinated tea and protection from diabetes, the results did suggest such an effect might exist.

The average coffee drinker in the United States consumes about three cups a day, according to the Coffee Research Institute.

NO CAUSE-EFFECT LINK YET

The latest work, reported in the Annals of Internal Medicine, is one of several studies linking coffee to healthier blood sugar. A separate report released in early 2004, for example, also found Swedish women who drank several cups of coffee a day were less likely to have diabetes than those who consumed less of the beverage.

Annika Rosengren, MD, professor, Sahlgrenska University Hospital, Göteborg, Sweden.
Coffee Research Institute.
Annals of Internal Medicine.

Although coffee's ability to lower the risk of diabetes has come up in several studies, how it does so is not clear. "Coffee contains several hundreds, if not thousands, of different compounds," says Dr. Annika Rosengren, a cardiologist at Sahlgrenska University Hospital in Göteborg, Sweden, who led the coffee study from that country. "It's very difficult to say which compound is the protective one."

In addition, over the short run coffee seems to impair, not improve, the body's sensitivity to insulin, the hormone that helps cells take up blood sugar. This effect is evidently transient, Rosengren says.

Some of the coffee drinkers studied have other unhealthy habits. They frequently smoke, drink alcohol and lead a sedentary lifestyle—a combination known to raise the risk of diabetes and heart problems. But the researchers found coffee consumption reduced the risk of diabetes despite these factors.

However, the researchers warn their study "cannot prove a cause-effect relationship" between caffeine consumption and a lower risk of diabetes. And, they add, "it is premature to recommend increased coffee drinking as a means to prevent type 2 diabetes." Other studies have shown that excess caffeine consumption can be a major contributing factor to heart disease, hypertension, stomach ailments, and sleep disorders.

info Try the Coffee Research Institute at *www. coffeeresearch.org.*

■ ■ ■ ■

Coffee Provides Boost Against Stress and Possibly Even Cancer

While that morning cup of coffee always seems to get you instantly stimulated, you might be surprised to find out that it has another plus side, according to a report from the Yale University School of Medicine.

When 20 people were given either caffeine or a placebo 90 minutes before physical exertion, the caffeine group showed higher levels of cortisol, an anti-stress hormone, and endorphins, the body's natural painkillers. The

placebo group showed only a small increase in cortisol and no increase in endorphins.

German researchers say they have found a highly active compound, called *methylpyridinium,* in coffee that may prevent colon cancer. Scientists have suspected for years that coffee may offer some cancer protection. This is the first study that's identified a specific, highly active anticancer compound in coffee.

"But until human studies are done, no one knows exactly how much coffee is needed to have a protective effect against colon cancer," says study co-leader Thomas Hofman, professor and head of the Institute for Food Chemistry at the University of Munster. "However, our studies suggest that drinking coffee may offer some protection, especially if it's strong."

Methylpyridinium is found almost exclusively in coffee and coffee products. It's formed during the roasting process and is not present in raw coffee beans.

Good News: Food that Helps Control Glucose Levels

Journal of Agricultural and Food Chemistry.
American Chemical Society news release.

Diabetics may have a surprising new ally in the fight to manage their condition—buckwheat.

Buckwheat is widely distributed in food stores and natural products outlets. It's most often seen as a dark flour, much grittier than regular wheat flour. Buckwheat pancakes are often a staple in southern cooking.

University of Manitoba (Canada) researchers found that buckwheat seed extracts fed to diabetic rats lowered their blood glucose levels by up to 19%.

"With diabetes on the rise, the incorporation of buckwheat into the diet could help provide a safe, easy and inexpensive way to lower glucose levels and reduce the risk of complications associated with the disease, including heart, nerve and kidney problems," says study leader Carla G. Taylor, an associate professor in the department of human nutritional sciences.

But she says that until studies are done on humans with diabetes, it's not clear how much buckwheat flour or extract a person would have to consume to affect glucose levels.

■ ■ ■ ■

How You Can Add Buckwheat to Your Diet

It is not too difficult to incorporate buckwheat into your diet. Following are a few recipes that can help get you started.

BUCKWHEAT PANCAKES

1 cup buckwheat flour

1 cup whole wheat flour

½ tsp salt

1 Tbsp brown sugar

2 tsp baking powder

1 Tbsp vegetable oil

2 eggs, beaten

2 cups milk

Mix dry ingredients. Add remaining ingredients and mix briefly.

BRAISED BUCKWHEAT KERNELS (KASHA)

1 cup medium buckwheat kernels (kasha)

1 egg

2½ cups boiling water

2 Tbsp butter or margarine

2½ tsp instant beef bouillon

¼ tsp salt

¼ tsp pepper

Mix buckwheat kernels and egg; cook in ungreased skillet over medium-high heat, stirring constantly, until kernels separate and brown.

Stir in water, butter, bouillon, salt and pepper; reduce heat. Cover and simmer until liquid is absorbed and buckwheat kernels are tender, about 5 minutes. Makes 6 servings.

info For more information about buckwheat, go to *www.foodsubs.com*. For more buckwheat recipes, try *www.recipegoldmine.com*.

Gastric Bypass Surgery May Reverse Diabetes

Annals of Surgery.
University of Pittsburgh Medical Center news release.

The weight-loss procedure called gastric bypass surgery, which has been gaining popularity recently, can improve or eliminate type 2 diabetes in people who are obese, according to Pennsylvania researchers.

Laparoscopic gastric bypass surgery makes the stomach smaller. Patients lose weight because their smaller stomach can't take in as many calories as before.

THE STUDY

A study by scientists at the University of Pittsburgh Medical Center found that 83% of obese patients with type 2 diabetes who underwent the operation saw improvement in, and even total reversal of, their disease.

"Most patients in the study with type 2 diabetes who underwent bypass surgery achieved excellent biochemical [blood sugar] control and were able to reap the clinical benefits of withdrawing from most, if not all, anti-diabetes medications, including insulin," says principal investigator Dr. Philip Schauer, director of bariatric surgery.

"Younger diabetes patients with less severe disease stand to gain more from the surgery by circumventing years of progressive, debilitating disease," Schauer adds.

THE PROCEDURE

Gastric bypass surgery is intended for the estimated 8 million Americans who are considered morbidly obese—100 pounds or more above their ideal weight.

Morbid obesity is believed to cut between 15 and 20 years off a person's life, according to the University of Arkansas for Medical Sciences.

Most people who have gastric bypass surgery lose approximately two thirds of their excess body weight during the first year after the procedure. Most are able to keep that weight off for years.

■ ■ ■ ■

Diabetes Epidemic

An estimated 18.2 million Americans, or approximately 6% of the adult population, have diabetes, but only 13 million have been diagnosed, according to the American Diabetes Association (ADA).

Between 90% and 95% of people who have diabetes have the type 2, or adult-onset, form of the disease, which is closely tied to excess weight. The incidence of type 2 diabetes has jumped 50% in the last decade, primarily due to the ever-growing number of overweight and obese Americans and the country's sedentary lifestyle.

People who have type 2 diabetes gradually lose sensitivity to insulin, a hormone that helps cells convert sugar into energy. Many of these patients require daily injections of insulin to make up for the problem.

In type 1, also called juvenile-onset diabetes, the insulin-producing cells in the pancreas die off early in life.

SYMPTOMS

Type 2 diabetes has some symptoms similar to type 1, including frequent urination, excessive thirst and hunger, dramatic weight loss, irritability, weakness and fatigue, and nausea and vomiting.

But there are also symptoms of type 2 diabetes that are exclusively its own, such as recurring or hard-to-heal skin lesions, gum or bladder infections, blurred vision, tingling or numbness in hands or feet and itchy skin.

Symptoms for type 2 diabetes usually occur gradually over a period of months or perhaps even years, and some people who have type 2 diabetes have symptoms that are so mild they go undiagnosed.

TREATMENTS

There are a number of different treatments for people who have type 2 diabetes, including drugs other than insulin.

Very often patients can control their sugar and glucose levels through a diet that is recommended by a physician, as well as an exercise plan and careful daily monitoring of their blood sugar levels.

info The US National Diabetes Education Program lists four steps to control diabetes on their Web site at *www.ndep.nih.gov/diabetes/control/4Steps.htm.*

'Miracle Molecule' Great News for Type 2 Diabetes

Joseph P. Grippo, PhD, vice president, metabolic diseases, Hoffman-La Roche Inc., Nutley, NJ.
Franz M. Matschinsky, MD, professor, biochemistry and biophysics, University of Pennsylvania School of Medicine, Philadelphia.
Science.

A recently discovered family of molecules could lead to more effective and sophisticated treatment for type 2 diabetes, the most common form of the disease, researchers say.

The molecules increase the activity of the gene that produces *glucokinase,* the most important member of a family of enzymes that maintain normal blood sugar levels in the body, says Joseph P. Grippo, vice president for metabolic diseases at the Hoffman-La Roche Inc.

The Hoffman-La Roche investigators' work was done in collaboration with Dr. Franz M. Matschinsky, a professor of biochemistry and biophysics at the University of Pennsylvania School of Medicine, who did much of the work to establish the importance of glucokinase.

Glucokinase acts in two distinct ways to keep blood sugar levels under control, Grippo explains. It is activated when blood sugar levels rise above normal after eating, thus increasing insulin secretion from the pancreas and stimulating the process of glucose metabolism in the liver. It is inactivated just as quickly, when blood glucose levels drop to normal.

"Thus, [if we could control the molecules in question], we could control two very important points in the process of blood sugar control," Grippo says.

The newly reported work is just the beginning of a long effort that may or may not produce a usable medication, Grippo says.

This medication would perform double-duty, unlike today's leading diabetes drug classes, all of which have a single mode of action. For example, the sulfonylureas, the most widely used medications to control blood sugar, are effective because they increase insulin production. Metformins reduce production of glucose. So, many patients must be given more than one drug to treat type 2 diabetes.

Like the sulfonylureas and other oral medications, the prospective new medications would be useful only for people with type 2 diabetes, whose bodies can still produce some insulin. Type 1 diabetics require insulin injections because the pancreas cannot produce the critical hormone.

Mood Can Affect Diabetes Control

Duke University Medical Center news release.

Depression and a demanding insulin regime can affect a diabetic's ability to control her disease, according to a recent study by scientists at Duke University Medical Center, Durham, North Carolina.

THE STUDY

The study, which looked at 1,000 people with diabetes, found that depressed diabetics who self-administer at least three insulin injections per day have a much greater risk of having poor control over their disease than diabetics who require less or no insulin.

The researchers note that depression only affects diabetes control in some patients. But they recommend that diabetics who require higher amounts of insulin pay close attention to symptoms of depression.

"We know that patients who require more insulin on a daily basis have less residual pancreatic activity and a more difficult time regulating their glucose levels," says Richard Surwit, vice chairman of research, department of psychiatry and behavioral medicine at Duke.

"Their metabolic control is going to be more vulnerable to disruption by behavioral and neuroendocrine factors. This means that diabetics who have more difficulty regulating their glucose levels are more likely to get thrown even farther off balance by depression," Surwit said.

Exercise Decreases Diabetes Danger

Diabetes.
Mayo Clinic news release.

Exercise is one of the pillars of diabetes prevention and control, and in fact, people who are more fit are less prone to the blood sugar disease.

But people older than 40 who rely on working out to avoid diabetes and its complications must exercise frequently, and must not skip too many days, to reap the benefits of physical activity, according to Mayo Clinic researchers.

Exercise can help diabetics use the insulin that they do produce more efficiently, However, middle-aged and older people can't sustain this increased insulin sensitivity generated by aerobic exercise, the study found. A decline in insulin sensitivity is normal as people age and that makes them more prone to developing diabetes.

THE STUDY

The Mayo Clinic study included 65 healthy, but mostly sedentary, men and women aged 21 to 87. They took part in a four-month aerobic exercise program where the intensity and length of training sessions increased over time.

Researchers measured participants' insulin sensitivity, abdominal fat and their key enzyme systems at the beginning of the study and again a few days after the final exercise session.

"The insulin sensitivity of younger people remained higher four days after exercising. But no increase was recorded in the middle-aged and older participants," says lead investigator and endocrinologist Dr. K. Sreekumaran Nair.

"The study found no close connections between increased insulin sensitivity in middle- and older-aged people and reduced abdominal fat or increased energy conversion," Nair says.

Both younger and older study subjects had reduced abdominal fat and increased enzymes involved in cellular production when they were evaluated after the exercise program.

"The [study] results may be helpful to prediabetic and diabetic patients and their healthcare providers as they plan more effective exercise regimens," Nair says.

info More information about diabetes is available from the American Diabetes Association Web site at *www.diabetes.org.*

■ ■ ■ ■

Early Warning: Prediabetes

In addition to people with full-blown diabetes, 20 million people have what's called prediabetes. They show signs of insulin trouble and abnormally high blood sugar that's not yet significant enough to be called diabetes.

But even if it's not actual diabetes, prediabetes carries its own risks. Even moderate blood sugar problems can seriously harm the heart, blood vessels, kidneys and other organs.

The good news, however, is that prediabetes doesn't have to become the real thing. Taking steps to improve blood sugar, such as exercising regularly, losing weight and quitting smoking can delay the evolution of diabetes or prevent it completely.

Smoking Raises Type 2 Diabetes Risk

Valdemar Grill, MD, professor, internal medicine, University of Science and Technology, Trondheim, Norway, and adjunct professor, Karolinska Institute, Stockholm, Sweden.

Nathaniel Clark, MD, national vice president, clinical affairs, American Diabetes Association.

Presentations, American Diabetes Association annual meeting, Orlando, FL.

Smokers who may be worried about their risks for lung cancer and heart disease now have another reason to quit—tobacco use raises the risk for type 2 diabetes.

"This increased risk for type 2 diabetes could be due to increased insulin resistance, which has previously been shown to occur after an acute episode of smoking," theorizes Dr. Valdemar Grill, a professor at both the University of Science and Technology in Trondheim, Norway, and the Karolinska Institute in Stockholm, Sweden.

Experts have long understood that smoking does serious damage to the arteries while also raising the risk of lung cancer. But Grill's study, as well as another study by Johns Hopkins researchers, suggest it may encourage the development of diabetes, too.

THE STUDY

Grill and his colleagues analyzed 11 years of health data on approximately 39,000 Norwegian adults.

They found that regardless of sex, age, weight, physical activity and alcohol use, people who smoked at least one pack of cigarettes a day faced a 64% higher risk of developing type 2 diabetes than nonsmokers.

According to Grill, previous studies have suggested that smoking contributes to insulin resistance. And since similar associations were found in people who used smokeless "snuff" tobacco, "it is likely that it is nicotine, the common substance in cigarettes and snuff, that is the culprit," he said.

"It is also possible that nicotine has a negative effect on insulin secretion," Grill added. "We have some data in animals to support this notion."

SECOND STUDY CORROBORATES FINDINGS

In another study, researchers who were led by Dr. Hsin-Chieh Yeh of The Johns Hopkins School of Public Health examined nine years of data on approximately 9,000 older American adults.

The team of researchers discovered that after adjusting for age, sex, race, weight and other factors, long-term smokers faced a 50% higher risk of developing diabetes compared with people who never smoked. The risk was even higher for people who smoked for longer periods of time.

Dr. Nathaniel Clark, the American Diabetes Association's (ADA) national vice president for clinical affairs, says, "When we usually list the risk factors for diabetes, smoking is never on that list. In that sense, this is new information," he said.

Although the findings are too preliminary to prompt any change in official ADA policy on preventing diabetes, Clark says quitting smoking should be a no-brainer.

"There are so many reasons not to smoke. I can't imagine that a fear of developing diabetes would trump dying from lung cancer or any of the other terrible things smoking does," he says.

Death? Taxes? Diabetes? How to Beat the Odds

K.M. Venkat Narayan, MD, chief, diabetes epidemiology section, US Centers for Disease Control and Prevention, Atlanta.

Tuan Tran, MD, fellow, endocrinology, Ochsner Clinic Foundation, New Orleans.

Robert Rizza, MD, professor, medicine, Mayo Clinic, Rochester, MN.

Journal of the American Medical Association.

Death, taxes, diabetes? A recent study has found that one in three Americans born in the year 2000 will contract the blood sugar disorder at some point in their life.*

Those startling numbers were higher than expected. "That estimate may even be a conservative one," says Dr. K.M. Venkat Narayan, lead author of the study, which details those sobering projections.

"We have all along known that diabetes is common and growing," says Narayan, chief of the diabetes epidemiology section at the US Centers for Disease Control and Prevention. "We knew [the probability of developing diabetes in a lifetime] would be high, but it was startlingly high."

*One in three people is not the same as one third of the population because not everyone will develop the disease at the same time. Nor does it mean that those people will develop the disease as children; it could happen at any point during their lifetime.

Adds Dr. Tuan Tran, a fellow in endocrinology at the Ochsner Clinic Foundation in New Orleans, "It's not very surprising, but it is alarming."

Diabetes has become a large and growing public health problem. In the last decade, the prevalence of this disease has increased 40%, from 4.9% of the US population to 6.9%.

Experts estimate that the number of Americans diagnosed with diabetes will increase by 165% by 2050. If not adequately controlled, the disease can cause people to lose limbs, eyesight, kidney function and, eventually, their lives.

Experts cite several reasons for this large increase, including the country's growing rate of obesity and Americans' sedentary lifestyles.

People diagnosed with diabetes have shorter life expectancies. The researchers estimate that a man diagnosed at age 40 will lose 11.6 years from his life, and even more "quality" years without serious illness.

THE STUDY

Narayan and his colleagues analyzed data on almost 360,000 individuals collected between 1984 and 2000 as part of the National Health Interview Survey. They calculated that the estimated lifetime risk of developing diabetes for males born in 2000 is 32.8%, and for females, 38.5%. Women had a higher lifetime risk at every age.

The highest risk was among Hispanic people, with males having an estimated lifetime risk of 45.4%, and females, 52.5%.

The risk of developing diabetes is equal to or higher than the risk of developing many other diseases. Compare the diabetes figures with the risk of developing breast cancer (one in eight for US women) and coronary heart disease (one in two for men and one in three for women).

TYPE 2 DIABETES IS AVOIDABLE

The data in Narayan's study didn't make a distinction between type 1 and type 2 diabetes, but the great majority of diabetes cases (approximately 95%) are type 2.

In type 1 diabetes, the body doesn't produce the hormone insulin, which is vital for proper control of blood sugar. In type 2 diabetes, the body doesn't make enough insulin or cells don't process the insulin adequately. These people are advised to lose weight, eat a healthy diet and exercise regularly. Some must take oral medication or inject insulin to manage blood sugar levels.

Type 2 diabetes can be prevented by exercising regularly and keeping slim, as obesity is a major risk factor for the condition. The disease can be kept in check by these lifestyle habits and with medication.

Adds Dr. Robert Rizza, vice president of the American Diabetes Association, "There are data that if you treat diabetes, you can substantially reduce the risks of adverse outcomes. If you have the disease and are not managing it, bad things happen."

info For more on type 2 diabetes, visit the National Diabetes Information Clearinghouse at *http://diabetes.niddk.nih.gov.*

Researchers Cure Diabetes in Mice

Denise L. Faustman, MD, PhD, director, Massachusetts General Hospital's Immunobiology Laboratory, Boston.

Science.

Researchers in Massachusetts say they have cured type 1 diabetes in mice— but the cure for human patients may require millions of dollars invested in research.

The researchers, led by Dr. Denise L. Faustman, director of Massachusetts General Hospital's Immunobiology Laboratory, are reporting that their technique—injecting spleen cells that transform into insulin-producing cells— also seems applicable to other autoimmune conditions, in which the body's immune system attacks its own tissue.

But the necessary human trials will be very expensive.

The animal studies have been financed primarily by the Iacocca Foundation. Automotive legend Lee Iacocca created the foundation to support diabetes research after his wife died of complications of the disease. But the foundation doesn't "have the resources to scale up to human clinical trials," Faustman says.

"There is a tremendous amount of momentum required that people don't appreciate in moving from raising $1 million a year to raising $20 million a year to get human trials started," she says.

The demand is there, however, for human trials of the technique, according to Faustman. "We must get 500 calls a month from people who want to be in clinical trials," Faustman says. "The enthusiasm of the patient population is impressive."

Those patients are responding to a series of progress reports at Faustman's laboratory about type 1 diabetes, a condition in which the immune system destroys insulin-producing islet cells. Type 1 diabetes generally appears early in life and is more difficult to treat than type 2 diabetes, where the body becomes less sensitive to the effects of insulin.

Insulin, a hormone, is needed to carry sugar from the bloodstream to the body's cells, which use the sugar—called glucose—for energy.

THE RESEARCH

The Massachusetts researchers' first step in the mice study was to stop the immune system attack on islet cells with injections of a naturally occurring protein known as *TNF-alpha.*

They injected spleen cells from healthy mice into the diabetic mice that had been treated with TNF-alpha.

The expectation was that the spleen cells would halt the autoimmune attack, so that transplants of islet cells would restore insulin production.

SURPRISING RESULTS

No transplants were needed, because normal islet cells appeared in the mice and started producing insulin. Some of those insulin-producing cells appeared as the few remaining islet cells in the mice multiplied—a regeneration process that was something of a surprise to the researchers.

But there was a bigger surprise. Some of the injected spleen cells had transformed into islet cells, "which was kind of amazing to us," Faustman says.

The transformation could help explain the existence of the spleen, she says. The organ, which acts as a filter against foreign organisms that infect the bloodstream, is not considered essential. People can live without a spleen as other organs will take over its function.

The important fact, Faustman says, is that adult cells can undergo this kind of transformation and regeneration. The idea of re-educating the immune system not to attack friendly tissue and then regenerating cells to restore normal function could be applied to other autoimmune diseases such as rheumatoid arthritis and multiple sclerosis—if the money was there, Faustman says.

info The Iacocca Foundation offers information on diabetes research at *www.iacocca foundation.org.*

New Devices Promise Pain-Free Diabetes Care

Richard Bergenstal, MD, executive director, International Diabetes Center at Park Nicollet, Minneapolis.

Wayman Wendell Cheatham, MD, senior vice president, medical and regulatory affairs, MannKind Bio-Pharmaceuticals, Danbury, CT.

Marcia A. Testa, PhD, senior lecturer, Harvard School of Public Health, Boston.

Study abstracts, American Diabetes Association annual meeting, Orlando, FL.

New devices that monitor blood sugar levels and deliver insulin may one day help ease the painful daily management of diabetes.

GLUCOSE MONITORING

Keeping a close eye on the body's blood sugar levels is critical to staying healthy. Right now, patients with type 1 diabetes (and many with type 2) draw blood up to four times each day to gauge their blood sugar levels.

"Good glucose control prevents eye, kidney and nerve problems, and seems to be associated with a lower risk of heart disease,"

says Dr. Richard Bergenstal, an endocrinologist and executive director of the International Diabetes Center at Park Nicollet in Minneapolis. Still, he adds, only 57% of people test even once a day.

One group of researchers is working on a device that measures levels of volatile organic compounds in human breath, eliminating the need for diabetics to prick their finger to test their blood sugar levels.

Another group of researchers described the HypoMon, a chest-belt transmitter that continuously takes glucose measurements on the surface of the skin.

One advantage that this system has is that it would be able to monitor glucose levels even during sleep. The downside is that movement and sweat could affect the readings.

Bergenstal stresses that short-term monitoring of blood glucose levels should not replace long-term monitoring with the *hemoglobin A1c test,* which measures all blood sugars for a two- to three-month period. In fact, the two should work together. "A1c has been best correlated to long-term complications," Bergenstal says.

INHALED INSULIN

Another important area of diabetes research is inhaled insulin. Although this is not yet approved, inhaled—as opposed to injected—insulin would be a great relief to millions of diabetics who hate needles.

This new technology would deliver insulin that's absorbed in 10 to 14 minutes, much faster than the 90 minutes it now takes.

"This methodology allows a person not to have to worry about taking insulin until they actually started eating, and then use an inhaler about the size of a pocket pager," says Dr. Wayman Wendell Cheatham, senior vice president of medical and regulatory affairs for Mann-Kind BioPharmaceuticals in Danbury, Connecticut, which is developing the technology.

EASIER INSULIN MAY BE USED MORE OFTEN

Currently, insulin is the therapy of last resort for type 2 diabetics, to be considered only after lifestyle changes and various other medications fail. "The one thing that you know will work is the last resort," says Marcia A. Testa, a senior lecturer at the Harvard School of Public Health.

"What's the reason for that? Not that it doesn't work…it's that people just don't like to inject," she says.

If insulin were less burdensome to take, Testa theorizes, it might be used earlier.

Mixing Meds Messy Business for Diabetics

Harlan M. Krumholz, MD, professor, medicine and epidemiology and public health, Yale University School of Medicine, New Haven, CT.
Kenneth Hupart, MD, chief, endocrinology, diabetes and metabolism, Nassau University Medical Center, East Meadow, NY.
Journal of the American Medical Association.

Many diabetics who have heart failure regularly take medications that improve their blood sugar problem at the expense of their heart condition, recent research suggests.

Specifically, *metformin* (*brand name:* Glucophage) and a class of medications called *thiazolidinediones* (*brand names:* Actose, Avandia)—both of which help control glucose levels in diabetics—may cause serious complications in patients with heart failure. These include retaining too much body fluid and gaining weight.

Part of the problem is that so many patients—especially those who have diabetes or heart disease—often have several other health conditions as well.

"The typical heart failure patients are patients who have many concurrent illnesses and complications and can end up on a lot of different medications," says study author Dr. Harlan M. Krumholz, a professor of medicine and epidemiology and public health at Yale University School of Medicine.

THE STUDY

Krumholz and his team at Yale examined the medical records of more than 25,600 Medicare recipients hospitalized with heart failure and diabetes from April 1998 to March 1999, and from July 2000 to June 2001. Some were discharged with a prescription for metformin, some with a prescription for a thiazolidinedione medication.

The study didn't ask how many people had adverse reactions, but simply how many patients were prescribed the drugs.

Because the study found fluid retention and weight gain when using thiazolidinediones, it's very important that they not be used in patients with known heart failure or, if necessary, that possible problems be monitored very carefully, says Dr. Sid Smith, who is director of the Center for Cardiovascular Science and Medicine at the University of North Carolina, Chapel Hill.

DOCTOR DISCONNECT

There's also the issue of whether physicians are paying attention to US Food and Drug Administration (FDA) "black box" warnings on medications. Such warnings are the most serious the agency demands on labels.

The black-box warning for metformin says it could cause lactic acidosis—acid in the blood—a potentially life-threatening problem for people with heart failure.

"There's a discordance between what the FDA is saying and what's going on in practice," Krumholz says. "We're potentially undermining the entire system."

Why this disconnect is happening is not clear, the researchers say. Physicians may simply not be aware of the dangers or they may think the benefits outweigh the risks. Or they may have decided that the rate of adverse events isn't as high as advertised.

And that's not just an issue for heart failure patients with diabetes.

"It raises the issue about the way that we deliver health care in this country," says Dr. Kenneth Hupart, chief of endocrinology, diabetes and metabolism at Nassau University Medical Center in East Meadow, New York.

info The American Heart Association's Web site, *www.americanheart.org,* has information on the connection between heart disease and diabetes.

Blood Sugar Control Spells Sweet Success for Diabetic Heart Patients

Roberto A. Corpus, MD, interventional cardiology fellow, Mid America Heart Institute, Kansas City, MO.

Om Ganda, MD, associate clinical professor, medicine, Harvard Medical School, and director, lipid clinic, Joslin Diabetes Center, Boston.

Journal of the American College of Cardiology.

Heart patients who have diabetes are likely to fare better after having blood-vessel-opening procedures, such as angioplasty or stent placement, if they control their blood-sugar levels, a study says.

People who have diabetes are known to be at greater risk than nondiabetics of experiencing restenosis, or a re-narrowing of an artery after an angioplasty or stent procedure.

Yet there's been little research into the role blood sugar plays in that re-narrowing.

The angioplasty procedure was first performed more than 20 years ago by Dr. Andreas Gruentzig as a less invasive way to treat coronary artery disease.

What he envisioned as an alternative to open heart bypass surgery in perhaps 5% of cases has increased in popularity and now is used to treat more than 50% of cases involving blocked arteries.

THE PROCEDURE

In the procedure, a cardiologist uses a balloon catheter to open the heart artery. The catheter is a small, hollow, flexible tube that has a balloon near the end of it.

Approximately 70% of the time, doctors also install a tiny metal structure known as a stent at the site of the blockage. The stent helps hold the artery open.

Of the estimated 1.5 million of these procedures performed globally each year, one quarter involve diabetic patients, the study authors say.

"No one has really looked at outcomes after angioplasty," says study author Dr. Roberto A. Corpus, an interventional cardiology fellow at Mid America Heart Institute in Kansas City, Missouri.

He hopes his study will provide an impetus for physicians to better manage their diabetic patients' blood sugar levels.

THE STUDY

The study, which was conducted at William Beaumont Hospital in Royal Oak, Michigan, looked at 239 patients who were having balloon angioplasty or stenting to open clogged arteries, including 179 people who have type 2 diabetes. Sixty nondiabetic patients were randomly selected as a control group.

Each patient's hemoglobin (Hb) A1c, a component of blood that is higher in diabetics who have poorly controlled blood sugar levels, was taken before catheterization.

The study used the American Diabetes Association's definition of optimal blood sugar control—an Hb A1c of 7% or less.

RESULTS SHOW GOOD BLOOD-SUGAR CONTROL IS IMPORTANT

Diabetic patients who maintain strict blood-sugar control had a significantly lower rate of repeat procedures within a year of the initial angioplasty or stenting procedure, compared with diabetics whose blood-sugar levels exceeded 7%.

Just 15% of patients with optimal blood sugar control required revascularization, compared with 34% of the group with suboptimal Hb A1c levels.

The well-controlled group also had lower rates of recurrent angina and cardiac-related rehospitalizations at the 12-month follow-up.

Dr. Ran Kornowski and Dr. Shmuel Fuchs of Rabin Medical Center in Petach-Tikva, Israel, say that 30% to 40% of patients who experience re-clogging of the arteries are diabetics. Reducing that rate would have a favorable impact on angioplasty and stenting results, they say.

info For more information on diabetes, visit the Joslin Diabetes Center at *www.joslin. harvard.edu.*

Warning: Some Diabetes Drugs May Cause Heart Problems

Abhimanyu Garg, MD, professor, internal medicine, University of Texas Southwestern Medical Center, Dallas. *Mayo Clinic Proceedings.*

Type 2 diabetics with mild heart disease or kidney problems could increase their risk of developing congestive heart failure by taking certain diabetes medications, recent research has found.

The study examines six cases of congestive heart failure in people taking *pioglitazone* (*brand name:* Actos) or *rosiglitazone* (*brand name:* Avandia) to help control their diabetes.

"We could not identify any other reason for the deterioration of their status," says the lead author of the study, Dr. Abhimanyu Garg, a professor of internal medicine at the University of Texas Southwestern Medical Center located in Dallas.

Because these medications are known to cause fluid accumulation, doctors discontinued them and gave the patients diuretics to help flush excess fluid from the body. All responded to this treatment.

The current study, he says, confirms what is already known about these medications.

THE CASES

The researchers studied the records of six men, between the ages of 66 and 78 years, with type 2 diabetes who had gone to the emergency room at Dallas Veterans Affairs Medical Center.

All six complained of shortness of breath, swelling of their feet, and weight gain, which are symptoms of congestive heart failure and pulmonary edema (fluid buildup in the lungs).

Congestive heart failure occurs when the heart can no longer pump enough blood to maintain adequate circulation. Because the heart doesn't pump properly, fluid often builds up in the lungs.

These drugs are not recommended for people with more advanced heart disease—the type that causes physical limitations.

Four of the six people in this study had chronic renal insufficiency, which means that their kidneys weren't functioning normally. Only two of the participants had any previous signs of heart disease. Four of the six had high blood pressure.

All of the study subjects had been taking the diabetes medications for between one month and 16 months. Three of the participants developed symptoms within one to three months after the dose of their diabetes drug had been increased.

The authors conclude that anyone with a history of congestive heart failure or chronic kidney disease should avoid taking these medications, and they suggest that further study be done on them.

"If somebody is taking these medications and they develop severe swelling or severe weight gain, they are not tolerating the medication," says Garg, who recommends seeing a doctor immediately if you or someone you know is experiencing these symptoms.

■ ■ ■ ■

What the Medications Are

Avandia and Actos are medications that are members of a newer class of diabetes drugs called *thiazolidinediones* or *glitazones*, which work to increase the body's sensitivity to insulin.

The first approved drug in that class, Rezulin, was taken off the market in 2000 after it was linked to dozens of cases of fatal liver disease.

At the time, the Food and Drug Administration (FDA) said Actos and Avandia were "safer alternatives in this important class of diabetes drug."

Watchdog groups like Public Citizen criticized the agency for not acting faster in withdrawing Rezulin and warned that the other drugs could cause problems, too.

info The National Institute of Diabetes & Digestive & Kidney Diseases offers information on diabetes at *www.niddk.nih.gov.*

Surgery Cuts Recurrence Of Foot Ulcers by 50%

Journal of Bone and Joint Surgery.
Washington University School of Medicine news release.

Surgery to lengthen the Achilles tendon significantly reduces the risk that people with diabetes will suffer return bouts of foot ulcers. A recent study showed that patients who had the operation cut their ulcer risk in half or more.

About 15% of people with diabetes develop ulcers on their feet. Even after treatment, these ulcers often come back.

"The return of these ulcers has been a key concern for patients and their clinicians," says principal investigator Michael J. Mueller, associate professor of physical therapy at Washington University School of Medicine, St. Louis.

"If these wounds don't heal, there's a greater risk that a patient will have to have a portion or all of the foot amputated," Mueller says. "This study shows that lengthening the Achilles tendon can have a dramatic effect on the problem of ulcer recurrence."

Limited ankle mobility is often a cause of foot ulcers, so lengthening the Achilles tendon, which allows greater movement, often resolves the problem of a recurrence. In addition, the cast immobilizes the foot, reducing the chances of getting an injury that may go unnoticed. Nerve damage in diabetics may cause them to lose sensation in their feet, allowing undetected injuries to occur and fester.

THE STUDY

The study included 64 people with diabetes who all had an ulcer on the ball of the foot. None had had an amputation. They were divided into two groups. The first group received a foot cast—the standard treatment—while the second group received both a cast and the surgery.

After seven months, the group that received the cast and the surgery was 75% less likely to have an ulcer recurrence than the group that received the cast only. After two years, the surgery group was 52% less likely to have an ulcer recurrence.

■ ■ ■ ■

How You Can Prevent Foot Ulcers

The American Diabetes Association (ADA) offers the following tips on how to prevent foot ulcers...

●**Check your feet every day** for signs of trouble, like red spots, cuts and blisters.

●**Wash your feet every day** and dry them carefully. Pay extra attention to the area between the toes.

●**Use lotion** to keep the skin on your feet smooth and soft.

●**Always wear shoes and socks.** Going barefoot increases your risk of injury.

●**Avoid temperature extremes,** like hot water or scorching sand. Don't stick your feet directly into a hot bath. Don't use electric blankets, heating pads or hot water bottles that can burn you without your knowledge.

●**Keep the blood flowing to your feet** and toes by moving them, even when sitting.

●**Quit smoking.**

●**Exercise regularly.**

info Try the American Podiatric Medical Association Web site at *www.apma.org/topics/diabetes.htm.*

Unexpected Finding May Change Treatment For Some Diabetics

David M. Harlan, MD, head, transplant and autoimmunity branch, National Institute of Diabetes & Digestive & Kidney Diseases, Bethesda, MD.
Journal of the American Medical Association.

Diabetics who receive a pancreas transplant seem to have lower survival rates than patients who remain on the donor waiting list and continue to receive conventional therapy.

Pancreatic transplantation is usually considered a "last resort" for individuals with intractable diabetes.

But because treatments for diabetes are advancing rapidly, stubborn diabetes may in fact be treatable with lifestyle changes and medication. As a result, transplantation is now a controversial issue.

Whereas most people who need a heart or liver transplant will die without it, people can live without a new pancreas.

Nevertheless, between 1995 and 2002, the annual number of pancreas transplants in people with diabetes increased fivefold.

PANCREAS TRANSPLANTS NOT WITHOUT RISKS

Patients who have a successful pancreas transplant are able to stop taking insulin. However, they need to take immunosuppressant drugs for the rest of their lives to make sure their bodies don't reject the donated organ.

"It's incorrect for a patient with diabetes to think, 'If I get this transplant, then that's that,'" says study author Dr. David M. Harlan, head of the transplant and autoimmunity branch at the National Institute of Diabetes & Digestive & Kidney Diseases (NIDDK).

"There's a tail to that treatment—and that tail is they have to take immunosuppressive drugs forever, and those drugs have significant toxicity. It's a real trade-off," he says.

THE STUDY

A recent retrospective study tried to sort out whether pancreatic transplantation offers any advantage over conventional therapy in terms of survival.

The researchers analyzed data on 11,572 patients with diabetes from 124 transplant centers in the United States. All of these patients were on waiting lists for pancreas transplants between 1995 and 2000.

Of this initial group, 6,595 received a new pancreas. Over a four-year follow-up period, those who had the transplant had a 57% increased risk of death compared with patients on the waiting list.

The absolute survival rates, however, were still high. One- and four-year survival rates for those people who received a pancreas were 96.5% and 85.2%, respectively.

IMPLICATIONS

Because it was retrospective, the study was subject to a number of limitations.

Nevertheless, the findings of this study do seem to indicate that a serious decision-making process between the doctor and the patient should be undertaken before choosing the operation.

THE KEY QUESTION PATIENTS MUST ANSWER

"Even though mortality was higher in the transplant group, the mortality is still low in absolute terms," Harlan says.

So he suggests patients ask themselves this question: "'Is the 85% or greater chance that I'll be able to come off insulin worth the somewhat higher chance that I won't survive it?' It's a tough decision."

■ ■ ■ ■

Where Diabetes Research Is Headed

The Centers for Disease Control and Prevention (CDC) identifies the following techniques with which scientists are working to find a cure for diabetes…

● **Islet cell transplantation.** Islet cells are located in the pancreas and produce insulin.

● **Artificial pancreas development.**

● **Genetic manipulation.** Fat or muscle cells that don't normally function to make insulin have a human insulin gene inserted. Then these "pseudo" islet cells that can produce insulin are transplanted into people who have type 1 diabetes.

"Each of these approaches still has a lot of challenges, such as preventing immune rejection, finding an adequate number of insulin cells, keeping cells alive, as well as others. But progress is being made in all areas," according to the CDC.

Key to Safer Driving for All Type 1 Diabetics

Daniel J. Cox, researcher, University of Virginia Health System, Charlottesville.

Kenneth Hupart, MD, chief, endocrinology, diabetes and metabolism, Nassau University Medical Center, East Meadow, NY.

Diabetes Care.

If you have type 1 diabetes, you may be at risk behind the wheel, say researchers from the University of Virginia Health System.

Type 1 diabetes develops when the pancreas can no longer manufacture insulin, the hormone necessary to move sugar out of the blood. To compensate, patients with type 1 diabetes must rely on an outside source of insulin, usually in the form of injections several times a day.

THE STUDY

The study involved 1,036 participants from seven diabetes specialty-care centers across the United States, as well as four centers in major European cities. At each center, people with either type 1 or type 2 diabetes, as well as their spouses (who did not have diabetes), were asked to fill out an anonymous questionnaire concerning both their driving record and their diabetes history for the two years prior to the survey.

According to Daniel J. Cox, the lead researcher, the questions included the number of automobile accidents and moving violations the patient has had, the number of times driving assistance was required because of low blood sugar, and how often the patient drove while experiencing severe low blood sugar.

The survey questioned the patients' knowledge of low blood sugar levels, and whether they routinely tested their blood sugar levels before getting behind the wheel.

"Type 1 diabetic drivers reported significantly more crashes, moving violations and episodes of hypoglycemic stupor [caused by extremely low blood sugar], and required assistance while driving, compared with type 2 diabetics or control subjects," says Cox. He concludes that type 1 diabetics are at "significant risk" for driving accidents compared with type 2 diabetics and nondiabetic drivers.

AS BLOOD SUGAR DROPS, ACCIDENTS MAY RISE

When insulin levels aren't controlled, blood-sugar levels can get too high or too low, and researchers believe that the drop in blood sugar commonly seen in type 1 diabetes may precipitate the driving dangers.

"There's always the concern that patients who experience low blood sugar—hypoglycemia—may be at greater risk when driving or performing other tasks that require mental concentration and high performance," says Dr. Kenneth Hupart, chief of endocrinology, diabetes and metabolism at Nassau University Medical Center in East Meadow, New York.

"If you're driving during a period of hypoglycemia, for example, your reaction time and judgment may be impaired," Hupart explains.

Hupart says the study results could help develop guidelines to reduce risks on the road.

For example, he says, doctors could determine levels of blood glucose that would be considered unsafe for driving, and then encourage patients who are at risk to pay attention to their own sugar levels before getting behind the wheel. But he also cautions against this or other similar studies being used to discriminate against those with diabetes.

7

Drug News

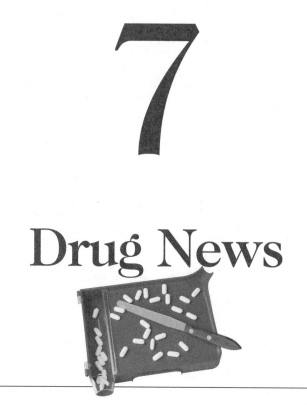

Medicine Mistakes— Read This Before You Take Another Dose...

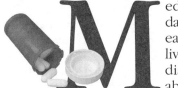edications can cure dangerous infections, ease pain and make living with a chronic disease more bearable. But medicines can also cause harm and even kill.

One in 20 prescriptions filled at a pharmacy has an error, according to the Institute for Safe Medication Practices. And a study in the *New England Journal of Medicine* found that 25% of 661 patients who responded to a survey had an adverse reaction to medications.

Many of these adverse reactions are preventable, health experts agree.

"The biggest mistakes are made by the prescribers," says Larry Sasich, a pharmacist and research analyst for the Public Citizen Health Research Group.

But a substantial number of errors are made by consumers. If consumers would take a few minutes to double-check basic information, they could greatly reduce the chances of errors.

HOW TO PREVENT ERRORS

"Know what medication you are taking and why you are taking it," says Edgar Arriola, a pharmacist and coordinator of the Drug Information Center at the University of California, Los Angeles Medical Center. "Also, know the proper dose."

Pay close attention to the exact name of the drug you're supposed to be taking. Confusion over drugs with similar sounding or similarly spelled names has resulted in serious problems.

For example, the thyroid medicine Levoxine has been confused with Lanoxin, a heart

Larry Sasich, PharmD, MPH, research analyst, Public Citizen Health Research Group, Washington, DC.

Edgar Arriola, PharmD, coordinator, Drug Information Center, University of California, Los Angeles Medical Center.

Peggy Han, PharmD, clinical coordinator, University of Southern California Community Pharmacies, and adjunct professor, clinical pharmacy, University of Southern California School of Pharmacy, Los Angeles.

medicine, leading to several deaths, according to federal health officials. Levoxine has been renamed Levoxyl.

Consumers should know what drugs they are allergic to, says Peggy Han, a pharmacist and clinical coordinator for the University of Southern California Community Pharmacies.

"Be sure [allergies are] written down in the chart. And don't assume if it is written into the chart it is seen" by your doctor or pharmacist, says Han.

Another tip: Make sure the doctor who is prescribing any new medicine knows about all your health problems as well as any other medications that you are already taking. Taken together, certain drugs can cause serious side effects.

People who are taking multiple medications often see several doctors—so they should be sure each doctor knows their entire list of medicines, experts say.

To further protect yourself, carry an index card listing all your medicines and the dose of each, Han suggests.

Ideally, all your medications should be filled at one pharmacy; if that's impossible, the index card is even more crucial.

GET ALL THE INFORMATION

Many pharmacies distribute patient information leaflets—the "plain English" information—in lieu of the package insert from the manufacturer, which carries highly technical language.

Sasich says his group advises consumers to ask for the package insert, since the US Food and Drug Administration (FDA) has approved it.

If they are difficult to read, Sasich recommends paying close attention to four areas listed on the insert: Approved uses, contraindications (situations in which the medicine should not be used), drug interactions and dose (to see if your dose is within the acceptable range for your weight and problem).

After starting a new drug, assume that any new symptom you develop is the result of the medicine until proven otherwise, and be sure to tell your doctor. And if your doctor decides to add a new drug, ask if any of your other medicines can be discontinued.

Finally, schedule a drug review—in which you go over all your medicines, the doses and what each is for—with your physician every three to six months.

info For details on keeping medicines safe, check with the Institute for Safe Medication Practices at *www.ismp.org.*

■ ■ ■ ■

How to Make Sure You're Using Your Drugs Correctly

Mixing over-the-counter with prescription drugs can present a number of problems.

The US Food and Drug Administration's Center for Drug Evaluation and Research offers the following information on making sure you're protecting not only yourself, but also the drugs you use.

GIVE YOUR MEDICINE CHEST A YEARLY CHECK-UP

To help organize information about your medications, list all the prescription and over-the-counter medicines, dietary supplements, vitamins and herbal supplements that you take. Bring this list with you when you have appointments with your doctor and any other health-care professional.

The list should include: The name of the medicine, the doctor who prescribed it, how much and how often you should take it, what it is taken for and any possible side effects.

It is also important to get rid of any expired medicines that you may have.

QUESTIONS FOR YOUR DOCTOR

Before you leave the doctor's office with a new prescription, ask…

●**What is the name of the medicine and what is it supposed to do?** Is there a less expensive alternative?

●**How and when do I take the medicine and for how long?**

●**Do I take it with water,** food or on an empty stomach? Do I take it at the same time as other medicines?

●**Can it be taken with over-the-counter medicines?**

●**What do I do if I miss a dose?**

●**Do I take the medicine before, during or after meals?**

●**What is the timing between each dose?** For example, does "four times a day" mean that I have to wake up to take it in the middle of the night?

●**What does "as needed" mean?**

●**Are there any other special instructions to follow?**

●**What foods, drinks, other medicines, dietary supplements or activities should I avoid** while taking this medicine?

●**Will any tests or any monitoring be required** while I am taking this medicine? Do I need to report back to the doctor?

●**What are the possible side effects** and what do I do if they occur?

●**When should I expect the medicine to start working?** How will I know if the medicine is working?

QUESTIONS FOR THE PHARMACIST

At the pharmacy, or wherever you get your medicines, ask…

●**Do you have a patient profile form for me to fill out?** Does it include space for my over-the-counter drugs as well as for my dietary supplements?

●**Is there written information about my medicine?** Ask the pharmacist if it's available in large print or in a language other than English if you need it.

●**What is the most important thing I should know about this medicine?** Ask the pharmacist any questions that may not have been answered by your doctor.

●**Can I get a refill?** If so, when?

●**How and where should I store this medicine?**

NSAIDs May Protect Against Parkinson's

Honglei Chen, MD, PhD, instructor, Harvard School of Public Health, Boston.
Diana Casper, PhD, assistant professor, department of neurosurgery, Albert Einstein College of Medicine, Montefiore Medical Center, Bronx, NY.
Archives of Neurology.

People who regularly use aspirin, ibuprofen and other *nonsteroidal anti-inflammatory drugs* (NSAIDs) may lower their risk of Parkinson's disease by approximately 45%, experts say.

An estimated 1 million Americans have Parkinson's disease, a serious disorder that affects nerve cells (called neurons) in the brain. The neurons that release *dopamine*—a chemical that transmits signals to your muscles to make smooth and controlled movements—are damaged or destroyed in patients who have this ailment.

Animal studies have suggested that NSAIDs may protect against Parkinson's disease and perhaps even Alzheimer's. But the latest research is the first to show the association in a large group of people.

THE STUDY

Dr. Honglei Chen, a researcher at Harvard School of Public Health and the leader of the work, looked at NSAID use and the risk of Parkinson's in 44,000 men and almost 100,000 women participating in two large health studies.

Of those, 415 developed Parkinson's during the 14-year studies.

Regular use of NSAIDs other than aspirin was uncommon, with 6.1% of men and 3.7% of women taking such drugs twice a week or more at the start of the study.

However, people in this group were 45% less likely to be diagnosed with Parkinson's disease as those who took the drugs less frequently, the researchers say. The risk of getting the disease also fell the longer a person took the NSAIDs.

Low daily doses of aspirin, taken to prevent heart attacks, didn't seem to prevent Parkinson's disease, yet higher doses did. Caffeine and smoking have been shown to lower the risk of Parkinson's, but the researchers found that the benefits of NSAIDs were independent of these effects, Chen says.

FURTHER RESEARCH NEEDED
BEFORE RECOMMENDATIONS MADE

According to Chen, "It is far too early to make public health recommendations based on one study."

Further research is necessary to determine which, if any, NSAIDs are more protective than others, at what dose and what the magnitude of the protection is, adds Chen.

"I think it's a very exciting opportunity because if NSAIDs [truly protect the brain], they might benefit people who already have Parkinson's disease and delay its progression," Chen says.

Experts caution that although NSAIDs are available without prescriptions, they are far from benign. The drugs can cause bleeding ulcers and other gastric problems that have been linked to approximately 16,500 deaths every year in this country.

According to Diana Casper, a brain researcher at the Montefiore Medical Center and the Albert Einstein College of Medicine in New York City, "Knowing that NSAIDs can play a role in protecting neurons provides important clues about the mechanism of neurodegeneration in Parkinson's disease and can lead to the design of better drugs to treat it, delay its progression and perhaps prevent it."

However, she cautions, "because of the risks associated with these drugs, they need to be studied further."

info For more on Parkinson's disease, visit the National Parkinson Foundation at *www.parkinson.org.*

■ ■ ■ ■

Here Are the Symptoms...

The National Institute of Neurological Disorders and Stroke offers the following information about Parkinson's disease...

WHO GETS PARKINSON'S?

In the United States, as many as 500,000 people are believed to have Parkinson's disease, and approximately 50,000 new cases are reported annually.

These figures are expected to increase as the average age of the population increases.

The disorder appears to be slightly more common in men than women. The average age of onset is approximately 60 years.

SYMPTOMS

Often, the first symptom of Parkinson's disease is a tremor (trembling or shaking) of a limb, especially when the body is at rest. The tremor often begins on one side of the body, frequently in one hand.

Other common symptoms of the disease include slow movement (bradykinesia), an inability to move (akinesia), rigid limbs, a shuffling gait and a stooped posture.

People with Parkinson's disease often exhibit reduced facial expressions and speak in a soft voice.

Occasionally, the disease may also cause depression, changes in personality, dementia, sleep disturbances, speech impairments or sexual difficulties.

The severity of Parkinson's symptoms tends to get worse over time.

THE CAUSES OF PARKINSON'S

Although there are many theories about the cause of Parkinson's disease, none of them has ever been proved. Until recently, the prevailing theory was that one or more environmental factors caused the disease.

Severe Parkinson's-like symptoms have been described in people who took an illegal drug contaminated with the chemical MPTP (1-methyl-4-phenyl-1,2,3,6-tetrahydropyridine) and in people who contracted a particularly severe form of influenza during an epidemic in the early 1900s.

Recent studies of twins and families who have Parkinson's have suggested that some people have an inherited susceptibility to the disease that may be influenced by environmental factors.

What Are the Odds? Some Parkinson's Drugs May Cause Gambling

Mark Stacy, MD, medical director, Parkinson's Disease and Movement Disorder Center, Duke University Medical Center, Durham, NC.

Jay Van Gerpen, MD, neurologist, Ochsner Clinic Foundation Hospital, New Orleans, LA.

Neurology.

A combination of some Parkinson's disease medications may produce a rare but potentially devastating side effect —addictive gambling behavior.

Researchers found nine pathological gamblers in a group of more than 1,000 people being treated for Parkinson's disease. These people said they hadn't had any gambling problems in the past.

THE STUDY

Dr. Mark Stacy, lead author of the study, says he began this study because he had two Parkinson's patients report huge gambling losses soon after Stacy had changed the doses of their medications. Stacy is the medical director of the Parkinson's Disease and Movement Center at Duke University Medical Center in Durham, North Carolina, but was at the Muhammad Ali Parkinson Research Center in Phoenix at the time of the study.

He and his colleague reviewed the charts of 1,184 of their patients with Parkinson's disease, and found seven other cases of problem gambling.

In all of the cases, the gambling was severe enough to cause financial problems. On average, the people with gambling problems had been diagnosed with Parkinson's disease 11 years before the start of their addictive gambling behavior.

PARKINSON'S DRUGS MAY BE INVOLVED

All nine people were taking *levodopa* and a *dopamine agonist* when their gambling problems began. Levodopa is a drug that changes into dopamine in the brain, and dopamine agonists help the body use the created dopamine. People with Parkinson's disease have low levels of dopamine, which is believed to help control smooth movement. Dopamine also appears to affect mood and personality.

Of those with a gambling problem, eight were taking a dopamine agonist called *pramipexole* and one was taking *pergolide*. None of the people who were taking levodopa alone reported problem gambling, and none of those taking a different dopamine agonist, *ropinirole,* reported any gambling problems.

Stacy says he's not sure how the medications cause addictive gambling behavior, but seven of the patients reported that their problems started within a month of when their dosage was increased. This suggests, Stacy says, that the higher doses of the dopamine agonists act as a catalyst for problem gambling behavior.

When their medications were switched, or the doses were lowered, most of the patients were able to control or stop their gambling behavior, according to the study results. Some of the patients also attended Gamblers Anonymous meetings.

DON'T BE SURPRISED BY SIDE EFFECTS

Dr. Jay Van Gerpen, a neurologist and movement disorder specialist from the Ochsner Clinic Foundation in New Orleans, says he was not surprised by this study's findings.

"Medicines for Parkinson's disease may elicit unwanted side effects relating to mood and personality," says Van Gerpen.

"These medicines are extremely useful, but they may produce unwanted effects. Dopamine agonists can be associated with changes in personality, such as sexual inappropriateness, and changes in sleep cycles. Patients need to be aware of these possibilities," he adds.

Stacy says although this side effect is rare, it's important for doctors and patients to know that higher doses of these medications may increase the risk of problem gambling.

info If you think you or someone you love may have a gambling problem, find out for sure with a self-test from the National Council on Problem Gambling at *www.ncpgambling.org.*

■ ■ ■ ■

Compulsive Gambling Symptoms Similar to Other Addictions

The US Government's Medline Plus archive offers the following information on gambling addiction...

SYMPTOMS

• **Occasional gambling becomes habitual.**

• **A person loses control over the amount of time spent gambling.**

• **Gambling continues until all money is lost** or the game is terminated.

• **Gambling persists until large debts are accumulated.**

• **Unlawful behavior** may occur to support the habit and pay debts.

The urge to gamble becomes so great that the tension it creates can only be relieved by more gambling.

Higher stakes and personal risks become involved, as well as neglect of other interests, family and work.

TREATMENT

Treatment for the person with compulsive gambling begins with the recognition that there is a problem.

As with any addiction, compulsive gambling is often associated with denial, so the person believes there is no need for treatment.

Most compulsive gamblers enter treatment under pressure from others, rather than a voluntary acceptance of the need for treatment.

Treatment programs include individual or group psychotherapy as well as support groups such as Gamblers Anonymous, a 12-step program similar to Alcoholics Anonymous.

Abstinence principles that apply to other types of addiction are also used in the treatment of compulsive gambling behavior.

Recently, antidepressants in combination with psychotherapy have been found to be beneficial in treating a gambling addiction.

Parkinson's Drugs May Cause Alzheimer's-Like Symptoms

Bill Thies, PhD, vice president, medical and scientific affairs, Alzheimer's Association, Chicago.
Allan I. Levey, MD, PhD, professor and chairman, department of neurology, Emory University School of Medicine, Atlanta.
Annals of Neurology.

Some drugs used to treat the symptoms of Parkinson's disease may be causing Alzheimer's-like dementia.

A study by Newcastle General Hospital and University College London, both in England, found that Parkinson's patients who take drugs that control tremors and bladder function also had the hallmark protein buildups of Alzheimer's disease. However, these protein buildups were much less dense than in Alzheimer's patients and the Parkinson's patients did not have clinical symptoms.

Parkinson's and Alzheimer's are both neurodegenerative diseases, meaning cells in particular areas of the brain gradually die off.

This cell death changes brain chemistry. To combat these changes, Parkinson's patients take drugs that block molecules called *acetylcholine receptors* to help ease some symptoms. However, these same drugs could exacerbate symptoms of dementia, which is marked by a loss of acetylcholine, according to the study.

"We know that a fair amount of dementia is attached to Parkinson's," says Bill Thies, vice president of medical and scientific affairs at the Alzheimer's Association in Chicago. "Often people [with Parkinson's] get demented and, for that matter, people with Alzheimer's often develop motor problems late in the course of the disease. So it is perhaps not entirely surprising that these drugs that block a particular type of acetylcholine receptor would lead to some damage to thinking processes."

THE STUDY

The study authors looked at the brains of 120 people older than 70 years who had died of Parkinson's disease. Specifically, they were looking for evidence of the protein buildups —or plaques and tangles—that are hallmarks of Alzheimer's disease.

Those subjects who had taken acetylcholine-blocking drugs for more than two years had more than twice as many plaques and tangles as patients who took the drugs for less than two years or not at all.

The density of the structures did not approach that found in Alzheimer's patients, however, and could not even be considered "definite Alzheimer's disease."

Also, none of the Parkinson's patients ever had symptoms severe enough to warrant an Alzheimer's diagnosis, the researchers say.

According to the study authors, people with Parkinson's have a dementia rate that is six times higher than in healthy individuals, although this is not always due to an Alzheimer-related pathology.

RESEARCH IMPLICATIONS

This study was observational, meaning it showed an association but could not determine a cause-and-effect relationship.

"Physicians who are treating people with Parkinson's should be aware of this study. Whether it revolutionizes the care, I think, is unknown," says Thies.

Dr. Allan I. Levey, chairman of the department of neurology at Emory University School of Medicine in Atlanta, says the study "probably doesn't change the immediate landscape, but it should make people more cautious" when using these drugs.

"These Parkinson's drugs are still prescribed way too widely," he adds. "If it turned out to be that long-term use enhanced the likelihood of developing Alzheimer's disease, that would be tragic."

Thies hopes, however, that the findings don't discourage the use of Parkinson's drugs. "But if a physician prescribes these drugs and sees a very rapid deterioration in a patient's cognitive function, he or she might want to examine whether the drugs are a component of that," he says.

Incontinence Drug Linked to Memory Loss

Jack Tsao, MD, DPhil, neurologist, Naval Hospital Jacksonville, Jacksonville, FL.

Michael Freedman, MD, geriatrician, New York University Medical Center, and the Diane and Arthur Belfer professor of geriatric medicine, New York University School of Medicine, New York City.

Daniel J. Watts, spokesman, Pfizer Inc., New York City.
New England Journal of Medicine.

A popular medication used to treat urinary incontinence may cause hallucinations and memory loss, especially in older patients.

A case study detailed how a 73-year-old woman taking the drug *tolterodine* had hallucinations and significant memory impairment. When she stopped taking the medication, the hallucinations stopped and her memory improved, according to the report by two physicians in Florida.

"The message we want to get across is that if people are on these medications and they are losing their memory, they should go to their doctor to be evaluated," says one of the article's authors, Dr. Jack Tsao, who is also a neurologist at Naval Hospital Jacksonville. "This is not going to affect everyone," he notes. "Many people do fine on this medication."

Tolterodine, sold under the brand name Detrol, is used to treat urinary incontinence caused by an overactive bladder. It works by stopping muscle contractions in the bladder.

THE CASE STUDY

Tsao says the elderly woman in the case study received a prescription for tolterodine from her primary-care physician. The prescription called for her to take 2 milligrams (mg) of the medication twice a day. It was not the extended release form of the medication.

Several weeks after she started taking the medication, she began to have hallucinations that she was talking with dead relatives. These hallucinations occurred only at night. She also reported having short-term memory problems, the study says.

Her physician attributed the symptoms to dementia and prescribed *donepezil* (Aricept), a memory-enhancing drug often prescribed for people with Alzheimer's disease. Tsao says after she began taking donepezil, the hallucinations went away.

For reasons not cited in the case study, the woman stopped taking tolterodine for a few months, and her memory improved. But her incontinence problems returned, so she began taking the drug again. Tsao says her memory problems then came back, although the hallucinations did not.

Tsao and his colleague, Dr. Kenneth Heilman from the Veterans Affairs Medical Center in Gainesville, administered tests to assess the woman's delayed recall and immediate learning abilities. She scored only in the first percentile (99% of people did better) on both tests while taking the medication.

She was again taken off tolterodine and, after two months, her memory improved significantly. Off the medication, she scored in the 50th percentile for recall and in the 75th percentile for immediate learning ability.

FINDINGS NOT SURPRISING

Dr. Michael Freedman, a geriatric specialist at New York University Medical Center, says he's not surprised by these findings.

Tolterodine is one of many different types of medications with an anticholergenic effect. That means the drug reduces the level of acetylcholine, a neurotransmitter that aids in memory. Other medications that have an anticholergenic effect include some tricyclic antidepressants and some antihistamines.

"If you give someone with borderline acetylcholine these drugs, you decrease acetylcholine even further, and they'll get much worse," he says.

While acknowledging that there have been a few reported cases of hallucinations associated with anticholergenic medications, Daniel Watts, a spokesman for Pfizer Inc., the maker of Detrol, points out, "These appear to be quite rare, and the definitive cause can be difficult to assess because patients often take various medications."

Tsao and Heilman recommend that before physicians prescribe medication for incontinence, they perform a screening test so they have a baseline memory score. If someone taking this type of medication is having problems with their memory, they should report it to their doctor immediately.

info To learn about how medications affect older people, visit the US Food and Drug Administration at *www.fda.gov.*

New Drug Could Aid Incontinence

Journal of Urology.
Boehringer Ingelheim news release.

Women bothered by urinary incontinence could soon get help from an antidepressant that is in the final stages of development.

THE STUDY

A recent study looked at 683 American and Canadian women 22 to 84 years old who had stress incontinence—accidental urine leakage due to an increase in abdominal pressure from laughing, sneezing or exercise. This condition affects an estimated one in three American women older than 18 years.

The medication, *duloxetine,* reduced the frequency of incontinence episodes by 50%, according to the study. In addition, 62% of the women who used the drug say it improved their lifestyle.

Duloxetine (*brand name:* Cymbalta) is an antidepressant that acts on two brain chemicals, *serotonin* and *norepinephrine.*

Urinary stress incontinence seems to have a connection to both serotonin and norepinephrine. The developers of Cymbalta—Eli Lilly and Company and Boehringer Ingelheim—say that it blocks the absorption and retention of these two chemicals in the spinal cord. This stimulates the contraction of the urethral sphincter, which is located at the opening of the bladder. This contraction helps prevent the leakage caused by activity.

■ ■ ■ ■

Types of Incontinence and Current Treatments

An estimated 13 million women and men in the United States suffer from urinary incontinence, according to the National Institutes of Health (NIH).

Women are twice as likely as men to develop the condition, thanks to the strain of pregnancy and childbirth, menopause and the anatomy of their urinary tract.

In addition to stress incontinence, the NIH identifies several other types of bladder control problems…

•**Urge incontinence.** Large quantities of urine are discharged at unexpected times, including during sleep.

•**Functional incontinence.** Ill-timed urination because of a physical disability, external obstacles or problems in thinking or communicating that prevent a person from reaching a toilet.

•**Overflow incontinence.** Small amounts of urine escape a full bladder.

•**Mixed incontinence.** Stress and urge incontinence, or other forms of leakage, combine.

•**Transient incontinence.** Temporary incontinence caused by a condition that will resolve, such as an infection or a side effect of medication.

There are a variety of treatments for urinary incontinence, ranging from biofeedback to exercise. As a first option, doctors often recommend Kegel exercises to strengthen the muscles in the pelvis and sphincter.

Electrical stimulation using temporary electrodes can also help strengthen the muscles in the pelvic floor.

In extreme cases, doctors may recommend surgery. Surgical procedures may involve reorienting the bladder or, less often, implanting an artificial sphincter that encircles the urethra.

info You can learn more about urinary incontinence from the National Kidney and Urologic Diseases Information Clearinghouse at *http://kidney.niddk.nih.gov.*

Viagra Pumps Up Hypertension Drug

Hossein A. Ghofrani, MD, researcher, University Hospital, Justus-Liebig-University Giessen, Giessen, Germany.
Bruce H. Brundage, MD, president, Pulmonary Hypertension Association, and medical director, The Heart Institute of the Cascades, Bend, OR.
Journal of the American College of Cardiology.

Viagra is best known for treating impotence, but the drug may soon be used to treat a very dangerous form of high blood pressure that strikes the lungs.

German scientists have found that Viagra helps patients with pulmonary hypertension (a type of high blood pressure) walk farther by relaxing the smooth muscle of blood vessels and increasing blood flow in the breathing organs.

THE STUDY

The researchers added Viagra to the standard therapy for pulmonary hypertension, a drug called *iloprost*.

Before taking iloprost, these patients could walk about 712 feet in six minutes. After the subjects took iloprost, they could walk 1,000 feet. After 18 months, however, the results declined to 840 feet, on average.

When Viagra was added after this decline, their six-minute walk distance increased to 1,135 feet.

RESULTS SURPASS EXPECTATIONS

These results exceeded expectations. "The best thing we expected to achieve was to stabilize the patients, but they stabilized and then improved," says Dr. Hossein A. Ghofrani, a physician at the University Hospital, Justus-Liebig-University Giessen in Germany, and leader of the research.

Patients with the condition who deteriorate even on long-term therapy are often considered urgent candidates for lung transplants. But the patients who took Viagra dropped off this list.

No serious adverse events were reported with the Viagra use, Ghofrani adds, including no reports of unwanted erections.

"The importance of this study is it is one of the first to report that two drugs are better than one" for pulmonary hypertension treatment, says Dr. Bruce H. Brundage, medical director of The Heart Institute of the Cascades in Oregon.

In addition to Viagra, there are now two other approved drugs for the treatment of impotence in men—Cialis and Levitra.

The German study doesn't address whether these medications would also be effective in treating pulmonary hypertension, but since they share a common mechanism of action, there's reason to think they will.

info For more on pulmonary hypertension, see the Pulmonary Hypertension Association at *www.phassociation.org.*

■ ■ ■ ■

Comparing the Drugs Used to Treat Impotence

All three drugs that are used to treat erectile dysfunction—Viagra, Levitra and Cialis—work by inhibiting the enzyme *phosphodiesterase 5* (PDE-5), which degrades an erection. All of the drugs carry warnings for men who have heart conditions. *But here are the major differences…*

Two major differences in the drugs are what is called the "window of opportunity" for sexual activity and the restrictions that are placed on food and alcohol.

●**Viagra.** Effects last one to four hours. Viagra should be taken on an empty stomach or after a low-fat meal because fatty foods can inhibit the absorption of the drug.

●**Levitra** takes effect quicker than Viagra (15 minutes) and lasts up to to five hours. Levitra has no food or alcohol restrictions.

●**Cialis** is effective for a longer period of time (30 to 36 hours) than either Viagra or Levitra. Cialis has no food or alcohol restrictions.

The three drugs are prescription medications and should not be used without consulting a physician.

Drug Combo Reduces Need for Prostate Surgery

Claus G. Roehrborn, MD, professor and chairman, department of urology, University of Texas Southwestern Medical Center, Dallas.

Jed Kaminetsky, MD, clinical assistant professor, urology, New York University School of Medicine, New York City.

New England Journal of Medicine.

Doctors routinely prescribe one of two drugs to treat men who have enlarged prostates, but a new study says that using both works even better.

Doxazosin and *finasteride* together reduce severe complications and the need for surgery to treat an enlarged prostate.

Because doxazosin and finasteride work by such different mechanisms, a combination approach "intuitively made sense," says study co-author Dr. Claus G. Roehrborn, chairman of the department of urology at the University of Texas Southwestern Medical Center in Dallas.

Doxazosin, an alpha blocker, relaxes the muscle at the opening of the bladder so urine can flow. Finasteride shrinks the prostate and eases the pressure on the urethra and bladder.

THE STUDY

The study followed up more than 3,000 men for approximately five years. The participants were randomly selected to receive either doxazosin alone, finasteride alone, a combination of the two or a placebo.

Doxazosin reduced the risk of overall progression of the condition by 39%; finasteride reduced the risk by 34%. The combination therapy reduced this risk by 66%.

SWITCH NOT LIKELY

Regardless of these positive results, doctors are not likely to switch to combination therapy based on this study.

One reason is that a trial earlier this year found that although finasteride reduced the risk of some types of prostate cancer, it also increased the risk of other cancers.

Roehrborn thinks men at high risk for their prostate enlargement to get worse could be given both drugs at once, but low-risk patients should take one or the other.

info For more on prostate enlargement, visit the American Academy of Family Physicians at *http://familydoctor.org*.

■ ■ ■ ■

What Happens When the Prostate Enlarges

Prostate enlargement affects more than half of American men older than 50 years. The prostate is next to the bladder and the urethra. When enlarged, it can pinch the urethra and disrupt the flow of urine. In extreme cases, it can even cause acute urinary retention (the inability to urinate), which may require surgery.

The Pressure's On To Find the Best Hypertension Drug

Carl J. Pepine, MD, chief, cardiovascular medicine, University of Florida School of Medicine, Gainesville.

Michael J. Alderman, MD, professor, medicine and epidemiology, Albert Einstein School of Medicine, Bronx, NY.

Journal of the American Medical Association.

A large new study provides support for using calcium channel blockers to control high blood pressure. However, one expert says the debate over which drugs are best for which patients will continue.

THE STUDY

The study included more than 22,000 patients who had coronary artery disease and high blood pressure. Researchers compared a drug regimen that included a calcium channel blocker with another regimen that included a beta-blocker. Both drugs lower blood pressure by relaxing arteries through different molecular mechanisms.

The percentage of patients who experienced "a primary outcome event"—death, a nonfatal heart attack or nonfatal stroke—during an average 2.7-year follow-up was almost identical in both groups.

The results directly contradict some earlier and much smaller studies suggesting that calcium channel blockers were not as safe and effective as other blood pressure drugs.

"What was apparent [from the earlier studies] was that there was not enough data to reach conclusions," says study author Dr. Carl J. Pepine, chief of cardiovascular medicine at the University of Florida School of Medicine. "What was clearly needed was a study of this magnitude."

TREATING HIGH BLOOD PRESSURE

Pepine's way of treating high blood pressure is to start with either a calcium channel blocker or beta-blocker "and build on that until you can get blood pressure under control," Pepine says. "Combination therapy may be what is needed because single-drug therapy is often not enough to achieve blood pressure control."

Most physicians would agree with that, says Dr. Michael J. Alderman, professor of medicine and epidemiology at Albert Einstein College of Medicine, but he prefers a different recipe.

Alderman starts patients on a diuretic, a drug that lowers blood pressure by removing fluid from the body, and then adds an artery-relaxing medication—a calcium channel blocker, beta-blocker or an angiotension-converting enzyme (ACE) inhibitor, which has yet another mode of action.

Alderman says debate about which drug combination is best should take a back seat to the fact that "the most important thing is to treat high blood pressure." Studies indicate that less than one third of Americans who have high blood pressure are getting any drug therapy to reduce their risk of heart attack and stroke, he says.

"Everyone would agree that the choice of drugs is a secondary issue," Alderman says.

And no single regimen is best for all patients, since there is no single cause of high blood pressure, he says. Approximately one third of all patients have high blood pressure simply because there is too much fluid in their arteries, Alderman says, and they will do best with a diuretic. But they will also tend to require some sort of medication that reduces blood pressure by widening blood vessels.

COST CONCERNS RAISED

"A diuretic costs a penny or so per day," Alderman says. "A calcium antagonist is a buck a day. I wouldn't base a medical decision on cost alone, but before we make the more expensive drug the first choice, we need better evidence that it is more effective.

"If we can just get the message out about controlling blood pressure, there are lots of ways to do it," he says

■ ■ ■ ■

The Dangers of High Blood Pressure

The National Institutes of Health estimate that one in every four American adults suffers from high blood pressure.

The condition increases your chance for getting heart disease or kidney disease and for having a stroke.

High blood pressure is especially dangerous because it often has no warning signs or symptoms.

Regardless of race, age or gender, anyone can develop high blood pressure, and once high blood pressure develops it usually lasts a lifetime.

The causes of high blood pressure vary, and may include narrowing of the arteries, a greater than normal volume of blood, or the heart beating faster or more forcefully than it should. Any of these conditions will cause increased pressure against the artery walls.

High blood pressure might also be caused by another medical problem. Most of the time, the cause is not known.

Although high blood pressure usually cannot be cured, in most cases it can be prevented and controlled.

info The US government's MedlinePlus has information on beta-blockers at *www.nlm.nih.gov/medlineplus*. Click on "Drug Information."

Heart Patients Live Longer With New Beta-Blocker

Richard A. Stein, associate chairman, medicine, Beth Israel Hospital, New York City.
The Lancet.

A newcomer to the beta-blocker drug family helps heart failure patients live longer than those who are prescribed an older version of the medication, European researchers have found.

THE STUDY

In one study, the difference was shown to be modest: Patients with heart failure who took *carvedilol* had about a 6% lower risk of death over a five-year period than those taking its older relative *metoprolol.*

Extrapolating from these study results, the researchers estimate that the patients taking carvedilol would have gained about 1.5 years of life over those who were taking metoprolol. They found no difference in the incidence of side effects, which was low for both drugs.

The research not only cements the value of beta-blocker treatment for heart failure, in which the heart gradually loses its ability to pump blood, but also "suggests that carvedilol may be a superior drug," says Dr. Richard A. Stein, associate chairman of medicine at Beth Israel Hospital in New York City and a spokesman for the American Heart Association.

"It is clear that beta-blockers are now the standard of treatment for [the type of] heart failure in which the left ventricle does not have an adequate ejection fraction," Stein says.

The left ventricle is the heart chamber that pumps blood to the body. The ejection fraction is the percentage of blood in the ventricle that is pumped with each beat.

Beta-blockers have emerged as a treatment for heart failure only in the last few years. This is a development that took many cardiologists by surprise. Previous thinking was that beta-blockers would worsen the condition, which has traditionally been treated with drugs that stimulate the activity of the heart. Beta-blockers slow the heart rate.

COST FACTOR

Cost is a potential issue in using carvedilol. Carvedilol, marketed as Coreg, is expensive compared with metoprolol, often sold as Toprol-XL, which is available as a generic. But the extra money is worth it, Stein says.

"A typical heart failure patient will have 1.8 hospital admissions a year, and the average cost of an admission is $20,000," he says. If you can reduce the number of admissions, Stein says, the extra cost of carvedilol may be well worth it.

info You can learn about heart failure from the Texas Heart Institute's Web site at *www.tmc.edu/thi*.

Drug May Save Lives of Heart Failure Patients

Andrew R. Marks, MD, chairman, physiology and cellular biophysics, Columbia University Medical Center, New York City.
Science.

Researchers say they have discovered a medication that corrects a cellular flaw that sometimes leads to death in heart failure patients.

The discovery is based on 15 years of research into the molecular mechanism of heart failure, says Dr. Andrew R. Marks, chairman of physiology and cellular biophysics at Columbia University Medical Center located in New York City.

Heart failure, which affects an estimated 4.6 million Americans and contributes to 300,000 deaths every year, is a progressive loss of the heart's ability to pump blood. Current treatments may include medications or more drastic measures, such as implanted defibrillators and heart transplants.

"We hope to develop a pill that millions of people could take at a cost that is relatively low compared to such measures," Marks says. Columbia University, which holds the patent on the new treatment, is talking to pharmaceutical companies about developing such a pill.

About half of the deaths related to heart failure are caused by arrhythmia, a fast and erratic heartbeat. The Columbia researchers discovered the cause of arrhythmia more than three years ago, according to Marks.

THE STUDY

In laboratory tests, the drug prevented arrhythmias in 10 mice that had the same molecular defect that is found in human heart failure. Eight of nine mice with the same defect who did not get the drug developed fatal arrhythmias.

"The next step is to optimize the drug and to test it in an animal model in preparation for a clinical trial," he said. "We would hope that we could move into patients, at least on an experimental basis, in a year or two."

info You can find out more about current treatment options for heart failure, including lifestyle changes, from the American Heart Association at *www.americanheart.org*.

Cholesterol-Lowering Drug May Relieve Leg Cramps and Fatigue

Circulation.
American Heart Association news release.

The cholesterol-lowering drug *atorvastatin* may help relieve leg pain and improve the walking ability of people with peripheral artery disease.

A common symptom of peripheral artery disease is *intermittent claudication*—cramping or fatigue in the legs and buttocks during activity. This fatigue usually eases when the person rests. Approximately 5% of people aged 60 and older have intermittent claudication.

THE STUDY

A recent study included 354 participants 60 years or older with intermittent claudication.

They received a daily dose of either a placebo, 10 milligrams (mg) of atorvastatin or 80 mg of atorvastatin.

After one year, the patients were tested to see how long they could walk on a treadmill, and how long they could walk without pain. The patients also answered a quality-of-life questionnaire to gauge their energy expenditure at work, at home and during leisure-time activities.

The maximum walking time did not vary greatly between the people in the three groups. However, the amount of time they could walk without leg pain improved by 63% for the patients taking the 80-mg dose of atorvastatin, compared with 38% for those taking the 10-mg dose and the placebo.

On the quality-of-life questionnaire, patients taking either dose of the drug showed improvement in physical activity over those taking placebo.

Nearly 8% of the patients who were taking the placebo experienced increased claudication or foot pain, or had to have a procedure to open clogged arteries. That figure dropped to 1.3% for the patients receiving either dose of the drug.

"The significance of the finding is that patients with claudication treated with a statin may experience an improvement in walking distance and lifestyle in addition to the known benefits of reduced risk for heart attack, stroke and death," says Dr. Mark A. Creager, senior author and director of the Vascular Center at Brigham and Women's Hospital in Boston.

■ ■ ■ ■

What Is Peripheral Artery Disease?

Peripheral artery disease (PAD) is a common cardiovascular disorder that affects the arteries in the body beyond the heart. According to the Vascular Disease Foundation, the disease affects 8 to 12 million Americans.

Arteries carry oxygen-rich blood from the heart to all areas of the body, and normally have a smooth lining that prevents blood clotting and promotes optimal blood flow.

In PAD, the arterial wall linings slowly become narrowed and rough due to a buildup of plaque. This allows clots to form. Consequently, the organs that depend on oxygen supplied by blood receive inadequate blood flow for normal function.

Despite its prevalence and cardiovascular risk implications, only 25% of those suffering from peripheral artery disease are undergoing treatment, according to the American Heart Association.

info The University of Maryland Medicine has more information about peripheral artery disease and intermittent claudication at *www.umm.edu/patiented*, where there is an alphabetical listing of conditions.

Eye Opener! Statins May Clear Up Vision Problems!

Michael F. Marmor, MD, professor, ophthalmology, Stanford University School of Medicine, CA.
Craig Greven, MD, professor and vice chairman, department of ophthalmology, Wake Forest University School of Medicine, Winston-Salem, NC.
British Journal of Ophthalmology.

Indirect evidence indicates that cholesterol-lowering drugs called statins may also prevent macular degeneration.

A study found patients who had macular degeneration were less likely to have filled a prescription for statins.

SOME EXPERTS URGE CAUTION

Other experts urged caution in interpreting the results, however, because no evidence was found that the drugs were the reason that the users were less likely to have eye trouble.

"This should not be put forward as a reason to go out and take these drugs," says Dr. Michael F. Marmor, an ophthalmology professor at Stanford University School of Medicine in California.

"The authors did not show a direct cause-and-effect relationship, only an association.

There are a number of theoretical explanations," he adds. For example, people taking statins may have had better lipid levels or may have been taking better care of themselves.

Macular degeneration, also known as *age-related maculopathy* (ARM), is the leading cause of irreversible vision loss among older adults in the United States. It is caused by the deterioration of light-sensitive cells in the part of the eye known as the *macula*. Older people, as well as people who smoke, appear to be more vulnerable to the condition, and there are few effective treatments.

In certain groups of people, antioxidants can slow the progression of the disease, says Dr. Craig Greven, vice chairman of the ophthalmology department at Wake Forest University School of Medicine.

Because cardiovascular disease and ARM may share some risk factors, there has been speculation that some of the same biological processes may be at work.

THE STUDY

The study authors looked at 550 people who recently had been diagnosed with ARM and compared them with 5,500 people who ostensibly did not have ARM. All of the participants were at least 50 years old.

People with ARM were 50% less likely to have received and filled a prescription for statins than the control group. This was true regardless of whether the person was taking statins or had taken them in the past.

In addition, the participants with ARM were more likely to also have diabetes, high blood pressure or vascular disease than the control group. However, the control group was just as likely to have arterial disease or lipid metabolism disorders as the group with ARM.

There may be some methodological problems with the study. "Two thirds of the people who were included in this study never had an eye examination to confirm whether they had macular degeneration. A lot of people in the control group may have had macular degeneration," says Greven. "I think that is a big problem."

The authors, as well as other experts, agree that the findings are extremely preliminary.

"It's an interesting observation, but certainly a lot more work and research into this needs to be done before any suggestion about statin use and macular degeneration can be made," Greven says.

info For more on this eye condition, visit the American Macular Degeneration Foundation at *www.macular.org*.

How to Put Unused Meds To Good Use!

Carol Kirschenbaum, MD, internist, president, North Carolina Committee to Defend Health Care, and board member, Physicians for a National Health Program, Durham.

Paul Patton, executive director, Tulsa County Medical Society, OK.

Tom Clark, RPh, director, policy and advocacy, American Society of Consultant Pharmacists, Alexandria, VA.

When Carol Kirschenbaum finished her chemotherapy several years ago, she had hundreds of dollars' worth of the antinausea medication Zofran left.

Rather than toss out the pills, which cost almost $30 each, Kirschenbaum gave them to her nurse. Her nurse then passed them on to another cancer patient who had no insurance to cover such a "luxury."

This type of exchange is not routine. However Kirschenbaum is a doctor as well as the president of the North Carolina Committee to Defend Health Care, which supports universal health coverage. The nurse trusted Kirschenbaum and was certain that the medication she gave her was still good.

COST CONCERNS

According to research done by the Health Law and Policy Institute at the University of Houston, up to $10 million worth of unused prescription drugs are flushed away each year in Oklahoma alone.

"If you multiplied that by the big states, we're talking about millions and millions of dollars," says Paul Patton, executive director of the Tulsa County Medical Society in Oklahoma, which started a program to salvage some of these drugs.

Although government and independent agencies, including the US Food and Drug Administration (FDA) and the American Society of Consulting Pharmacists (ASCP), have guidelines on the use of leftover drugs, the regulations usually are formulated on a state-by-state basis. Most states require that they be destroyed.

SAFETY CONCERNS

"When you start looking into the issue to see how we can safely reuse medicines, it's a lot more complicated than people realize because there is the issue of safety," says Tom Clark, director of policy and advocacy for the ASCP. The agency would support the return of unused drugs to the original dispensing pharmacy, but only if stringent safety measures were taken. But, Clark admits, verifying that every pill is safe is a time-consuming and labor-intensive project.

Health officials in Tulsa County are finding out just how complex that task is. But their breakthrough plan also is showing how it is possible.

THE PLAN

There were several obstacles to overcome. "The bureaucracy that is in place to protect us is prepared to protect us whether it kills us or not," Patton says.

It became clear to Patton and his colleagues that the FDA "rules" that people were afraid of actually were only position statements. They were able to persuade state legislators to change existing statutes to allow some recycling of drugs from nursing homes to the county pharmacy, and the program was on its way.

In the trial program, when a nursing home has extra medication (from a resident who has discontinued that drug, moved or died), it calls the county pharmacy. The pharmacy sends one of four retired physicians to pick up the pills, which the pharmacy then freely distributes to citizens who can't afford to have their prescription filled.

New Drug Calms Nausea Caused by Chemo

Journal of Clinical Oncology.
American Society of Clinical Oncology news release.

A drug called *aprepitant*—the first in a new class of medications that interferes with the vomiting reflex—helps reduce chemotherapy-induced nausea and vomiting in cancer patients, according to two international studies.

THE FIRST STUDY

The first study found that adding aprepitant to standard therapy to control nausea and vomiting helped reduce these symptoms on the day that patients received chemotherapy and for the following several days.

"Aprepitant should change the standard of care for the treatment of chemotherapy-induced nausea and vomiting," says lead researcher Dr. Paul J. Hesketh, of the Caritas St. Elizabeth's Medical Center in Boston.

THE SECOND STUDY

The second study discovered that the benefits of aprepitant extend over multiple cycles of chemotherapy.

Previous research had found that cancer patients experience increasingly severe nausea and vomiting over the course of several cycles of chemotherapy. Standard therapy to control the nausea and vomiting becomes less effective as chemotherapy cycles progress.

This study found that after six cycles of chemotherapy, 59% of the patients who took aprepitant along with the standard therapy reported no nausea or vomiting, compared with 34% of the patients who received standard therapy alone.

■ ■ ■ ■

What Chemotherapy Does

Chemotherapy destroys cancer cells by using drugs that stop these cells from growing or multiplying. *According to the National Cancer Institute, chemotherapy can be used to...*

●**Rid the body of cancer cells.**

●**Keep the cancer from spreading** by slowing the cancer's growth and killing cancer cells that may have spread to other parts of the body from the original tumor.

●**Relieve any symptoms that the cancer may cause.**

However, healthy cells can also be harmed, and this is what causes side effects.

Cells that divide quickly are most likely to be affected, including those in the digestive tract, reproductive system and hair follicles. Blood cells forming in the bone marrow can also be affected. Some anticancer drugs also may affect the cells of vital organs, such as the heart, kidney, bladder, lungs and nervous system.

The most common side effects of chemotherapy are nausea and vomiting, fatigue, pain, hair loss, diarrhea or constipation, anemia and infection.

■ ■ ■ ■

How to Reduce Nausea From Chemo

The National Cancer Institute recommends that patients experiencing nausea or vomiting from chemotherapy treatments…

●**Drink liquids at least an hour before or after mealtime,** instead of with meals.

●**Eat small meals throughout the day,** instead of one, two or three large meals.

●**Eat foods cold or at room temperature** so you won't be bothered by strong smells.

●**Chew your food thoroughly to make digestion easier.**

●**Drink cool, clear, unsweetened fruit juices,** such as apple or grape juice or light-colored sodas such as ginger ale that have lost their fizz and do not have caffeine.

●**Try to distract yourself by chatting with friends or family members,** listening to music or watching a movie or TV show.

●**Use relaxation techniques.**

●**Try to stay away from odors that bother you,** such as cooking smells, smoke or perfume.

●**Avoid sweet, fried or fatty foods.**

●**Rest but do not lie flat** for at least two hours after you finish a meal.

●**Avoid eating for at least a few hours before treatment** if nausea usually occurs during chemotherapy.

info You can learn more about chemotherapy from the American Cancer Society's Web site at *www.cancer.org.*

Doubling Up on Osteoporosis Drugs Weakens Bones

New England Journal of Medicine.

Combining osteoporosis drugs may do more harm than good, according to two studies.

The studies sought to prove that combining *alendronate* and *parathyroid hormone* would work even better than using the drugs separately. Instead, it proved exactly the opposite, researchers say.

Alendronate, sold by Merck as Fosamax, helps stop bone loss. Parathryoid hormone helps build bone.

THE STUDIES

The first study looked at the drug combination in 238 women with untreated osteoporosis. Some got one drug, some got the other and some got both.

The study, which was conducted at several major hospitals nationwide for a year, found "no evidence of synergy" when both drugs were used. In fact, Fosamax reduced the effects of parathyroid hormone.

The second study, done at Massachusetts General Hospital, targeted 83 men with brittle bones. It, too, found that Fosamax canceled the effects of the parathyroid hormone.

Women should talk to their doctors about whether to take Fosamax alone.

■ ■ ■ ■

About Osteoporosis

Osteoporosis is a major health risk for 28 million Americans, according to the National Institutes of Health (NIH). In the United States today, 10 million people already have osteoporosis and 18 million more have low bone mass, placing them at increased risk for this disease.

Osteoporosis is a skeletal disorder characterized by compromised bone strength. The disease leads to an increased risk of fracture and is the underlying cause of most fractures in older people.

The condition usually remains silent and undetected until a fracture occurs. Your doctor may recommend that you have your bone mass measured, which can detect whether you have low bone density and a greater chance of experiencing a fracture in the future. Some bone mineral density tests measure bone density in the spine, wrist and hip, while others measure bone density in the heel or hand.

Osteoporosis is responsible for more than 1.5 million fractures annually, including 300,000 hip fractures, approximately 700,000 spinal fractures, 250,000 wrist fractures and more than 300,000 fractures at other sites, according to the NIH. Fractures that are due to osteoporosis can happen from normal lifting and bending, as well as from falls. Furthermore, osteoporotic fractures, particularly vertebral fractures, can be associated with disabling pain.

Hip fractures have the greatest impact on health and well-being. One in five patients dies within one year of an osteoporotic hip fracture, the NIH reports. Fifty percent of those people experiencing a hip fracture will be unable to walk without assistance, and 28% will require long-term care. The burden of health care costs due to osteoporotic fractures is estimated to be $10 to $15 billion per year.

American women are four times more likely to develop osteoporosis than men. One of every two women and one in every eight men older than 50 years will have an osteoporosis-related fracture in her or his lifetime.

A number of factors can contribute to osteoporosis, including...

● **Accelerated bone loss** because of aging or menopause.

● **Bone growth that is below normal during childhood and adolescence,** which results in a failure to reach peak bone mass.

● **Bone loss caused by disease,** eating disorders or certain medications and medical treatments.

info Learn more about bone loss and its treatment from the National Osteoporosis Foundation at *www.nof.org.*

Herb and Drug Combo Battles Malaria

The Lancet, article and news release.

Combination drug therapy using a common Chinese herbal medicine, in addition to antimalarial drugs, may offer the best hope for treating malaria.

The main barrier for treating the millions of people who are affected by malaria worldwide is drug resistance.

An extract of sweet wormwood, also known as artemisinin, could solve this problem. Researchers say a derivative of artemisinin, called *artesunate,* was found to be highly effective in treating the disease when added to other antimalarial drugs.

THE STUDY

The study involved approximately 6,000 patients in 16 randomized trials. The addition of artesunate decreased treatment failure by approximately 80% and doubled the rate of successful treatment when compared with standard malaria treatment with antimalarial drugs, according to research conducted by the International Artemisinin Study Group.

■ ■ ■ ■

Malaria: How You Can Get It, How to Treat It

According to the Centers for Disease Control and Prevention, malaria is a serious, sometimes fatal, disease caused by a parasite. Malaria occurs in more than 100 countries and territories, including large areas of Central and South America, Haiti and the Dominican Republic, Africa, the Indian subcontinent, Southeast Asia, the Middle East and Oceania.

The World Health Organization estimates that 300 million to 500 million cases of malaria occur annually, with more than 1 million people dying from the disease. Approximately 1,200 cases of malaria are diagnosed in the United States each year, mostly in immigrants and travelers returning from high-risk areas.

Humans get malaria from the bite of a malaria-infected mosquito.

Malaria often brings on a fever and flu-like illness, with symptoms that include chills, headache, muscle aches and tiredness. Nausea, vomiting and diarrhea may also occur. Malaria may cause anemia and jaundice because of the destruction of red blood cells.

Malaria can be cured by using prescription drugs. The type of drugs and length of treatment depend on which kind of malaria is diagnosed, where the patient was infected, the age of the patient and how severely ill the patient was at the start of treatment.

info Learn more about malaria from the Centers for Disease Control and Prevention Web site at *www.cdc.gov/malaria.*

Breathe Easy: SARS Vaccine on the Horizon

Andrea Gambotto, MD, assistant professor, departments of surgery and medicine, division of infectious diseases and the Molecular Medicine Institute, University of Pittsburgh School of Medicine.

Scott Winram, PhD, product development project officer, National Institute of Allergy and Infectious Diseases, Bethesda, MD.

The Lancet.

An experimental vaccine against *severe acute respiratory syndrome* (SARS) has succeeded in protecting monkeys from the deadly virus, according to scientists from the University of Pittsburgh.

Although a human vaccine to protect against SARS is probably still years away from the market, the researchers say the tested vaccine looks promising.

"Many other groups are working on similar approaches, but this is the first [SARS] vaccine study reported in a peer-reviewed journal," says Dr. Andrea Gambotto, assistant professor in the departments of surgery and medicine at the University of Pittsburgh School of Medicine and the project leader.

THE STUDY

Gambotto's team, working with colleagues from the US Centers for Disease Control and Prevention, immunized six rhesus monkeys and administered a placebo vaccine to two control animals. Second doses were given after 28 days.

Six weeks later, the researchers evaluated whether the monkeys had an antibody response, which shows protection against the disease. All six animals that got the vaccine had detectable antibody levels, but neither control animal did.

"These animals don't get SARS [in the same was as humans], but they do have an antibody response," Gambotto says. "This antibody response was a very strong response. What we are now doing is following up the animals to monitor their long-term response, to see how long the response will last."

The animals that received the vaccine also had detectable levels of T-cells, which is a type of white blood cell involved in the immune system response to foreign invaders.

"The results are interesting and it is very encouraging," states Scott Winram, a project officer at the National Institute of Allergy and Infectious Diseases.

Winram notes that many other groups of scientists are also researching a SARS vaccine and are taking other approaches. Which vaccine will eventually prove best? "We'll have to wait and see," he says. "None are yet in clinical trials."

Before its containment, the SARS epidemic of 2003 sickened about 8,098 people worldwide and killed 774 of them, according to the World Health Organization.

Longer Anthrax Treatment May Be Necessary

Ronald Brookmeyer, PhD, professor, biostatistics, Johns Hopkins University Bloomberg School of Public Health, Baltimore, MD.
Stephen Fienberg, PhD, professor, statistics and social science, Carnegie Mellon University, Pittsburgh, PA.
Proceedings of the National Academy of Sciences.

The conventional 60-day course of antibiotics to treat people exposed to anthrax might be half as long as optimal, researchers have learned.

"Sixty days of antibiotic treatment may not be enough to confer protection," says Ronald Brookmeyer, professor of biostatistics at Johns Hopkins Bloomberg School of Public Health and a member of the research team. "If the exposure to anthrax spores is high, we may need to double that, to four months."

THE STUDY

"This [treatment] is not one size fits all," says Brookmeyer, adding that research is meant to add to the growing body of knowledge about how to handle a bioterrorist attack.

Brookmeyer and his colleagues used a competing-risks model, often used by biostatisticians, to determine the best length of antibiotic therapy. The research team found that 60 days of antibiotic therapy is probably adequate if the exposure to the spores that cause the disease is low. However, if the exposure is high and the treatment is stopped too soon, some spores may remain and cause illness.

The study report is aimed at convincing people that they need to take the full course of antibiotic treatment prescribed.

"There were some people in the 2001 attack who did not take the full 60-day course," says Brookmeyer. The adherence rates in the 2001 outbreak were only 64%, 61% and 31%, respectively, in the Washington, DC, New Jersey and Florida cases.

"This study really gives us a sensible time frame for treatment for low and high exposure," says Stephen Fienberg, a professor of statistics and social science at Carnegie Mellon University.

■ ■ ■ ■

Three Types of Anthrax Present Different Symptoms

Anthrax disease is caused by exposure to *Bacillus anthracis,* a bacterium that forms spores. These spores can live in the soil for many years and then infect people who work with infected farm animals or who inhale the spores from the air. Anthrax spores have also been used as a biological weapon. A powder form was distributed via the US Postal Service in 2001, causing 22 cases of anthrax disease.

Early treatment with antibiotics can cure most cases of *cutaneous* anthrax (skin is exposed to spores), according to the Centers for Disease Control and Prevention (CDC). Other forms—*gastrointestinal* (spores are ingested) and *inhalation* (spores are inhaled)—are more serious. In 2001, half the cases of inhalation anthrax were fatal.

Symptoms vary depending on the form of contraction. The first symptom of cutaneous anthrax is often a small sore that becomes a blister. Nausea, loss of appetite and fever can be the initial symptoms of gastrointestinal anthrax. Inhalation anthrax symptoms mimic a cold or flu. Symptoms for all types of anthrax can occur within seven days, but inhalation anthrax symptoms may appear up to 42 days after exposure, the CDC reports.

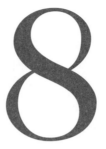

8

Emotional Well-Being

Don't Get Even—Get Mad And Live Longer

If you're mad and you show it, you just might live longer than other people who say nothing and just sit and seethe, according to a study of elderly priests, brothers and nuns. Researchers found that people who bottled up their anger were twice as likely to die over a five-year study period.

Some may find it odd to study anger in priests and nuns, but "the Catholic clergymen and nuns feel the full range of emotion that everybody else feels," says Robert S. Wilson, a professor of neuropsychology at Rush University Medical Center in Chicago. And they live in almost identical social and economic circumstances, he adds, which also makes them good study subjects.

THE STUDY

Wilson and his colleagues examined the medical records of 851 subjects from 1994-2002.

More than two thirds were women, and their average age when the study started was 75 years. When one of the subjects died—164 of them did—the researchers looked back at the tests measuring the subject's level of negative feelings and their ability to express it.

The goal was to examine how the expression—or suppression—of anger affects a person's life span, Wilson says. "From the time of the ancient Greeks, people have thought that personality and the way you express your emotions are related to health. There's a long history of studying that in medicine."

Studies have shown that depression is related to shorter life spans and heart disease, but there's less research into how people cope with negative emotions such as anger, Wilson says.

THE RESULTS

Over an average of five years, the 10% of the subjects who had the greatest tendency to

Robert S. Wilson, PhD, professor, neuropsychology, Rush University Medical Center, Chicago.

John E. Morley, MD, professor, gerontology, Saint Louis University, St. Louis, MO.

American Journal of Epidemiology.

keep their negative emotions bottled up were twice as likely to die as the 10% on the other end of the scale. The people who lived longer were those who said, *I get angry and I slam a door. I curse a lot,* Wilson says.

For now, it's still unclear how anger management—or the lack thereof—affects health. "There are studies that suggest negative emotions have been related to cardiovascular disease, and it's possible the mechanism could be through that," Wilson says. "They've also been connected to immune function and hormonal changes in your brain."

EXPERT ADVICE

Dr. John E. Morley, a professor of gerontology at Saint Louis University, says emotional outbursts "remain a better coping mechanism than internalizing and continuing to fret about the reason you are angry." Even so, he adds, people can find healthier ways of releasing their emotions.

"It is much better to be able to talk things through, but the old *Saturday Evening Post* cartoon of the husband yelling at the mother who yells at the kid who kicks the dog who bites the cat who claws the mouse remains a classical American coping strategy, no matter how nonpolitically correct it may be," he says.

info If you'd like to know more about healthy ways to release your anger, visit the American Psychological Association at *www.apa.org/pubinfo/anger.html.*

■ ■ ■ ■

How to Control Your Anger

Most medical experts agree that expressing anger can be beneficial. But letting your anger get out of control is not a good thing.

Anger is a normal, healthy emotion that only becomes a problem when it is expressed in a way that hurts you or others, or when it is the only feeling you allow yourself to experience.

If anger is not channeled or expressed in a healthy manner, it can sometimes lead to destructive behavior.

Learning how to express your anger in an appropriate way helps you improve your physical and emotional health, and also helps you

work more effectively with people at your job and at home.

The US government's National Institutes of Health (NIH) offers some suggestions on managing your anger…

THINGS TO DO WHEN YOU GET ANGRY

● **Try to understand why you are angry** and take responsibility for dealing with it in an appropriate and constructive way.

● **Walk away from a situation** that is escalating your anger.

● **Consider other options** you may have for dealing with anger.

● **Use conflict resolutions skills.**

● **Express how you are feeling with "I" statements.**

● **Express your emotions with someone who can empathize.**

● **Remember that your actions can have lasting consequences.**

● **Ask for help.**

Avoid Anger and Protect Your Own Health

Cardwell C. Nuckols, PhD, author of *Healing an Angry Heart.* Health Communications. *Bottom Line/Tomorrow.*

Anger is a powerful force that can be positive or negative. Handled well, anger can spur us to do something constructive about a problem. Handled badly, it can do serious damage to our relationships.

Example: A friend says something to you that hurts your feelings. Depending on how you handle anger, you might say something hurtful back…quietly seethe and act cold toward your friend…yell…avoid the other person…or tell him/her that his comments hurt you and why.

The last response is likely to have a positive result—building understanding and strengthening the friendship. Each of the other reactions undermines the friendship by keeping anger alive without resolving the conflict.

Chronic anger not only hurts relationships, it can affect your health.

One study of men over 60 years found that those with the highest hostility scores on a personality test had three times the average risk of heart attack and fatal heart disease. *Following are some ways to help recognize and control anger…*

UNDERSTANDING ANGER

Most anger stems from a feeling of losing control of our lives. By getting angry, we are able to temporarily regain a feeling of power.

Example: A father gets angry when his grown children fail to follow his advice. For him, it's easier to get angry than to accept that they need to learn from their own mistakes. By yelling at his children and making them feel guilty, he momentarily feels in charge again.

Anger is fueled even further by the negative comments we make to ourselves about things that happen to us. Often, we are not even aware of these self-defeating statements.

Example: While driving to an important meeting, you have a flat tire. Your first thought is, *Why does this always happen to me?* Your resentment builds as you struggle with the jack. You think, *No one is stopping to help… people are so uncaring.* You picture yourself arriving late at the meeting and making a terrible impression. You get so worked up that when another driver does stop, you snap, *It's about time!*—and he drives away. *That just proves what jerks people are,* you say to yourself. When you get to the meeting, you make a terrible impression—not because you are late, but because you are so hostile.

RECOGNIZING ANGER

You can handle anger in a constructive way if you can try to interrupt the automatic, negative spiral of thoughts and emotions. *Cooling-off techniques…*

●**Keep a journal.** Carry a small notebook with you. The next time you get angry, imagine you are a newspaper reporter collecting facts. Immediately after the incident, write down exactly what occurred…who you were with…where you were…and the thoughts that went through your mind before, during and after you got mad.

Do this in a private place so that you can think clearly.

Observing and recording details enables you to use rational powers of objectivity and analysis, rather than just relying on impulse and emotion.

●**Know the early warning signs.** Pay attention to the physical and mental symptoms of your anger.

Examples: Your face feels hot…your heart rate speeds up…you assume the worst about other people's motives…you get a general sense that things aren't right.

Write these signals down in your notebook. At first, you may not recognize them until after you have gotten mad. Over time, you'll notice them earlier and earlier.

●**Look for patterns.** What situations provoke you? Try to identify common themes, such as being criticized, having your authority challenged or feeling ignored. Ask yourself whether these themes remind you of other times in your life—especially childhood and adolescence, when many of our habitual reactions are formed.

Example: One woman noticed that she got angry at anxious people. Upon reflection, she remembered that her parents expected her to be poised and confident as a teen, and in fact, made fun of her when she appeared nervous. She also realized that now, as an adult, she tended to act hostile whenever she felt anxious herself.

Exploring the roots of your anger can help you to be more objective, so that you are no longer at the mercy of your habitual response. Some people find counseling useful in uncovering deeper sources of anger.

MANAGING ANGER

●**Create a safety plan.** On an index card, write down four things you can do that will help you calm down when you begin to get mad. Common techniques include breathing deeply, walking around the block, counting to 10 or calling a friend. Carry the card with you.

●**Call a time-out.** The moment you notice any of your warning signs, take a break and put your safety plan into action. If you are with other people, politely excuse yourself from the situation.

Example: I know this issue is important to you. Let's take a break and continue this conversation in 15 minutes.

Important: Keep your "exit strategy" simple. A scripted excuse is useless if you can't remember it under pressure.

●**Change what you are saying to yourself about the situation.** By changing the negative statements we make to ourselves, we can change our emotions.

Example: Replace *Why does this always happen to me?* with *I know that I can cope with this situation.*

●**Learn assertiveness and problem-solving skills.** After learning why you become angry, you may want to clarify a misunderstanding or correct a wrong by using rational thought—not rage. You can do this by using assertive communication, negotiation and problem-solving techniques.

Example: Clearly stating how you feel... acknowledging the other person's point of view...assessing and weighing options for action...agreeing on a trial period for change.

Courses in communication and negotiation skills are offered at some YMCAs, community colleges and as part of many adult education programs.

●**Develop spiritual strengths.** Coming to terms with anger requires making peace with the fact that we can't control many parts of life—not layoffs, illness or other people's reactions.

Spiritual connectedness can help us accept our limitations and embrace our need for the help of others.

This doesn't necessarily mean adopting a religion. Many find spiritual solace in nature... exploring meditation...opening up to friends and family about fears and concerns...helping others by volunteering or mentoring.

Finally, if you have trouble understanding and managing your anger, consider psychological counseling.

Meditate Your Way to Much Better Health

Stephan Bodian, author of *Meditation for Dummies.* John Wiley & Sons.
Bottom Line/Health.

If someone told you that you could lower your blood pressure or cholesterol level, reduce stress and curb chronic pain without taking expensive medications or exposing yourself to possible side effects, wouldn't it be worth a try?

With all the recent scientific evidence touting the mental and physical health benefits of meditation, more people than ever want to try this ancient practice.

But it's common for beginners to feel intimidated, bored, frustrated or confused. They often quit—before they can begin to reap the health benefits.

Good news: With the right approach, anyone can learn to meditate—and stick with it.

Dozens of well-designed studies have demonstrated the health benefits that are associated with meditation.

THE STUDY

Researchers working at the University of Wisconsin have actually used new brain-imaging technology to show how meditation affects the brain.

For this study, 25 volunteers enrolled in an eight-week meditation program. Each participant showed an increase in activity in the left side of the brain's frontal region—an area associated with positive emotions. Participants also reported a reduction in anxiety, anger and other negative feelings. A control group registered no such changes.

The participants who meditated also had a more vigorous immune response than the controls, which may help protect against infection and possibly even cancer.

CAN YOU ENJOY MEDITATION?

Even if you are aware of the long-term value of meditation, you are unlikely to do it on a regular basis unless you start to experience some real benefits.

Most people who meditate find it rewarding. They're more relaxed, think more clearly, appreciate the break from the stress and turmoil of everyday life and return to their ordinary activities refreshed. But it may take time.

Meditation can seem difficult and frustrating until you get the hang of it. In fact, you may even doubt whether it's worth the effort.

Helpful: Meditate daily. If you do it just once or twice a week, you'll be unlikely to experience any noticeable benefits.

Although you can certainly meditate on your own, it's often much easier to get started with the help of a group. Nowadays, many community colleges, adult-education programs and even hospitals offer classes.

HOW TO MEDITATE

There are several forms of meditation, but they all come down to one thing—focused awareness. This means directing your attention to an image, an object, a thought or a set of physical sensations, such as breathing.

What to do: Find a comfortable sitting position, close your eyes and take a few deep breaths, exhaling slowly.

Inhale and exhale through your nose (unless this is difficult or unpleasant). While maintaining a natural rhythm, allow your attention to focus on the sensation of your breath coming and going through your nostrils or the rising and falling of your belly as you breathe.

Your mind will inevitably wander off, and you might become engrossed in planning, thinking or fantasizing. As soon as you realize that you're doing this, bring your attention back to your breath.

Another widely practiced type of meditation involves repeating a word or phrase (called a *mantra*) to yourself, over and over. It may be helpful to coordinate the repetition with your breath, saying the mantra silently as you exhale.

You may choose a mantra that has personal, perhaps even spiritual, significance, such as "I trust in God," "May all beings be happy" or "May peace prevail."

Although most people meditate in a sitting position—in a firm chair or on a cushion, with straight backs and hands folded in laps

or resting on knees—you can also do it lying down, standing or walking.

If you're a beginner, start off slowly—10 to 15 minutes daily—and then lengthen the time period as you feel more comfortable to 20 minutes, 30 minutes or even an hour. Meditating for a longer period of time gives you more opportunity to settle into a focused, relaxed state of mind. Consider setting an alarm clock so you don't have to look at a clock or check your watch repeatedly.

Many people find it helpful to meditate at the same time every day, perhaps soon after rising or after things quiet down in the evening hours.

DEALING WITH DIFFICULTIES

If you're like most people, you may become discouraged before you've begun to experience the benefits of meditation. *Here's how to overcome the most common obstacles...*

●**Perfectionism.** This may be the biggest barrier. We have an idea of what we think meditation is supposed to be like, and the experience just doesn't measure up. Instead of peace and calm, our minds are full of chaotic thoughts. We may think, *What's the use...I'm just not good at this...This isn't working for me.*

Helpful: Realize that there isn't any wrong way to meditate. Simply making the effort and returning your mind to its focus is all that's required. Be aware of the mental chaos you are experiencing—then simply resume your breathing and/or mantra.

●**Physical restlessness.** During meditation, it's common to feel fidgety. Sitting still makes you aware of all the nervous energy and stress that is normally masked by the seemingly constant activity that happens in many people's daily lives.

It's not necessary to be completely still. If you need to fidget or adjust your position, do so. Many people find that restless feelings diminish after the first few minutes. As you become more experienced in meditation, you may want to simply observe the restlessness without acting on it.

Helpful: Walking meditation—very slow, mindful walking—allows you to move while focusing on your breath or a mantra.

•**Boredom.** You may become bored when your mind is not focused on its usual thinking and planning. Virtually all meditators experience this from time to time.

Helpful: Simply allow this boredom to exist. If you have patience and continue meditating, it will probably diminish over time.

•**Difficult emotions.** Some people experience anger, anxiety or other unpleasant emotions when they begin a meditation. It's hard to stay put when such feelings surface.

Helpful: Treat these emotions in the same way you do thoughts—notice them without getting caught up in them. How does anger and anxiety feel in your body?

The more regularly you meditate, the better able you'll be to deal with these emotions when they arise.

info For more information on meditation techniques and concepts from around the world, visit The Meditation Society of America at *www.meditationsociety.com*.

Yoga Eases MS Symptoms

Oregon Health & Sciences University news release.

Performing yoga can significantly improve the daily lives of patients who have multiple sclerosis (MS), a potentially crippling disorder that can leave people unable to move without assistance.

That finding comes from an Oregon Health & Science University study, the first randomized controlled trial of yoga in people with MS.

The researchers concluded that yoga was as effective as a traditional aerobic exercise program in improving fatigue, a common and potentially disabling symptom of MS. Six months of yoga eased tiredness, but the exercise regimen did not have any effect on alertness, attention or other measures of cognitive function, the study found.

The 90-minute yoga classes used in this study were held once every week. Participants were taught up to 19 yoga poses and also did breathing, visualization and meditation exercises. They were encouraged to practice each day at home.

Another group of MS patients took part in weekly aerobic exercise classes and were also asked to do aerobics at home each day.

People in both the yoga and aerobic exercise groups had reduced MS-related fatigue symptoms. One of the study authors says any kind of exercise seems to help, though it's not clear why. Regular exercise reduces fatigue "whether the regular exercise is yoga, swimming, using a stationary bicycle or any other physical activity. Sometimes the effects are quite dramatic, and other times they are less so. But everyone with MS who exercises regularly reports a benefit," says study co-author Dr. Dennis Bourdette, a professor of neurology and director of the Multiple Sclerosis Center of Oregon.

■ ■ ■ ■

The Different Types of Multiple Sclerosis

Multiple sclerosis (MS) is the name for a family of diseases that strike the body's central nervous system, which includes the brain, spinal cord and optic nerves.

Nerves in the central nervous system are covered by a fatty substance called *myelin* that helps them transmit electrical signals. In MS, the myelin erodes, leaving nerves vulnerable to damage and complete destruction.

Different forms of MS take different clinical courses, according to the National Multiple Sclerosis Society (NMSS).

Roughly 85% of people with MS are diagnosed with the *relapse-remitting* form of the disease, marked by periodic flare-ups that get better with time.

Approximately one in 10 people who have MS have the *primary-progressive* form. They have a gradual but progressive worsening of symptoms.

An estimated 50% of patients who have relapsing MS then go on to develop the *secondary-progressive* form of the disease within

10 years of diagnosis. In this form of MS, symptoms come and go, until these patients slip into a steady decline.

Finally, approximately 5% of MS patients have *progressive-relapsing* symptoms in which they steadily get worse and also experience periodic flare-ups.

Regular exercise, including yoga, is an important part of living with MS, according to the NMSS. Sedentary patients are at greater risk of heart disease, muscle weakness, fractures linked to poor bone density and breathing trouble.

info The National Multiple Sclerosis Society has more information about exercise and MS at *www.nmss.org.*

'Til Death Do Us Part— And that Might Be a While

Psychosomatic Medicine.
Health Behavior News Service news release.

Relationships with family and friends may help protect older women against death, and marriage may be the most beneficial relationship of all, a study says.

Married women, aged 65 and older, who are more socially active may live at least one to two years longer than more isolated women. Having large social networks significantly reduced the women's overall risk of earlier death, even when other factors such as diabetes, body weight, high blood pressure and other medical conditions were taken into account, the study found.

Among the strongest protectors were individual indicators of social networks, such as whether the women had anyone to talk to about important decisions, and whether anyone helped them with the cooking, cleaning or shopping.

"Most—though not all—of the benefits of social networks in this sample seemed attributable to marriage. Both marriage and larger social networks might provide a protective effect independently, whereas the combination of the two seems to be most beneficial," says researcher Thomas Rutledge of the University of Pittsburgh.

SIMILAR VIEW

David Ribar, a researcher for the department of economics at George Washington University in Washington, DC, came to some similar conclusions in a previous study about how marriage benefits the entire family.

Ribar examined quantitative research about the benefits of marriage on children's well-being, adults' earnings and adults' physical health and mortality.

The study considered different theories of how marriage might directly affect these outcomes, and offered various alternative explanations for why well-being appears associated with marriage.

Ribar's conclusion: "Consistent with the findings of previous reviews, there is evidence throughout the literature that marriage is associated with positive outcomes for the couple and for their children."

So, being married is better for men, too?

"Yes," according to Dr. Marty Sullivan, a heart specialist with Duke University Medical Center located in Durham, North Carolina. Dr. Sullivan says that once a man puts on that wedding ring, his health tends to improve and his life expectancy increases, even if it's an unhappy marriage.

However, for a woman to see any health benefits, she requires happiness in her marriage. Otherwise, she's better off alone.

According to Sullivan, it's not clear why these gender differences exist, but additional studies are planned to investigate and determine the cause.

info Information about social networks and other issues that affect the health of older women can be found at the National Library of Medicine's Medline Plus Web site at *www.nlm.nih.gov/medlineplus/womenshealth issues.html.*

Is Successful Marriage a Numbers Game?

Kristin Swanson, PhD, adjunct research assistant professor, applied mathematics, University of Washington, Seattle.

Catherine Cohan, PhD, assistant professor, human development and family studies, Pennsylvania State University, State College.

Kandi Walker, PhD, associate professor, communications, University of Louisville, KY.

Presentation, American Association for the Advancement of Science, Seattle.

Is it possible for a mathematical formula to predict which married couples are going to get divorced and which will stay together? A team of mathematicians and a psychologist say "yes."

"Using the mathematical model, we can predict dissolution or divorce with 90% accuracy over four years," says Kristin Swanson, an adjunct research assistant professor of applied mathematics at the University of Washington.

The leader of the team, psychologist John Gottman, has been working on marriage formulas for approximately 15 years.

"Before this model was developed, divorce prediction was not very accurate," says Gottman, "and we had no idea how to analyze what we call the masters and disasters of marriage—those long-term happily married couples and those divorced couples."

THE FORMULA

But after studying hundreds of videotaped conversations between spouses, the researchers came up with a mathematical formula to gauge the stability of the relationships. They give each person points—or take them away—depending on how they react to their own emotions and those of their spouses. "Something like showing contempt would be scored a negative-four, while making your partner laugh would [be scored] a plus-two," Swanson says.

After the conversation is over, researchers plot the points on a chart. "You'll see something that looks like a Dow Jones Industrial Average of positives and negatives," she says.

According to the researchers, the marriage is in trouble if the ratio of positive-to-negative interactions is less than 5-to-1.

"When the masters of marriage are talking about something important, they may be arguing, but they are also laughing and teasing and there are signs of affection because they have made emotional connections," Gottman says.

"But a lot of people don't know how to connect or how to build a sense of humor, and this means a lot of fighting that couples engage in is a failure to make emotional connections. We would not have known this without the mathematical model," he adds.

IDEAL SPOUSES CONSISTENT RESPONDERS

The researchers also discovered that ideal spouses consistently respond to each other in similar ways, but tend to keep their own individual emotions in mind, too, Swanson says. "If someone is reacting to every single subtlety of a partner, it's going to be hard to maintain," she says.

If the tests show that a relationship is troubled, researchers can make hypothetical revisions to the conversations, changing how the spouses react to each other, and then see if it changes the overall picture, Swanson says. Counselors can then make suggestions to the couple on the basis of the results.

"It's a balance, finding a balance for people for how much they respond to their own emotions versus how much they respond to their spouses," Swanson says.

EXPERT REACTION

Two experts say they're intrigued by the team's findings. Catherine Cohan, an assistant professor of human development and family studies at Pennsylvania State University, likes how the research analyzes not just positive and negative statements by spouses but also the interaction.

"Gottman's team has shown that some couples start a conversation on a positive note and continue to get more positive as the conversation goes on. Some couples start a conversation on a negative note and continue to get more negative as the conversation ensues," she says. "It is a particularly interesting pattern when the conversation starts out negative but one of the spouses says something positive, and the other spouse follows suit. They turn the direction of the conversation around and it becomes positive."

Gottman's "preliminary research has made it into texts on relationship and communication almost as soon as he spoke the words," says Kandi Walker, an associate professor of communications at the University of Louisville in Kentucky. "I find this work interesting and quite groundbreaking. I believe human interactions are the basis for much of a person's happiness, and Gottman has cleverly found a way to give us a prescription for a good marriage."

info For more tips on how to live a happy married life, visit the comprehensive page on family and marriage from Trinity University at *www.trinity.edu/mkearl/family.html*.

Family and Friends Can Be Good Medicine

Jaak Panksepp, PhD, professor emeritus, Bowling Green State University, Bowling Green, OH, and head, affective neuroscience research, Falk Center for Molecular Therapeutics, Northwestern University, Evanston, IL.
Matthew Lieberman, PhD, assistant professor, psychology, University of California, Los Angeles.
Science.

Researchers at the University of California at Los Angeles (UCLA) have found that emotional pain and physical pain stimulate the same parts of the brain, and experts now suggest that to avoid pain, people take better care of the social and emotional sides of their lives.

"Emotional pain is an undesired psychological state of affairs, and the less there is of that in social networks, the more harmoniously people will interact," explains Jaak Panksepp, a professor emeritus with Bowling Green State University.

THE STUDY

In the UCLA research, 13 participants were hooked up to *functional magnetic resonance imaging* (fMRI) equipment while they played a ball-tossing video game called Cyberball. The fMRI monitors blood flow to different parts of the brain.

The experiment involved three scenarios. In the first, the participant was allowed only to watch, not play. In the second scenario, the participant played ball with two other "players" (actually the computer). In the third and final scenario, the two computer-generated players threw the ball only to each other, intentionally excluding the study participant.

When a player was intentionally excluded from playing with the other players, the blood flow changes to the brain were the same as if the person had been physically injured.

"For human beings, and mammals more generally, being socially connected is just as important [as avoiding physical harm]. You are more likely to die as a result of social exclusion than of physical pain," says Matthew Lieberman, senior study author and an assistant professor of psychology at UCLA.

The next step would be to look at how social support systems can mitigate the painful emotions people experience.

"It would be important to see how social comfort actually changes pain-induced distress, and which types of pain it can modulate," Panksepp says.

info To find out how you can help someone who is depressed, visit *www.healthy place.com*.

■ ■ ■ ■

Dealing with Emotional Pain

Emotional pain can result from an abusive relationship, childhood or adult trauma or loss of a loved one. Left untreated, emotional pain can lead to depression, a psychological condition that changes how you think and feel, and also affects your social behavior and sense of physical well-being.

Other ways to seek relief from emotional pain could include seeing a therapist or talking to a friend. People with severe emotional pain should ask a doctor about appropriate medications.

Longer Treatment Needed For Bipolar Patients

American Journal of Psychiatry.
University of California, Los Angeles, news release.

The standard treatment for the depression that accompanies bipolar disorder may need to be reconsidered. A recent study suggests that people with the disease may need to take antidepressants twice as long as previously prescribed.

About 3.5% of Americans have bipolar disorder, which is characterized by alternating cycles of depression and mania. Symptoms of depression may include prolonged periods of sadness, irritability, anxiety, pessimism, indifference and persistent lethargy. Some symptoms of mania may include inflated sense of self-esteem or self-importance, inappropriately elevated mood, decreased need for sleep, racing thoughts and impulsive behavior.

CURRENT COURSE OF TREATMENT

Current guidelines recommend that during a depression cycle, patients be given antidepressants in conjunction with a mood-stabilizing medication. These drugs are usually discontinued within the first six months after the symptoms of depression are under control.

But researchers at the University of California at Los Angeles (UCLA), found that patients treated according to these guidelines relapsed at almost twice the rate of those who continued to take antidepressants for the first year after remission of their depression. The study authors also saw no increased risk of manic relapse in the patients who continued the antidepressant for a year.

THE STUDY

Researchers examined 84 people with bipolar disorder whose depression symptoms eased with the addition of an antidepressant to an ongoing mood stabilizing medication, such as lithium. The study compared the risk of depression relapse between the 43 people who stopped taking antidepressants within six months of remission and the 41 who continued taking antidepressants.

"The common clinical practice of discontinuing antidepressant use in bipolar patients soon after remission of depression may actually increase the risk of relapse," says study author Dr. Lori Altshuler.

"Long-held concerns regarding the risk of switching into mania may actually interfere with establishing effective guidelines for treating and preventing a relapse of bipolar depression," according to Altshuler.

"Guidelines that are more similar to those of maintenance treatment of unipolar depression may be more appropriate for those individuals with bipolar depression who respond well to antidepressants. A controlled, randomized study is needed to address these questions," Altshuler says.

■ ■ ■ ■

A Professional Is Often Needed to Diagnose Bipolar Disorder

Bipolar disorder, also called manic depression, causes very dramatic mood swings —from overly "high" and/or irritable to sad and hopeless, and then back again. In between these swings, there are often periods of a normal mood.

Severe changes in energy and behavior go along with these changes in mood.

The periods of highs and lows are called *episodes* of mania and depression.

The following information from the National Institutes of Mental Health (NIH) describes some types of behavior that indicate professional help may be needed.

MANIC EPISODE

A manic episode is diagnosed if an elevated mood occurs with three or more of the following symptoms most of the day, nearly every day, for a week or longer period of time. If the mood is irritable, four additional symptoms must be present.

●**Increased energy and activity levels,** often accompanied by restlessness.

●**Racing thoughts and talking very fast,** jumping from one idea to another.

●**Distractibility,** can't concentrate well.

•**Little sleep needed.**

•**Unrealistic beliefs in one's abilities and powers.**

•**Poor judgment.**

•**Spending sprees.**

•**A lasting period of behavior that is different from usual.**

•**Increased sex drive.**

•**Abuse of drugs,** particularly cocaine, alcohol and sleeping medications.

•**Provocative,** intrusive or otherwise aggressive behavior.

•**Denial that anything is wrong.**

DEPRESSIVE EPISODE

A depressive episode is diagnosed if five or more of these symptoms last most of the day, nearly every day, for a period of two weeks or longer.

•**Sad,** anxious or empty mood.

•**Feelings of hopelessness** or pessimism.

•**Feelings of guilt,** worthlessness or possibly helplessness.

•**Loss of interest or pleasure in activities once enjoyed,** including sex.

•**Decreased energy,** a feeling of fatigue or of being "slowed down."

•**Difficulty concentrating,** remembering, making decisions.

•**Restlessness or irritability.**

•**Sleeping too much or can't sleep.**

•**Change in appetite** and/or unintended weight loss or gain.

•**Chronic pain** or other persistent bodily symptoms that are not caused by physical illness or injury.

•**Thoughts of death or suicide,** or suicide attempts.

Chronic Depression Is Easily Overlooked

Michael E. Thase, MD, professor of psychiatry at University of Pittsburgh Medical Center, PA.
Bottom Line/Health.

Virtually everyone has occasional moods when life seems dreary and pointless and nothing brings much pleasure or satisfaction. These normally pass, and a few hours or days later, you're feeling fine.

For some people, however, such feelings do *not* pass. They're not so down that they can't work or see friends, but life has lost its sparkle. Although this chronic, low-level depression—known as *dysthymia*—affects approximately 3 million Americans, it often goes undetected by the sufferers themselves, their families and even their doctors.

Unlike grief—a natural reaction to a death or other loss that gets better over time—dysthymia has no apparent reason and may keep your spirits low for the greater part of most days. Sadness might predominate your emotions, or the feeling may be one of apathy, emotional numbness or an inability to enjoy the things you once did.

Caution: If untreated, you run a 90% risk of experiencing an episode of major depression within the next several years. Even if your symptoms haven't lasted long, you may well benefit from medication and/or therapy.

Whether or not you opt for professional assistance, you can help manage the symptoms of your condition by reevaluating and changing how you *think* and *act*.

YOU CAN CHANGE

Many scientists believe that chronic depression is linked to a tendency, perhaps inherited, for brain chemicals to get out of balance.

Stress or trauma early in life can also play an important role as well as chronic health or personal problems in adulthood. But no matter where it comes from, a major part of the condition is a negative way of thinking that generates unpleasant emotions.

It's normal to think negative thoughts approximately 20% of the time, but for depressed people these thoughts consume more than 70% of their inner monologue.

Changing these patterns can make a difference in how you feel. *Here's how...*

●**Substitute optimism for pessimism.** The outlook of the "half-empty glass" condemns you to live in a world where nothing seems likely to work out well.

Pessimistic people tend to *generalize* from unpleasant events, believe distressing circumstances are *permanent* and *personalize* bad experiences.

A more realistic view—that most difficulties are limited in scope, temporary and impersonal—can prevent you from getting into the depressive spiral.

Example: You're shortchanged by a grocery clerk, who is rude when you bring it to her attention. You immediately think, *Everyone is out to cheat me.*

More realistic: This person is just a jerk.

To combat this negative way of thinking, start monitoring your thoughts. Whenever you find yourself thinking globally and personally, get down to specifics to limit the pain you cause yourself.

Example: When your inner voice says, *Nothing goes my way,* try, *This week has really been tough.*

●**Schedule pleasurable activities.** Depression slows you down and saps your energy. It's a vicious cycle—the less you do, the more you think about your problems.

Something as simple as going to a movie, having lunch with a friend, gardening or listening to music can provide a small but real lift to your spirits.

Think of enjoyment as a *prescription.* Plan at least one or two potentially pleasurable activities every day—*even if you're not in the mood to do them.*

Helpful: In a journal, rate from one to 10 how much you are expecting to enjoy a concert, dinner out, massage, etc. Afterward, rate the actual experience. You may get more pleasure than you expected.

●**Force yourself to exercise.** It releases endorphins and balances other brain chemicals to reduce tension, frustration and stress... raises your energy level...and distracts your attention from negative thoughts.

Helpful: Start with stretching exercises or strolling just 15 minutes a day. Gradually build up to brisk walking, biking or any exercise you like. Do it for at least 20 minutes, four to six times a week, strenuously enough to accelerate your pulse and break a light sweat.

WHEN TO GET HELP

If you've done what you can on your own but still feel down, it's time to seek expert assistance. Both medication and psychotherapy have been shown to work quite well for chronic depression.

A good therapist will help you understand how your thinking habits, social skills and relationship difficulties contribute to your depression, and support your concrete steps to change them. Just three months of such therapy can be effective.

The same antidepressant medications used for severe acute depression work with chronic low-level forms as well. Among the most commonly used antidepressants are *sertraline* (Zoloft), *fluoxetine* (Prozac), *bupropion* (Wellbutrin) and *venlafaxine* (Effexor).

Each is effective 50% to 60% of the time, so it may take some trial and error to find the drug that works best for you.

If you're reluctant to try an antidepressant, ask your doctor about taking the herb St. John's wort (900 to 1,200 milligrams [mg] daily for four to six weeks).

■ ■ ■ ■

Symptoms of Depression

If you have been bothered by three or more of the following symptoms for two years or longer, you may have dysthymia and should seek help from a health professional...

●**Unusually increased or decreased appetite and/or sleep.**

●**Feelings of inadequacy,** guilt or perhaps low self-esteem.

- **Trouble concentrating** or trouble making decisions.
- **Irritability.**
- **Lack of energy.**
- **Pessimistic brooding.**
- **Avoidance of social situations.**
- **Suicidal thoughts.***

Depression Drugs Risk: Is It Worth It for Kids?

Tim Kendall, MD, co-director, National Collaborating Centre for Mental Health, London, and consultant psychiatrist, Sheffield, UK.

Marvin Lipkowitz, MD, chairman, psychiatry, Maimonides Medical Center, New York City.

The Lancet.

Newer antidepressants may not be the best treatment for children with depression…and may even be harmful, according to a recent British study.

The research found that when data from both published and unpublished trials were combined, the risks for children taking *selective serotonin reuptake inhibitors* (SSRIs) or another drug, Effexor, appear to outweigh the benefits from these medications. The only exception to this was *fluoxetine,* marketed under the brand name Prozac, which had a favorable risk–benefit profile, meaning the benefits of taking the medication outweigh any potential risks.

"I'm not sure these drugs are any better than placebo," says study co-author Dr. Tim Kendall, who is also co-director of the National Collaborating Centre for Mental Health in London. "I'm not sure it's worth using SSRIs, and it may even be dangerous, with the exception of fluoxetine."

THE STUDY

The United Kingdom's Medicines and Healthcare products Regulatory Agency (MHRA)

*If you have thoughts of killing yourself, or your problems put your job or personal relationships in jeopardy, seek professional help immediately.

required drug companies to provide Kendall and his colleagues with the results of their unpublished studies.

The researchers reviewed 12 studies—six that were published, six that were unpublished —that compared the use of various SSRIs to treatment with a placebo.

While Prozac had a favorable risk–benefit profile, other SSRIs didn't fare as well.

Paroxetine (Paxil) and *sertraline* (Zoloft) had a slightly favorable risk–benefit profile when only the published data was examined. But when the unpublished data was added, the risks of taking these medications outweighed the potential benefits. Both *citalopram* (Celexa) and *venlafaxine* (Effexor, which is not an SSRI) also had unfavorable risk–benefit profiles.

Kendall believes legislation should require drug manufacturers to make unpublished data available. He says it's often difficult to get negative results published, and the drug manufacturers who financially support the study are under no obligation to make the results of unfavorable studies known.

DEFENDERS SPEAK OUT, URGE RESTRAINT

However, the SSRIs do have their defenders. "These drugs have done a lot of good. You don't want to throw the baby out with the bath water," says Dr. Marvin Lipkowitz, chairman of the psychiatry department at Maimonides Medical Center in New York City. "But you can't just count on the pills alone. This is not like treating a sore throat."

Lipkowitz recommends that any child taking antidepressant medication be monitored while they're on the drug.

Lipkowitz adds that most of the studies examined contained a relatively small number of children. When a study has only several hundred children, one or two adverse events can skew the data.

Kendall says in the absence of any convincing evidence, he believes parents whose children are depressed should try cognitive behavioral therapy first. If there's a need for an antidepressant, he says fluoxetine seems to be the safest choice. But, he adds, "You really do need to think carefully about these drugs, and I think it would be unwise to prescribe these drugs for children at risk of suicide."

Experts caution that no one should abruptly stop the use of these medications because serious withdrawal symptoms can occur. If you're concerned about your child, discuss the use of SSRIs with a psychiatrist.

info To learn more about children and depression, go to the American Academy of Family Physicians' Web site at *www.aafp.org.*

ADHD Drugs May Slow Growth

James Swanson, PhD, psychologist and professor of pediatrics, University of California, Irvine.

Ernest Krug, MD, medical director, Center for Human Development, William Beaumont Hospital, Royal Oak, MI.

Pediatrics.

Children who have *attention deficit hyperactivity disorder* (ADHD) could find their height stunted by the medications used to treat this condition.

The results of a study and two years of follow-up research by scientists at the University of California, Irvine, found that stimulant medications used to treat ADHD are effective, but they may slow growth in height a bit.

THE STUDY

The randomized clinical trial, which lasted 14 months, compared the use of the stimulant medication Ritalin with behavioral therapy. Both Ritalin alone and behavioral therapy alone were also compared with a combination of two and with no treatment at all.

Researchers found that the children who received medication or medication in conjunction with behavioral therapy had fewer symptoms than those who received no medication. Children on medication also grew slightly less than their nonmedicated peers.

James Swanson, a psychologist and professor of pediatrics at the University of California, Irvine, and his colleagues then followed up with 540 children with ADHD who had participated in the trial.

After 24 months, the researchers interviewed the children and the parents and found that both the effects of medication and the effects of behavioral therapy were fairly consistent throughout this time period.

They also confirmed that the children who were on medication showed a slight reduction in height, but according to Swanson, the effect was less pronounced at 24 months, amounting to approximately one centimeter less per year than the children who were not taking medication.

MEDICATIONS SAFE, BUT QUESTIONS REMAIN

"Stimulant medications are really extremely safe with very few side effects," says Swanson. "I do not think this is necessarily a cause for great alarm in parents. The effect we saw was rather modest."

Swanson also notes that many questions remain unanswered.

For example, researchers don't know if children on ADHD medications will have a growth rebound later.

He adds that many children who have ADHD are larger than average for their age, so the slight growth reduction for those on medication may just put them back into the normal height range.

Dr. Ernest Krug, medical director of Beaumont Hospital's Center for Human Development in Royal Oak, Michigan, says, "Growth suppression is something we always monitor in kids on medication. This study reinforces the importance of careful follow-up of children when they're on medication. It's a good idea for these children to be seen every three to four months."

With any medication, parents should be convinced that the drug is providing beneficial effects for their children without causing unreasonable side effects, Krug says.

info To learn more about ADHD, visit the Children and Adults with Attention Deficit/Hyperactivity Disorder (CHADD) Web site at *www.chadd.org.*

Bored? Restless?
Can't Get Organized?

Edward M. Hallowell, MD, instructor of psychiatry, Harvard Medical School, Boston, and director, Hallowell Center, Sudbury, MA.
Bottom Line/Health.

Up to 10 million American adults have *attention deficit disorder* (ADD), but only about 10% know it. *Following are some of the myths about ADD in adults...*

Myth #1: People with ADD can't sit still or focus properly.

The Diagnostic and Statistical Manual of Mental Disorders, the "bible" of psychiatrists, refers to attention deficit *hyperactivity* disorder. The term isn't entirely accurate because hyperactivity (having trouble sitting through movies, for example, or frequently tapping your fingers or feet) may or may not be present.

The other important symptoms of ADD are *inattention* and *impulsivity.*

Examples of inattention include reading a book and spacing out or staring at someone's lips while they're talking to you but not taking in what they're saying.

Examples of impulsivity include taking unnecessary risks or having trouble waiting in line. Most adults suffer from only one or two of the three primary symptoms—hyperactivity, inattention and impulsivity.

Even the term *attention deficit* is misleading. Most people with ADD can focus intensely when necessary.

Myth #2: ADD is a learning disability.

Most adults who have ADD have normal IQs. They read and absorb new information as well as people who don't have the disorder—though they may have to make adjustments for their ADD symptoms.

Example: High-energy adults with ADD often avoid careers that are detail-oriented, such as accounting, bookkeeping and secretarial work. They like to work on multiple projects at the same time to stave off boredom. These individuals create systems (calendars, notes, etc.) to stay organized.

Myth #3: Poor parenting causes ADD.

This is totally false. People with ADD have a physical problem that they're born with, but it is often not diagnosed until adulthood. The exact cause still isn't known, but ADD is believed to be primarily due to genetics.

Most people with ADD have at least one relative with the disorder. Adults whose mothers smoked cigarettes, took illegal drugs or drank alcohol during pregnancy are at an increased risk for ADD, according to recent research. People who have been exposed to environmental toxins, such as dioxins and polychlorinated biphenyls (PCBs), are also at an increased risk.

Many people with ADD have more challenging careers than those without it.

Consider David Neeleman, CEO and founder of JetBlue Airways. He has found ways to compensate for his ADD. For example, he takes a physical approach to his job, frequently going out onto the tarmac and checking up on his airplanes because he gets bored sitting in the office. An assistant helps keep his schedule.

I know many doctors, professors and other professionals with ADD. Research shows that one in three adults with ADD becomes an entrepreneur by their 30s.

People who have ADD also tend to be creative, intuitive and highly energetic. In my own case, I have three kids, have written 11 books and do 60 lectures a year. I don't think I would have the energy for all that if I didn't have ADD.

Myth #4: ADD cannot be diagnosed with any degree of accuracy.

There isn't a single test for ADD, any more than there's a single test for anxiety or depression. But it can be diagnosed objectively by a psychiatrist, psychologist or neurologist.

First, a careful medical history is essential for an accurate diagnosis. Before ruling out ADD, doctors also should discuss the patient's symptoms with a family member. People with ADD are poor self-observers. A second point of view often reveals things that patients overlook.

To see if the patient exhibits the criteria representative of ADD, psychiatrists usually use a checklist—a sense of not meeting goals, trouble getting organized, frequent procrastination, etc.

A relatively new test known as *quantitative electroencephalography* (QEEG), which provides physical data by looking for slow brain waves in the frontal lobes, also should be administered. This test is 90% accurate in diagnosing ADD.

Myth #5: Stimulant drugs are really the only course of treatment.

Many patients do get better when they take stimulant drugs, such as *methylphenidate* (Ritalin) and *dextroamphetamine* (Dexedrine).

These drugs don't cure ADD, but they reduce many of the symptoms, such as hyperactivity, inattention and impulsivity.

The medications also stimulate the inhibitor neurons, which stop much of the incoming and outgoing stimuli, allowing the patient to be more focused.

A new drug, *atomoxetine* (Strattera), is the first nonstimulant medication approved by the FDA for adults with ADD. It works differently but just as effectively as stimulants, promoting higher brain levels of *norepinephrine,* a neurochemical that helps people focus and stay calm.

Nondrug treatments also are essential. *All ADD sufferers should…*

●**Exercise for at least 20 minutes every day.** Any exercise that you enjoy, that is convenient for you and can be added to your daily routine, will be beneficial. Physical activity increases brain levels of the neurotransmitter *dopamine* and helps people who have ADD release nervous energy.

●**Get a lifestyle coach.** Many psychiatrists refer ADD patients to professionals who are trained to help them make lifestyle adjustments. A coach will come to your home and suggest ways to improve everything from your work area and habits to your family dynamics.

●**Talk to a psychotherapist.** A directed, focused regimen of psychotherapy can be helpful in dealing with feelings that are often experienced by adults with ADD, such as low self-esteem and self-doubt.

info To find a therapist, contact the Attention Deficit Disorder Association at 484-945-2101 *or www.add.org.*

ADHD Not Just for Kids

Historically, attention deficit hyperactivity disorder (ADHD) has been used to describe a condition in children. However, recent research has found that it affects 30% to 50% of adults who had ADHD in childhood.

The main symptom of ADHD is a lack of inhibition, according to the American Academy of Family Physicians. This can lead to inattention, distractibility and impulsiveness.

"The 'on the go' drivenness seen in many ADHD children is replaced in adults with restlessness, difficulty relaxing and a feeling of being chronically 'on edge,'" write researchers with the Family Medicine of St. Louis Residency Program in St. Louis, Missouri, in an article published in *American Family Physician.*

"Appointments, social commitments as well as deadlines are frequently forgotten," the researchers continue. "Impulsivity often takes the form of socially inappropriate behavior, such as blurting out thoughts that are rude or insulting."

"While many of the symptoms are reported by others in the patient's life, the problem often expressed by adults with ADHD is frustration over the inability to be organized. Prioritizing is another common source of frustration. Important tasks are not completed while trivial distractions receive inordinate time and attention," according to the researchers.

Diagnosis of adult ADHD is complicated by the overlap of its symptoms with the symptoms of other common psychiatric conditions, such as depression and substance abuse, the researchers in St. Louis found.

Also, press coverage of adult hyperactivity has led many people to believe they suffer from hyperactivity when in fact they do not, the researchers say.

"Studies of self-referral suggest that only one third to one half of adults who believe they have ADHD actually meet formal diagnostic criteria," they write. "While family physicians are knowledgeable about childhood ADHD, there is a noticeable absence of guidelines for primary care evaluation and treatment of adults with symptoms of the disorder."

info You can learn more about ADHD from the National Institute of Neurological Disorders and Stroke at *www.ninds.nih.gov.*

ADHD May Predict Alcoholism in Adults

Alcoholism: Clinical & Experimental Research.
University of Regensburg, Germany, news release.

Adult attention deficit hyperactivity disorder (ADHD) and alcoholism are connected, according to a recent study.

The researchers identified a distinct profile of adults who have ADHD and who are also alcoholics. But despite previous research that suggests a common genetic cause of ADHD and alcoholism, this study found no such evidence when it examined two specific genes.

"Our results indicate that individuals with persisting ADHD symptoms in adulthood seem to be at high risk of developing an alcohol-use disorder. Moreover, there is evidence for a highly increased severity of alcohol dependence in subjects with ADHD," says the study author Dr. Monika Johann of the University of Regensburg in Germany.

The study included 314 adult alcoholics and 220 healthy control patients. They were all assessed for such psychiatric disorders as substance abuse (including alcoholism), ADHD and *antisocial personality disorder* (APD).

The study findings indicate a distinct profile of adults who have ADHD and alcoholism. The adult alcoholics with ADHD in this study drank more alcohol per day and per month, became dependent on alcohol at an earlier age, had a greater frequency of suicidal thoughts, as well as a higher occurrence of APD and had been in court more times.

So, even though the study did not find a common genetic predisposition, "this data show once again that to have ADHD means to be at high risk for developing alcohol dependence," Johann says.

Same Genetic Defect Seen In Manic Depression, Schizophrenia

Sabine Bahn, MD, PhD, clinical lecturer, University of Cambridge, England.
Kenneth L. Davis, MD, dean, Mount Sinai School of Medicine, New York City.
The Lancet.

Two mental health disorders—schizophrenia and manic depression—appear to have the same underlying genetic defect, according to a study by scientists at the University of Cambridge in England.

THE STUDY

A study of the preserved brains of people who had either schizophrenia or *bipolar disorder*—the medical name for manic depression—discovered that there was a flawed performance of the genes that produce the protective coating around brain cells.

The protective coat consists of fatty molecules called myelin, held together by proteins. The study of gene activity in the preserved brains shows that "those proteins appear to be abnormal," study author Dr. Sabine Bahn, a clinical lecturer at the University of Cambridge, says.

The finding adds evidence for a growing belief by scientists that "these conditions are not as different as has been commonly thought," Bahn says. "The diagnosis is often imprecise, and it can take months or years to arrive at the correct diagnosis."

Together, the two conditions affect about 2% of the population.

HOPE FOR DIAGNOSTIC TEST

It's possible that this research could lead to better treatment for the illnesses, but that is a long-range hope, Bahn says.

A more immediate goal is a quicker and more accurate diagnostic test to help psychiatrists prescribe the best treatment.

Even that goal will not be easy to achieve, she says. The newly reported finding is based on the study of just 45 brains at the Stanley

Library of Brain Research in Bethesda, Maryland—15 of deceased patients who had schizophrenia, 15 of patients who had bipolar disorder and 15 of people who were free of mental disease.

Bahn's studies are being expanded, to look first at samples from another 150 preserved brains, and eventually to examine more than 20,000 postmortem tissue samples, she says. The idea is to determine exactly what is going wrong in the psychotic brain.

CHANGE IN FOCUS

The study is an important marker of "a sea change in what we in the field think is the likely culprit in psychosis," says Dr. Kenneth L. Davis. He did some of the earliest work on myelin abnormalities as head of the department of psychiatry at the Mount Sinai School of Medicine in New York. He is now the dean of the school.

Until recently, research on mental disorders focused almost entirely on how signals are transmitted between the synapses at the ends of nerve cells, Davis says.

The change in focus means that possible links can be seen between mental illnesses and physical diseases such as multiple sclerosis, which involve myelin abnormalities, Davis says.

info You can learn about bipolar disorder from the National Institute of Mental Health at *www.nimh.nih.gov.*

New Schizophrenia Drugs Show Promise

Dilip Jeste, MD, professor, psychiatry and neurosciences, University of California, San Diego, and the VA Medical Center, San Diego.

Hiten Patel, MD, psychiatrist, William Beaumont Hospital, Royal Oak, MI.

American Journal of Psychiatry.

The new generation of schizophrenia drugs appears to greatly reduce violent behavior in people with the disease who undergo treatment at community-based centers, according to a Duke University Medical Center study.

THE STUDY

The two-year study of 229 people found that schizophrenia patients who consistently took one of these newer drugs, called *atypical antipsychotics,* had less than one third the incidence of fighting or violence toward others, compared with schizophrenia patients who took older antipsychotic medications.

The Duke researchers say this is the first study to examine the long-term impact of treatment with this newer class of antipsychotic drugs—such as *clozapine, risperidone* and *olanzapine*—on violent behavior in real world (not laboratory) settings.

The study was funded by Eli Lilly and Co., which makes olanzapine. The drug is sold under the brand name Zyprexa.

MOST DON'T TAKE MEDICATIONS AS DIRECTED

Although drugs can help schizophrenics lead more normal lives, as many as 60% of patients don't take these medications as directed.

And that noncompliance leads to higher medical costs, according to another study.

"We looked at adherence to antipsychotic medications because they form the backbone of treatment for schizophrenics," says study co-author Dr. Dilip Jeste, a professor of psychiatry and neurosciences at the University of California, San Diego. "These medications are good, but they only work when taken properly."

For this study, Jeste and his team reviewed claims and eligibility data for 1,619 people with schizophrenia who were receiving treatment between 1998 and 2000.

Most of the study subjects were between the ages of 30 and 59 years—the average age was 42 years. Fifty-six percent were men.

Only 41% of the people studied took their medication as prescribed. Twenty-four percent of the subjects were nonadherent, meaning they filled less than 50% of their antipsychotic medication prescriptions, Jeste says. Seventeen percent were partially adherent, which means they filled between 50% and 80% of their prescriptions.

What surprised the researchers was the number of "excess fillers" they discovered. Nearly 20% of the people studied filled prescriptions for more medication than they needed.

Not surprisingly, psychiatric hospitalizations were much higher for those who didn't take their medications as prescribed. People who were nonadherent were 2.5 times as likely to be hospitalized for psychiatric reasons. Those who were partially adherent or excess fillers were 80% more likely to be hospitalized.

Even hospitalizations for nonpsychiatric reasons were higher for those patients who didn't follow their drug regimen.

Those who were noncompliant or excess fillers were 70% more likely to be hospitalized for medical reasons than people who adhered to their drug schedule. Those who were partially compliant were 30% more likely to have a medical hospitalization.

Hospital costs were three times higher for those people who didn't take their medication properly than for those who did. Costs for people who were partially adherent or excess fillers were about 2.5 times higher.

Dr. Hiten Patel, a psychiatrist at William Beaumont Hospital in Royal Oak, Michigan, says the study's findings are not surprising. "We know that there is a very high degree of noncompliance in people who have schizophrenia," he says.

Jeste says the researchers weren't able to discern the reasons for noncompliance from the available data. They did find that younger patients and substance abusers were less likely to take their medication as directed. People living with family or in assisted-living settings were more likely to follow prescriptions.

info To learn more about schizophrenia and ways to treat it, visit the American Psychiatric Association at *www.psych.org*.

■ ■ ■ ■

The Faces of Schizophrenia

Schizophrenia is a chronic mental ailment that affects approximately 1% of the US population, according to the National Institute of Mental Health.

Symptoms can include hallucinations, delusions, paranoia, disordered thinking and difficulty expressing emotions.

Symptoms of the disorder, which may be inherited, usually appear in late adolescence or early adulthood.

The precise causes of schizophrenia aren't clear, but probably involve some combination of alerted brain chemistry, as well as environmental triggers, according to the US Department of Health and Human Services.

Approximately six in 10 people who have schizophrenia respond well to treatment. Drugs can control the most troubling symptoms of the disease—including psychosis, hallucinations and delusions—while psychotherapy and self-help groups can improve social skills, coping and other important aspects of dealing with mental illness.

Silver Cars May Be Safer

Sue Furness, research fellow, University of Auckland School of Public Health, New Zealand.

Russ Rader, spokesman, Insurance Institute for Highway Safety, Bethesda, MD.

British Medical Journal.

Choosing a color when you are purchasing a car may be more than just a reflection of your tastes and style. It also may affect how likely you are to be injured in an accident.

Researchers in New Zealand report that car color can have an impact on your chances of being injured in a road accident—and silver is the safest.

THE STUDY

After analyzing the statistics from a two-year study of more than 571 auto accidents in Auckland, epidemiologists at the University of Auckland found that the risk of having a serious injury was 50% lower in silver cars than in white, yellow, gray, red or blue vehicles.

The study also found that there was "a significant increased risk of a serious injury" in brown vehicles and a slightly increased risk in black and green cars.

"Our conclusions are valid for the location where the study was done," says Sue Furness, a research fellow working at the School of Public Health at the University of Auckland. But, she adds, "how valid they are for other settings is questionable because studies haven't been done elsewhere."

"Silver cars are becoming more popular with new-car buyers," she says. "Increasing the proportion of silver cars could be an effective passive strategy to reduce the burden of injury from car crashes."

SHOULD WE TAKE THIS SERIOUSLY?

The study was reported in the traditional Christmas issue of the *British Medical Journal* that is devoted to research that is decidedly off the beaten track. For example, another study is an analysis of how elderly and disabled pedestrians are depicted on road signs in 119 countries.

Russ Rader, a spokesman for the US Insurance Institute for Highway Safety, is skeptical of the study—to say the least.

"The claim that car color could have this effect in reducing automobile accidents is preposterous, but there will be those people who read stories about this and actually think that it reflects reality," Rader says.

Vehicle color sometimes has been taken seriously in regard to highway safety. Some communities have the fire engines painted yellow rather than the more traditional red in the belief that they are more easily seen and identified, Rader acknowledges.

However, he adds, "There is no evidence that color has the kind of effect that the authors are finding. They have left out things like the driver's sex, vehicle engine size, vehicle age and ambient light conditions," all of which can affect auto safety, Rader says.

info You can get real model-by-model—but colorless—auto safety statistics from the National Highway Traffic Safety Administration at *www.nhtsa.dot.gov/cars/problems*.

Car Accidents Cause Post-Traumatic Stress Disorder

J. Gayle Beck, professor, psychology, The State University of New York at Buffalo.

After the Crash: Psychological Assessment and Treatment of Survivors of Motor Vehicle Accidents, by Edward Blanchard and Edward Hickling. American Psychological Association.

Car accidents are a leading cause of post-traumatic stress disorder (PTSD), according to a book titled *After the Crash: Psychological Assessment and Treatment of Survivors of Motor Vehicle Accidents.*

PTSD is a common psychological ailment, affecting as many as 5 million Americans each year, according to the National Institute of Mental Health.

Symptoms of PTSD include reliving the traumatic incident through flashbacks or nightmares, sleep problems, depression, anxiety, irritability and anger.

The authors, psychologists Edward Blanchard, from the the State University of New York (SUNY) at Albany, and Edward Hickling, in private practice in Albany, New York, provide information from a new study of motor vehicle accident survivors and PTSD.

THE STUDY

The researchers followed up 161 car crash survivors for five years after they had their accident. The study subjects were at least slightly injured and sought medical attention after their accident.

In this group, 110 subjects were diagnosed with PTSD, and 60% of them also experienced major depression.

Practically all—95%—of the crash survivors had become anxious when driving and many avoided certain situations, such as driving at night or highway driving.

J. Gayle Beck, a professor of psychology at SUNY Buffalo who specializes in treating PTSD after an automobile crash, says those are common behaviors for people who have lived through a serious accident.

"These people tend to refuse to drive or are unbelievably nervous drivers," Beck says.

And, she notes, a serious accident doesn't necessarily have to be one in which someone was seriously injured.

Any accident that scares someone or makes him/her believe they might die has the potential to cause PTSD, she says, recalling a patient whose car rolled over. He was not seriously injured, but during the accident, he believed that he was going to die, and those memories haunted him.

According to Beck, PTSD isn't easy to diagnose. Many PTSD symptoms are not obvious. The most common symptom, for example, is having recurrent and intrusive thoughts about the accident. This may make the person appear to be unable to concentrate. Beck says people suffering from PTSD often are hyperactive and have trouble sleeping.

Clearer signs that someone may need help after they've been in an accident is refusing to drive or exhibiting very nervous or altered driving behavior.

Although these signs can be common right after an accident, if any symptoms persist for more than six months, it's time to get treatment, Beck says. The experts agree that cognitive behavioral therapy is helpful for many people, as is supportive psychotherapy. Beck says researchers are experimenting with new ways to treat PTSD. In her lab, she is using virtual-reality driving simulations as a way to get people with PTSD driving again.

info To learn more about PTSD, visit the National Center for Post-Traumatic Stress Disorder at *www.ncptsd.org.*

■ ■ ■ ■

Post-Traumatic Stress Disorder More Common in Post-9/11 World

Post-Traumatic Stress Disorder (PTSD) was first introduced into the American lexicon in the 1970s when it was used to describe some Vietnam veterans' inability to readjust to civilian life.

The National Institute of Mental Health offers the following information about PTSD…

PTSD is an anxiety disorder that can develop after exposure to a terrifying event in which grave physical harm occurred or was threatened. Traumatic events that may trigger PTSD include violent personal assaults, natural disasters, accidents or military combat.

SIGNS AND SYMPTOMS

People with PTSD have persistent frightening thoughts and memories of their ordeal. They may experience sleep problems, feel detached, emotionally numb or be easily startled.

PTSD affects about 5.2 million adult Americans. Women are more likely than men to develop PTSD. It can occur at any age, and there is some evidence that susceptibility to PTSD may run in families.

The disorder is often accompanied by depression, substance abuse or one or more other anxiety disorders. In severe cases, the person may have trouble working or socializing.

Not every traumatized person experiences PTSD. It is diagnosed only if the symptoms last more than a month. In those who do develop PTSD, symptoms usually begin within three months of the trauma. The course of the illness varies—some people recover within six months; others have symptoms that last much longer. Occasionally, the illness doesn't show up until years after the traumatic event.

Effective treatments for PTSD are available, including medications and carefully targeted psychotherapy.

Dental Pain Memory May Be 'All in Your Head'

University of Florida news release.
Journal of Pain.

The pain you remember from your last visit to the dentist may not have been all in your teeth; a lot of it may be in your head.

A University of Florida College of Dentistry study found that a person's long-term memory of pain intensity may be influenced by how stressed the person was during the experience.

THE STUDY

The study included 52 men and 48 women, some of whom participated in a stressful situation—giving a speech about difficult social issues to a live audience and in front of a video camera.

The other group experienced a stress-free situation in which they read magazines about gardening or travel.

Researchers assessed the participants' stress levels during both sessions.

After each session, participants were asked to rate the severity of pain of an "ice-cream headache" caused by holding a bag of crushed ice against their foreheads.

Six months later, the study researchers interviewed 68 of the participants about their memories of that pain.

THE RESULTS

"We found that nearly everyone we spoke to remembered more pain at six months than they reported at the time of their experience," says researcher Henrietta L. Logan, director of public health services at the UF College of Dentistry.

People who were in the stressful situation remembered nearly 10% more pain than those who were in the non-stress situation.

The emotional state of the participants at the time they had their six-month follow-up interview also influenced their memory of the pain intensity.

"Clearly, many dental and medical procedures are anxiety-provoking, fear-provoking and uncomfortable in general," says researcher Jeffrey J. Gedney, a pain behavior research fellow at UF College of Dentistry.

"We found that emotional factors became a better predictor of what people would recall over a period of time than what their level of pain actually was during their experience," Gedney explains.

info The American Dental Association has information about dental anxiety at *www.ada.org/public/topics/anxiety.asp.*

Emotional Stress Taxes the Heart

Willem Kop, PhD, assistant professor, psychology, US Uniformed Services University of Health Sciences, Bethesda, MD.

J. Michael Gaziano, MD, associate professor, medicine, Harvard Medical School, Boston.

Archives of Internal Medicine.

Circulation.

The kind of stress that is encountered in everyday life can trigger abnormal heart rhythms in vulnerable people, recent research has found.

"This is the first study to demonstrate that mental stress alone can induce specific heartbeat irregularities that identify patients with high vulnerability to arrhythmias," says Willem Kop, an assistant professor of psychology at the US Uniformed Services University of Health Sciences.

It has long been known that physical stress can precipitate arrhythmias, abnormal heartbeats that can sometimes be fatal. Putting high-risk patients through "the mental equivalent of an exercise stress test" shows that emotional stress can have the same effect, he says.

THE STUDY

The test group examined 17 people who had a heart malfunction that was serious enough to require implanted defibrillators. These devices give an electric jolt to restore normal heart rhythm when it goes awry.

The 17 heart patients and 17 control subjects with healthy hearts underwent both exercise and mental stress testing.

One of the mental tests was having the participants recall recent incidents that angered them. Another was the bothersome task of subtracting multiples of the number 7 from a four-digit number while they were occasionally interrupted without warning and pestered to improve their performance.

The heartbeat irregularities occurred much faster in the defibrillator users during the mental stress tests than during the physical stress tests, Kop notes. It took an increase of 53.3 beats per minute during the exercise to cause irregularities. But those irregularities were triggered after an increase of just 9.7 beats per minute during part of the mental stress testing, he says.

"Now we need to find out two things—whether we can predict future events, and are there subgroups of patients at particularly high risk of developing arrhythmias, such as those with type A personalities," Kop says.

One group clearly at higher risk consists of "people who do not exercise much any more," a growing percentage of the American population, he says.

The study wasn't designed to offer advice on ways to lessen the health risks for people who are prone to stress in daily situations. But they could try some well-established stress management techniques, Kop says.

info For more information about stress and how to handle it, visit the American Psychological Association at *www.apa.org*.

Lower Stress in 5 Minutes or Less

Dawn Groves, author of *Stress Reduction for Busy People* and *Massage for Busy People* and *Yoga for Busy People*. New World Library.
Bottom Line/Personal.

No time to relax? Don't be so sure. *It can take only five minutes to unwind and refresh your mind…*

•**Move around.** Take a quick trip through the halls of your home or workplace—or simply around the block. Walk up and down a flight of stairs. Do 15 jumping jacks.

•**Stretch while seated.** Lace your fingers under your knee, and draw it to your chest. Repeat with the other knee. This stretches the leg and lower back.

Next, stretch your arms above your head, palms up and fingers interlaced.

Drop your hands to your sides, then raise your right shoulder to your right ear, keeping your head vertical. Repeat with the left shoulder.

Finally, bend back the fingers of each hand. This is especially important if you use a computer for long periods.

•**Take 10 long, deep breaths.** Your belly should expand as you inhale and contract as you exhale.

•**Massage your eyes and ears.** Place your palms over your eyes. Slowly spiral your palms while applying gentle pressure. Do the same for your ears.

Blocking out sights and sounds, even for just a few seconds, is psychologically refreshing.

•**Try aromatherapy.** Put a drop of lemon-lime or orange essential oil in a saucer. These gentle scents relax you without making your home or office smell like an incense store.

Great resource: *www.aromaweb.com.*

Rise in Stress Hormones Not Related to End-of-Life Pain

Dick Swaab, MD, PhD, director and professor, neurobiology, Netherlands Institute for Brain Research, Amsterdam.
Annette Carron, DO, director, palliative care services, William Beaumont Hospital, Royal Oak, MI.
Neuropsychopharmacology.

Losing a loved one is painful, but knowing that the person didn't suffer in the last moments can be a comfort to family and friends. So a new study may offer solace to the bereaved.

Researchers from the Netherlands have discovered that levels of the stress hormone cortisol rise just before death as a result of the failure of bodily functions, and not because of fear or pain.

"The levels of cortisol, our stress hormone, are strongly rising in the blood and cerebrospinal fluid in the last phase of our life," says study author Dr. Dick Swaab, director of neurobiology at the Netherlands Institute for Brain Research in Amsterdam.

Cortisol, Swaab explains, protects the body and the brain in stressful circumstances and it helps to make energy available for the body to react to danger.

Swaab says researchers wanted to know if fear or suffering were responsible for the increased cortisol levels.

THE RESEARCH

To answer this question, Swaab and his colleagues compared cortisol levels from 85 Alzheimer's patients with levels in 52 other people without dementia after their death. They also looked at cortisol levels in 19 control patients and 54 Alzheimer's patients who were given a high-dose of a painkiller with morphine during the last two weeks of their lives.

The cortisol levels were consistently higher in the people with Alzheimer's. In the control group, those treated with morphine had slightly lower levels of cortisol, but the Alzheimer's patients who were given morphine had higher levels of cortisol than those who didn't receive morphine.

That means, Swaab says, that the psychological stress or the fear of dying isn't the cause of the cortisol rise, because the Alzheimer's patients didn't know they were going to die. It also means that physical pain isn't the cause of the cortisol rise either, because patients on high doses of morphine had high increases in their levels of cortisol.

REASSURING FINDING

The higher levels of cortisol simply may be a protective physiological response that occurs as different body functions start to fail.

"This study shows that patients don't necessarily recognize the stress of dying. It is more physiological than psychological," says Dr. Annette Carron, director of palliative care services at William Beaumont Hospital, located in Royal Oak, Michigan. "It's nice for families to believe that they're not suffering."

The American Academy of Hospice and Palliative Medicine regards sedation as a valid, ethically sound, and effective modality for relieving symptoms and suffering in some patients reaching the ends of their lives. Sedation is reserved for those in whom suffering is not helped by appropriate palliative care measures. Those measures can include pain relief, non-pain symptom management, mental health care and spiritual counseling.

info The Medical College of Wisconsin discusses the benefits of end-of-life care at *http://healthlink.mcw.edu.*

■ ■ ■ ■

The Facts About Hospice Care

The Hospice Association of America offers some clarification about how hospice works and who qualifies...

Fiction: Hospice is a place where the terminally ill go to die.

Fact: Hospice is not a place, but a concept of care. More than 90% of the hospice services provided in this country are based in the home. Care provided in the home allows families to be together when they need it the most, sharing the final days in peace, comfort and dignity. However, when home care is not an option, in-patient care can be available through a contracting hospital, skilled nursing facility or the hospice's own in-patient facility (if available). In addition, in-patient care is available in emergency situations to those receiving home care or when family members need respite care.

Fiction: Hospice only serves persons diagnosed with cancer.

Fact: Other frequent admission diagnoses include diseases of the circulatory system; infectious and parasitic diseases, including human immunodeficiency virus (HIV); diseases of the nervous system and the sense organs, including Alzheimer's, Parkinson's, meningitis, etc.; and diseases of the respiratory system.

Fiction: A patient needs Medicare or Medicaid to afford hospice services.

Fact: Although insurance coverage for hospice is available through Medicare and in 44 states under Medicaid, most private insurance plans, HMOs and other managed care organizations include hospice care as a benefit. In addition, through community contributions, memorial donations and foundation gifts, many hospices are able to provide patients who lack sufficient funds with free services. Other programs charge patients in accordance with their ability to pay.

Fiction: A physician decides whether a patient should receive hospice care and which agency should provide that care.

Fact: The role of the physician is to recommend care, whether hospice or traditional curative care. It is the patient's right and decision to determine when hospice is appropriate and which program suits his or her needs. Before entering a hospice, however, a physician must certify that a patient has been diagnosed with a terminal illness and has a life expectancy of six months or less.

Fiction: Hospice services are very expensive because 24-hour on-call services are provided to patients.

Fact: Generally, hospice costs less than care in hospitals, nursing homes or other institutional settings. When in a hospice, the patient will pay only for those services that he or she or the family cannot provide and that are not covered by insurance.

Fiction: To be eligible for hospice care, a patient must already be bedridden.

Fact: Hospice care is appropriate at the time of the terminal prognosis, regardless of the patient's physical condition. Many of the patients served through hospice continue to lead productive and rewarding lives. Together, the patient, family and physician determine when hospice services should begin.

Fiction: After six months, patients are no longer eligible to receive hospice care through Medicare and other insurances.

Fact: The Medicare hospice program says services may be provided to terminally ill Medicare beneficiaries with a life expectancy of six months or less. However, if the patient lives beyond the initial six months, he or she can continue receiving hospice care as long as the attending physician recertifies that the patient is terminally ill with a limited life expectancy of six months or less.

Fiction: Once a patient elects hospice, he or she can no longer receive care from the primary care physician.

Fact: Hospice reinforces the patient–physician relationship by advocating either office or home visits. Hospices work closely with the primary physician and consider the continuation of the patient–physician relationship to be of the highest priority.

Fiction: Once a patient elects hospice care, he or she cannot return to traditional medical treatment.

Fact: Patients always have the right to reinstate traditional care at any time, for any reason. If a patient's condition improves or the disease goes into remission, he or she can then be discharged from a hospice and return to aggressive, curative measures, if so desired. If a discharged patient wants to return to hospice care, Medicare, Medicaid and the majority of private insurance companies and HMOs will allow readmission.

Fiction: Hospice means giving up hope.

Fact: When faced with a terminal illness, many patients and family members tend to dwell on the imminent loss of life rather than on making the most of the life that remains. Hospice helps patients reclaim the spirit of life. It helps them understand that even though death can lead to sadness, anger and pain, it can also lead to new opportunities for reminiscence, laughter, reunion and hope.

9

Family Health

The Life-Saving Vaccination 53% of Population Doesn't Have!

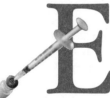

Even if you're careful about your health and schedule regular checkups and tests, you probably don't get one vaccination that could save your life. More than 53% of adults living in the United States are not protected against tetanus or diphtheria because they have failed to get the booster shot that is recommended once every 10 years, according to guidelines from the Centers for Disease Control and Prevention (CDC).

The National Foundation for Infectious Diseases (NFID) is conducting a public awareness campaign about the importance of getting a booster shot every decade.

"Probably the greatest obstacle to people getting their diphtheria and tetanus booster is that they do not know they are supposed to get it," says Dr. Susan Rehm, president of the NFID, as well as a staff physician at the Cleveland Clinic.

"There's been a lot of emphasis on childhood vaccines," Rehm says, but much less on the adult immunizations to curtail tetanus and diphtheria.

BACTERIAL DISEASES

Tetanus often is called lockjaw and it's a bacterial disease that affects the nervous system. It is contracted when the bacteria, found in soil, dust and manure, gets into a cut or wound. An infected person can have such severe muscle spasms that their jaw "locks," making it impossible to open the mouth, swallow and may lead to death by suffocation.

Diphtheria also is a bacterial disease, but it usually affects the tonsils, throat, skin or nose. It's passed through saliva—usually by breathing in the diphtheria bacteria after an infected person coughs or sneezes. Drinking from a glass used by an infected person can spread

Susan Rehm, MD, president, Board of Directors, National Foundation for Infectious Diseases, staff physician, Cleveland Clinic, OH.

155

the bacteria, too, warns the NFID. The condition leads to breathing problems, heart failure and paralysis.

Both potentially deadly diseases are rare in the United States. The average number of tetanus cases per year from 1998 to 2000 was 43, and there are an average of two or three cases of diphtheria in the United States each year, according to the CDC.

However, diphtheria is present in 87 countries, according to the NFID, and tetanus can be contracted while gardening. Rehm treated a man who fell ill with tetanus after getting a splinter from a packing crate.

"When I immunize someone, I try to emphasize that they are going to have to keep this up every 10 years for the rest of their life," Rehm says.

She encourages adults to think of some way to remember easily when their next immunization is due—perhaps on a "zero" birthday (like 30 or 40) or a special anniversary.

Once symptoms begin, treatment for tetanus can include a shot of tetanus immune globulin to neutralize the bacteria's toxin. For diphtheria, antitoxin and antibiotics are given.

If people still have doubts about the importance of the immunization, the case history of Rehm's patient who got tetanus from a splinter should convince them. He survived, but he was on a hospital ventilator for six weeks, she says.

"It doesn't take something dramatic [to get tetanus]," Rehm says. It can occur after what appears to be a trivial injury, she adds.

info The National Foundation for Infectious Diseases has immunization fact sheets on tetanus and diphtheria at their Web site, *www.nfid.org/factsheets.*

■ ■ ■ ■

Tetanus and Diphtheria: Rare, but Deadly

Although tetanus and diphtheria are diseases that now rarely occur in the United States, at one time they were scourge, often fatal and indiscriminate in their aggression.

The National Institutes of Allergy and Infectious Diseases offers the following information about both maladies…

TETANUS

A tetanus infection begins when the spores are introduced into an injury or wound.

The illness often begins with mild spasms in the jaw, neck and facial muscles. Stiffness then rapidly develops in the chest, back, abdominal muscles and sometimes the laryngeal muscles (which then interferes with breathing). Spasmodic contractions might be so powerful that they tear the muscles or cause compression fractures of the vertebrae.

Without treatment, one out of three people with tetanus dies. With proper treatment, less than 10% of infected patients die.

The incubation period of tetanus is five days to 15 weeks, with seven days as the average. About 100 cases of tetanus occur every year in the US, the vast majority in unimmunized individuals or those whose last immunization was no longer current.

DIPHTHERIA

There are two types of diphtheria: One type affects the nose and throat. Symptoms can include sore throat, low-grade fever and enlarged lymph nodes in the neck. The other type of diphtheria causes skin lesions that may become painful, swollen and red.

Diphtheria is transmitted through close contact with discharge from an infected person's nose, throat, skin, eyes and lesions.

Symptoms usually appear two to four days after infection, and people who are infected may be contagious for up to two weeks, but seldom more than four weeks. If the patient is treated with appropriate antibiotics (penicillin or erythromycin), the contagious period can be limited to less than four days.

Although it is extremely rare in the United States, if diphtheria goes untreated, serious complications such as paralysis, heart failure and blood disorders may occur. Death occurs in approximately 5% to 10% of all cases.

The diphtheria vaccine is usually combined with the tetanus vaccine and the acellular pertussis vaccine to form a triple vaccine known as DTaP. This vaccine should be given to children at two months of age, four months, six months, between 12 and 18 months, and between four and six years. Older children and adults should get a combination of the tetanus vaccine and the diphtheria vaccine (Td) every 10 years to maintain immunity.

Vaccines—Not Just for Kids

Ben Schwartz, MD, epidemiologist, National Immunization Program, US Centers for Disease Control and Prevention, Atlanta.

David Neumann, executive director, National Partnership for Immunization, Alexandria, VA.

Many adults believe that, other than the occasional flu shot, vaccines are strictly kid stuff. That attitude could cost you —or even kill you.

Each year in the United States, up to 60,000 adults die from vaccine-preventable diseases or their complications, according to the National Coalition for Adult Immunization (NCAI), a network of more than 130 organizations that includes professional associations, advocacy groups, vaccine manufacturers and government health agencies.

"The vast majority of deaths from vaccine-preventable diseases occurs in adults," explains Dr. Ben Schwartz, an epidemiologist with the National Immunization Program of the Centers for Disease Control and Prevention (CDC).

It's easy to forget as you move into adulthood and grow older that you're still susceptible to many of the same infectious diseases that you were protected against when you were a child, says David Neumann, executive director of the National Partnership for Immunization.

"People get past adolescence and, particularly if they're in good health, they don't see a physician until they're in their 30s or 40s or 50s," Neumann says.

The most common vaccinations are for the influenza and pneumococcal infections, Neumann says. Other adult vaccinations can include hepatitis B, measles/mumps/rubella and diptheria/tetanus.

GREATEST DANGER

The people who should be the most concerned about getting their vaccinations are 65 years and older, and those with chronic diseases, such as heart or lung problems or diabetes, Schwartz says.

For these people, an inoculation against a virulent disease such as pneumonia can mean the difference between life and death.

Pneumococcal disease accounts for an estimated 500,000 cases of pneumonia each year in the United States, as well as 6,000 cases of bloodstream infection and 3,300 cases of meningitis, he says.

SPECIFIC VACCINE NEEDS VARY

However, the need for specific vaccinations can vary from person to person, Schwartz points out. "In hepatitis B, for example, the risk factors include drug use and multiple sex partners—not a problem for many older adults," Schwartz says.

The majority of adults should get a flu shot once a year after turning 50, according to the CDC. They should also get a tetanus/diphtheria booster once every 10 years. Experts recommend that people who are in high-risk groups should be getting all other vaccinations on a regular basis.

Consult your doctor about which vaccinations are appropriate. "It's difficult for people to keep track of different recommendations for different vaccines, but doctors are there to sort it all out," Schwartz says.

FLU VACCINE

Another reason to get vaccinated is to keep yourself from spreading a disease among your family and friends. This is particularly true of influenza, which kills an average of 36,000 people in the United States each year.

"Influenza is very easy to transmit," Schwartz says. "People are contagious for about a day prior to suffering any symptoms."

Approximately 20% of the American population becomes infected with influenza during a typical flu season, according to the CDC, and 114,000 people will be hospitalized.

You can avoid this by joining the annual march to your doctor's office for a flu shot.

"By getting the flu shots themselves, they're protecting their family and friends and community from getting the disease," Neumann says. "Inoculated people [are far less likely to] spread disease."

Vaccines can cause side effects in some individuals, and you should discuss those with your doctor. For example, people who are allergic to eggs should not get a flu shot because the influenza vaccine is produced from chicken eggs, Neumann says.

Some common side effects of inoculation are a sore arm or a low fever. There are very small risks that serious problems could occur after getting a vaccine. But doctors stress that the potential risks associated with the diseases these vaccines prevent are much greater than the potential risks associated with the vaccines themselves.

info For more on adult vaccinations, visit the National Coalition for Adult Immunization at *www.nfid.org/ncai*.

New Flu Vaccine Is Painless

James King, MD, professor, pediatrics, University of Maryland School of Medicine, Baltimore.

For some people, the threat of catching the flu is easier to bear than the fear of the needle that can protect them.

But if you are in good health and between the ages of five and 49 years, there's a painless alternative for the flu season—a vaccine in a nasal spray.

FluMist, approved in 2003 by the US Food and Drug Administration, isn't for everyone. It's not recommended for older people who run the risk of developing other diseases—such as pneumonia—if they get the flu. And it's not appropriate for people who have compromised immune systems, such as AIDS or cancer patients.

FluMist also isn't recommended for children younger than five years or adults 50 and older;

for those sensitive to any component of the vaccine, particularly eggs; for children or teens on aspirin therapy; for pregnant women; and for those with Guillain-Barré syndrome, asthma or immune deficiencies.

Good candidates for the spray are healthy individuals who typically suffer through four or five miserable days of fever, headache, sore throat, congestion, tiredness and body aches that characterize influenza.

FLU EPIDEMIC

"So many people get [the flu] that whole aisles in the drugstore are full of flu medicines. And it costs about $3 billion annually in lost workdays," says Dr. James King, a University of Maryland pediatrician. "Furthermore, schools are a breeding ground" for the virus.

By receiving the nasal vaccine in a doctor's office, King says, families that would otherwise miss work and school should be able to sail through the flu season, which runs from November through April.

King, who describes himself as "very biased" in favor of getting the vaccine, headed up the clinical trials for FluMist, which is manufactured by MedImmune Inc., located in Gaithersburg, Maryland.

EASY TO GIVE, EASY TO TAKE

King says the vaccine is easy to administer —one spray in each nostril—and has very few side effects other than a runny nose, scratchy throat or a mild cold that last only a day or so. The Centers for Disease Control and Prevention (CDC) concurs.

What's more, he adds, this new vaccine is a pain-free alternative for children who can't stand shots. "Children giggle. They don't cry," he says.

FluMist is a live virus that has been weakened so it won't grow in the body, but will stimulate antibodies in the nose, as well as the rest of the body. The traditional flu shot vaccine contains a dead virus that is injected into the muscles to stimulate antibodies in the blood, King says.

FluMist's one drawback is its high cost— approximately $45 compared with $7 to $10 for a flu shot. What's more, it isn't covered by insurance. And children who are younger than 9 years must get two doses the first time they get the vaccine, meaning two trips to the doctor's office.

But since CDC statistics that say only 13% of healthy Americans ages 5 to 49 get an annual flu shot, FluMist's manufacturers think their product is a medication whose time has come.

Health officials says the best time to get a flu vaccine is October or November, although getting vaccinated in December or later can still protect you against the flu.

info For more information about the flu, visit the National Institute of Allergy and Infectious Diseases at *www.niaid.nih. gov/factsheets/flu.htm.*

Pneumonia After-Effects Deadly Even in Midlife

Grant Waterer, MD, PhD, senior lecturer in medicine, University of Western Australia, Perth.
American Journal of Respiratory and Critical Care Medicine.

Pneumonia is one of the leading killers of the infirm, who do not have the ability to withstand this severe lung infection. But even middle-aged people who manage to fight off the disease appear to be at an increased risk of death over the next two or three years, researchers have found.

"The message is that if you're young—under age 40—an episode of pneumonia is just bad luck," explains Dr. Grant Waterer, a senior lecturer in medicine at the University of Western Australia located in Perth and leader of the study. "If you are over 40, it may be an indication that all is not well, and your physician needs to look closely to see if there are any underlying illnesses that may not have been previously recognized."

THE STUDY

Waterer and his team looked at patients with community-acquired pneumonia who were admitted to Methodist Healthcare Memphis Hospitals in Tennessee and survived until they were discharged.

They were mainly interested in discovering whether pneumonia reduces long-term survival rates in otherwise healthy patients.

The researchers found that more than one third of the patients who they had data on died, on average, three years after discharge.

Other health conditions—especially heart disease and stroke, an altered mental state, anemia and poorly controlled diabetes—also were shown to be predictors of mortality after discharge for patients who had been hospitalized for pneumonia.

People 41 to 60 years old who had no previous illness were particularly vulnerable, the study found. That group's mortality rate was approximately six times greater than expected, according to Waterer.

Pneumonia victims aged 61 to 80 years who had no other observed illnesses died at approximately twice the rate that was expected for their age group.

Younger adults, aged 18 to 40 years, were at no increased risk of death after discharge, the study found.

PATIENTS, FAMILIES MUST STAY ON GUARD AFTER DISCHARGE

These findings add to a growing body of evidence indicating that people who have pneumonia can expect a modestly to substantially increased death rate up to four years after hospitalization, says Dr. Scott Dowell, of the Centers for Disease Control and Prevention's International Emerging Infections Program.

Dowell suggests that patients and their families remain vigilant after a bout of pneumonia and pursue preventive health measures. For example, he says, "The prognosis for modern-day patients who recover from a first bout of pneumonia may be substantially improved by offering an effective smoking cessation program, influenza vaccine and pneumococcal vaccine."

info Learn more about pneumonia from the American Lung Association Web site at *www.lungusa.org.* Click on "Diseases A to Z."

Hospital Injuries Cause More Than 32,000 Deaths per Year

Chunliu Zhan, MD, PhD, senior service fellow, Agency for Healthcare Research and Quality, Rockville, MD.
Paul Gluck, MD, obstetrician and member, National Patient Safety Foundation, Miami.
Journal of the American Medical Association.

Medical injuries that happen in hospitals claim more than 32,500 lives in the United States each year, a recent study has found. These complications—ranging from blood infections and bad reactions to transfusions and botched surgeries—lead to at least 2.4 million extra days on the wards and up to $9.3 billion in added costs.

Of course, some complications are the unavoidable risks of treating desperately ill patients, while others are obviously caused by physician error. "This study won't be able to tell you how much is preventable," says study leader Dr. Chunliu Zhan, a senior fellow at the Agency for Healthcare Research and Quality. "But some are more preventable than others."

Zhan's agency, a division of the US Department of Health and Human Services, has used a system for identifying medical injuries that relies on hospital billing records. The method is more cost-effective than sifting through medical records, which has been the gold standard of patient safety studies.

For the latest study, Zhan and his colleagues looked at nearly 7.5 million billing records from the year 2000. The cases covered 994 hospitals in 28 states, representing approximately 20% of all the nation's hospitals.

The researchers limited their study to 18 categories of complications, called Patient Safety Indicators. These included blood infection, adverse reactions to transfusions, mishandled surgeries and trouble during the birth of a baby. They tallied the extra days of hospital care attributable to the problems and the associated costs.

THE MOST SERIOUS COMPLICATIONS

Serious blood infection, or *sepsis,* following surgery was the most severe complication,
leading to an average of nearly 11 extra days in the hospital at a cost of more than $57,000 per patient. Almost 22% of patients who suffered postsurgery sepsis died of the infection.

The second most serious medical injury that the researchers found was a ruptured surgical wound. These patients spent an average of nine additional days in the hospital, resulting in an average of $40,000 in extra costs, and nearly 10% died of the injury.

Infections that were caused by medical care rounded out the top three, adding more than nine days to the hospital stay at a cost of nearly $39,000 per patient, with a risk of death at just over 4%.

At the bottom of the list, delivery trouble typically added no days or dollars to a hospital stay—at least for mothers who delivered vaginally without the assistance of any instruments—and had no additional risk of death. Injuries in women who required instrument help during labor were the most common complication in hospitals, occurring in approximately 22% of such patients—a "surprisingly high" rate, Zhan says. Again, however, deadly events were rare.

SIGNIFICANT COSTS

Overall, according to the researchers, the 18 types of patient injuries could account for 2.4 million extra hospital days, between $4.6 and $9.3 billion in added costs and roughly 32,500 deaths each year. Future studies may be able to flesh out how many of these truly are preventable, Zhan says.

PATIENT INJURIES A PROBLEM

Dr. Paul Gluck, an obstetrician located in Miami who sits on several committees at the National Patient Safety Foundation, says some experts may quibble with the safety measures that the researchers used. But because mounting evidence indicates that patient injuries are a problem, "we have to pay attention to that."

Estimates have put the share of preventable injuries at between 50% and 75% of all injuries. The problem is figuring out what the total truly is, Gluck says. One way to do that, he adds, is a confidential, nonpunitive reporting system for medical errors modeled on the system used in the airline industry.

info For more on the quality of the nation's health-care system, try the Web site produced by the Agency for Healthcare Research and Quality at *www.ahcpr.gov.*

'Keyhole' Appendectomies Easier on Patients

Ulrich Guller, MD, surgical resident, University of Basel, Switzerland.

Bruce McIntosh, MD, surgeon, William Beaumont Hospital, Troy, MI.

Annals of Surgery.

If you must have your appendix removed, *laparoscopic* surgery—also called keyhole surgery—appears to be the best choice for most patients, a study says. Laparoscopic surgery is performed through small incisions with the use of cameras and special cauterizing, cutting and stapling instruments.

The study found that people who had the laparoscopic procedure tended to have shorter stays in the hospital, a lower risk of infection and fewer complications than people who had standard surgery.

THE STUDY

Dr. Ulrich Guller, a surgical research fellow at Duke University at the time the study was conducted, looked at data from more than 43,000 people who had appendectomies. A little more than 17% of the people who had their appendix removed had laparoscopic surgery, the study says.

The average stay in the hospital for people undergoing laparoscopic surgery was 2.06 days, compared with 2.88 days for those who had open surgery. Subjects undergoing laparoscopic surgery had approximately half the risk of infection as open surgery patients, and approximately a 20% reduced risk of complications.

People who had undergone the laparoscopic procedure were also more than three times as likely to be discharged home, rather than to

a nursing home or home health care, according to the study.

"This study really puts laparoscopic surgery in a very favorable light," says Guller.

"People should know that laparoscopic appendectomy exists and they might have a quicker hospital stay with this procedure compared with the open procedure," he says. "We also found that laparoscopic surgery seemed to have advantages even if an abscess or perforation was present."

Dr. Bruce McIntosh, a surgeon at William Beaumont Hospital in Troy, Michigan, says this finding was particularly interesting because surgeons often will not consider a laparoscopic approach on someone with a perforation or abscess.

COST FACTOR

McIntosh says it would be helpful to see a cost analysis for both procedures, because although laparoscopic surgery may be more expensive than the open procedure, overall costs may be the same if the hospital stay is shorter.

info To learn more about appendicitis, visit the National Digestive Diseases Information Clearinghouse at *http://digestive.niddk. nih.gov.* Click on "Digestive Diseases."

Minor Surgery More Risky In a Doctor's Office

Hector Vila, Jr, MD, assistant professor, oncology and anesthesiology, H. Lee Moffitt Cancer Center, Tampa, FL.

Archives of Surgery.

Having plastic surgery, endoscopies and other minor surgeries in a doctor's office is risky, a study says.

"Our research compared adverse outcomes and deaths in physicians' offices with those in ambulatory surgical centers," explains study author Dr. Hector Vila, Jr, assistant professor of oncology and anesthesiology at the H. Lee

Moffitt Cancer Center in Tampa, Florida. "We found a much higher death rate and a much higher injury rate when surgery was done in the physician's office," he adds.

THE STUDY

Vila and his colleagues studied all the deaths and injuries during surgery in doctor's offices reported to the Florida Board of Medicine from 2000 through 2002. They looked at similar data from ambulatory surgical centers during 2000, reported to the Florida Agency for Health Care Administration.

The study included all types of outpatient surgeries. Vila says most surgeries were plastic surgeries and endoscopies, a procedure using a fiber optic scope to look at the intestinal tract.

Vila's team found that the injury rate in doctors' offices was 66 per 100,000 operations, compared with five per 100,000 surgeries in ambulatory surgical centers. For death, the corresponding numbers were nine per 100,000 in doctor's offices and less than one per 100,000 in ambulatory surgical centers.

The researchers note that if all procedures had been done in surgical centers, approximately 43 injuries and six deaths would have been prevented each year. Vila believes this problem is not confined to Florida.

CHECK THEIR CREDENTIALS

There are many reasons for the dramatic difference in death and injury rates, Vila says, including a lack of equipment and personnel, a lack of set procedures, and the inability to deal with emergencies. "Sometimes it's the [lack of] credentials of the people performing the procedure or administering the anesthesia," Vila adds.

"To work in a hospital, a physician has to apply for privileges, but a private physician can do whatever he or she wants in their office," Vila says. "You don't have to show anyone that you are able to do the procedure. You just open your office and do it."

Vila believes this is a new problem in medicine, and it relates to money. Office surgeries are much cheaper than those done in ambulatory surgery centers. In addition, "physicians who can't get privileges in a hospital, because

they are not board-certified or don't have the credentials to do the procedure, do it in their office because it's the only place they can do it," Vila says.

Patients concerned with safety need to ask several questions before deciding to have surgery in their doctor's office, Vila advises.

"You should ask your doctor if he has the same standards as those used in the hospital or ambulatory surgical center. Are the physicians board-certified in the specialty that normally performs this procedure? Do they have the same equipment? Do they have emergency resuscitative equipment? Who is going to be giving the anesthesia? And, where will you be taken if there is an emergency?"

"If you are unsure, then you should consider having your surgery in an ambulatory surgical center," Vila says.

info The American College of Surgeons offers more information about surgical procedures and risk at *www.facs.org*. Click on "Public Information."

■ ■ ■ ■

Read This Before You Have Outpatient Surgery

Few things in the medical field have changed more radically in the past 20 years than the location where people go for surgery.

More than 1,500 different surgical procedures that previously were performed only on an in-patient basis, including the removal of cataracts and colon polyps, now can be performed on outpatients who enter a facility in the morning and leave later the same day.

Although outpatient surgeries are cheaper and often safer (largely because of significantly lower infection rates), a successful outcome typically depends on the type of outpatient facility you choose for your procedure. *Charles Inlander, a health care consultant and president of the nonprofit People's Medical Society, suggests these key points to consider...*

●**Doctors' offices.** You are not paying the high overhead that is associated with a hospital or free-standing surgical center. Therefore, procedures performed in a doctor's office can cost up to 50% less than those in the other settings—but they come with greater risk. That's because doctors' offices are not accredited by any private or government oversight agency.

In fact, under current state laws, any licensed doctor (physicians must be licensed by the state in which they are practicing) can perform just about any surgical procedure in his/her own office without any special approval. Because of this, insurance companies and Medicare may not pay for a procedure performed in a physician's office. Check to see if your insurer will pay for the procedure you need with the doctor you are considering. If not, ask the company for a list of doctors' offices approved for payment.

●**Free-standing surgical centers.** Often called "surgi-centers," these usually are a better choice than a doctor's office.

These facilities, often independently owned by physicians or entrepreneurs, tend to be better regulated. Most states require that they be licensed, usually by the state health department. That means they are inspected and must meet certain standards for safety, infection control and other quality-related factors. They also can be accredited by the Accreditation Association for Ambulatory Healthcare or the Joint Commission on the Accreditation of Healthcare Organizations. Although accreditation is voluntary for surgi-centers, it's smart to choose a facility that is accredited by one of these organizations.

●**Hospital-owned outpatient facility.** This usually is your best choice for outpatient surgery. Because it is a part of a hospital, it must meet the same regulatory standards and accreditation requirements as the rest of the hospital (even if it is not located at the hospital site). These standards and requirements are much more strict and comprehensive than for other settings.

Unlike a doctor's office or a surgi-center, hospital-owned outpatient facilities collect important data, such as infection rates. Many hospitals now are making that information publicly available. Ask for the annual surgical and outpatient report. If it's not available, consider another facility.

Skip Mouth-to-Mouth When Doing CPR

Paul Pepe, MD, MPH, professor and chairman, emergency medicine, University of Texas Southwestern Medical Center at Dallas.

Wally Ghurabi, MD, medical director, Emergency Center at Santa Monica–UCLA Medical Center, Santa Monica, CA.

In a major change for emergency medicine, experts now suggest that 911 emergency dispatchers tell callers who are untrained in cardiac-pulmonary resuscitation (CPR) to skip the mouth-to-mouth part of the procedure and go directly to chest compressions.

Dr. Paul Pepe, medical director of the City of Dallas Emergency Medical Services and professor and chairman of emergency medicine at the University of Texas Southwestern Medical Center helped organize a conference for a group of physicians who, like himself, are the medical directors of emergency medical services for some of the country's largest cities, including Chicago, Los Angeles, New York, Philadelphia, San Francisco and Seattle.

At the conference, the group decided "this is the best way" for people untrained in CPR to save lives.

As these medical directors implement the new approach in their respective cities, it will mean that when people call 911 for help in a medical emergency, the dispatcher may skip directly to instructions for chest compressions, the process of pushing down repeatedly on the chest to mimic a steady heartbeat. "It takes too long to explain mouth-to-mouth," according to Pepe.

"We're not giving up on mouth-to-mouth," Pepe adds. The technique is still taught as part of CPR classes. But when people call 911 to report a heart attack, breathing problems or other medical emergencies, many are not trained or are too nervous to remember their CPR training, Pepe says.

OTHER STUDIES
SUPPORT RECOMMENDATION

In a May 2000 study, University of Washington researchers compared the outcomes of 241 patients who got chest compression alone with the outcomes of 279 people who received both chest compression and mouth-to-mouth from people fairly inexperienced at CPR. The survival rates up until they were discharged from the hospital were better among people who received chest compression only.

The researchers concluded that chest compression alone "may be the preferred approach for bystanders inexperienced in CPR."

Also, since September 2000, the American Heart Association has recommended compression-only CPR when the rescuer is unwilling or unable to perform mouth-to-mouth rescue breathing. "But this recommendation wasn't widely adopted," Pepe says.

"It's common sense versus dogma," explains Dr. Wally Ghurabi, who is medical director of the Emergency Center at Santa Monica–UCLA Medical Center in California. "If the rescuer is well-trained, [he or she can] go ahead and give mouth-to-mouth." If not, the compression-only instructions are better, he says.

But Ghurabi urges all people to take a CPR class. "Every three to five years, go get recertified," he advises. The investment of time—a few hours—is modest, compared with the potential payoff of saving someone's life.

info The University of Virginia Health System has more information on CPR at *www.healthsystem.virginia.edu.*

Narrowing Down the Causes of Heart Disease

Alan R. Dyer, PhD, professor of preventive medicine, Northwestern University Feinberg School of Medicine, Chicago.

Umesh N. Khot, MD, cardiologist, Indiana Heart Physicians, Indianapolis.

Journal of the American Medical Association.

Looking at the records of almost 400,000 people involved in three major studies, researchers at Northwestern University report that a majority of people who had a heart attack or "major coronary event" had at least one of four well-established risk factors —high cholesterol, high blood pressure, cigarette smoking or diabetes.

And analysis of data on more than 122,000 patients in 14 international trials shows essentially the same relationships, cardiologists at Indiana Heart Physicians report.

CONFIRMS FINDINGS

The American Heart Association as well as other health organizations have been declaring the dangers of these risk factors for years, so why are these findings such a big deal?

The reason these results are important is because "a lot of people out there have been saying you can have CHD [coronary heart disease] in the absence of these risk factors," says Alan R. Dyer, a professor at Northwestern's Feinberg School of Medicine and a member of one research team.

Papers have been published in medical journals saying that up to 50% of coronary events can occur in people who have none of these risk factors, he adds.

This latest report is being published "to refute that notion," he says.

THE STUDIES

And the numbers provide an easy refutation. In the Chicago Heart Detection Project in Industry, the Multiple Risk Factor Intervention Trial and the Framingham Heart Study, anywhere from 87% to 100% of the participants who died of heart disease had at least one of the four risk factors.

Those risk factors, which are well-known, include a blood cholesterol level of 240 or higher, blood pressure of 140/90 or higher, diabetes or cigarette smoking.

In the 14 international studies examined by Dr. Umesh N. Khot and colleagues, 84.6% of women and 80.6% of men with CHD also had at least one of the risk factors.

THE FIFTH FACTOR

Approximately 12.6 million Americans have CHD, which often results in a heart attack, according to the National Institutes of Health (NIH). An estimated 1.1 million Americans have a heart attack every year—approximately 515,000 of these heart attacks are fatal.

"Smoking particularly plays a major role in the development of premature heart disease," says Khot, who conducted the study while at the Cleveland Clinic Foundation and now is with Indiana Heart Physicians.

And there is another risk factor that actually underlies the other three factors, Khot explains—obesity, which is a contributing factor in diabetes as well as in high cholesterol and high blood pressure.

Like Dyer, Khot is at a loss to explain why so many ordinary people and physicians deprecate the role of the four major factors.

For both patients and doctors, the lesson of these studies is clear, Dyer says: "We must try to focus on these four risk factors when we try to reduce the risk of coronary heart disease."

info An overview of coronary risk factors is given by the Texas Heart Institute at *www.texasheartinstitute.org/riskfact.html.*

Scans Show Smoking Damages More than Just Lungs

Proceedings of the National Academy of Sciences.
Brookhaven National Laboratory news release.

The damage from smoking isn't just confined to the lungs—it also affects many of the body's organs, according to recent study results.

Researchers have discovered evidence of reduced levels of a critical enzyme, *monoamine oxidase B* (MAO B), in the kidneys, heart, lungs and spleen of smokers.

This enzyme breaks down neurotransmitters and dietary amines. Too much or too little of it can adversely affect a person's health and even personality.

"When we think about smoking and the toxicity of smoking, we usually think of the lungs. Here we see a very marked effect of smoking on one of the major enzymes in the body, and we see that this effect extends far beyond the lungs," says researcher Joanna Fowler.

Previous research by Fowler and her colleagues found that the levels of MAO B were lower in smokers' brains.

WIDESPREAD EFFECTS

"Since smoking exposes the entire body to the tobacco compounds that inhibit MAO B, we believed that it had the potential to limit MAO B activity throughout the body," according to Fowler.

She says the health consequences of these reduced MAO B levels need to be studied in greater detail.

■ ■ ■ ■

If You Smoke, Quit!

An estimated 46.2 million adults who are 18 years of age and older in the United States are smokers, according to statistics from the Centers for Disease Control and Prevention (CDC).

The number of smokers has declined only slightly over the past decade, from 25% of the population to 22.8%. During that period, smoking among adult men declined from 27.7% to 25.2%, while adult female smoking declined from 22.5% to 20.7%.

Cigarette smoking is the single most preventable cause of premature death in this country, according to the CDC.

Each year, more than 400,000 Americans die from the effects of cigarette smoking. In fact, one in every five deaths that occurs in the United States is smoking-related.

In the United States, smoking kills more than 276,000 men and 142,000 women every year. Between 1960 and 1990, deaths from lung cancer among women increased by more than 400%—exceeding breast cancer deaths in the mid-1980s. The American Cancer Society estimated that in 1994, 64,300 women died from lung cancer while only 44,300 died as a result of breast cancer.

The CDC offers a number of tips for smokers who want to quit. *They include…*

•**Don't smoke any number or any kind of cigarette,** even those promoted as low-tar and low-nicotine.

•**Write down why you want to quit,** to give yourself a concrete understanding of what your motivations are.

•**Be aware that it will take effort to quit smoking,** and that nearly all smokers experience some form of nicotine withdrawal when they try to quit.

•**Remember that half of all adult smokers have quit,** representing millions of people alive today who have learned to face life without a cigarette.

•**Get help if you need it,** from the many groups that offer written materials, programs, and advice to help smokers quit for good. Your doctor or dentist is also a good source of help and support.

info Learn more about the dangers of smoking from the American Cancer Society at *www.cancer.org.*

Low-Tar Cigarettes No Safer than Others

Norman Edelman, consultant, scientific affairs, American Lung Association.

Michael Thun, MD, head, epidemiologic research, American Cancer Society, Atlanta.

British Medical Journal.

If you still think you're doing your lungs a favor by smoking low-tar cigarettes, think again. A study found that the risk of lung cancer was the same among participants who smoked medium-tar, low-tar or very low-tar filtered cigarettes.

"There is still a huge increase in death rates from cancer if you smoke those supposedly safe cigarettes. There is no safe cigarette, and there is no way to hedge your bets," explains Dr. Norman Edelman, consultant for scientific affairs for the American Lung Association.

Previous studies had never compared cigarettes with so many different tar ratings.

"What has been missing is a large, well-conducted study of lung cancer risk that compares a regular cigarette with brands that have lower tar ratings," says study co-author Dr. Michael Thun, head of epidemiologic research at the American Cancer Society in Atlanta.

THE STUDY

Thun and his colleagues compared the risk of lung cancer among smokers of very low-tar (7 milligrams [mg] or less) filtered, low-tar (8 to 14 mg) filtered and high-tar (22 mg or more) nonfiltered cigarettes with the risk of lung cancer among smokers of conventional medium-tar (15 to 21 mg) filtered brands.

A total of 364,239 men and 576,535 women 30 years or older were followed up for six years to try to determine if there was a relationship between the type of cigarette that was smoked and death from lung cancer. The participants were nonsmokers, former smokers or current smokers.

All of the smokers had a higher risk of lung cancer than people who had never smoked or who had quit. The subjects who smoked very low-tar and low-tar brands had the same risk as the subjects who smoked medium-tar brands.

Men and women who smoked nonfiltered cigarettes with high-tar ratings had higher risks of lung cancer.

RESULTS CORRELATE WITH OTHER STUDIES

Previous studies have shown that regular smokers of low-tar brands often inhale more deeply, cover up ventilation holes or hold the smoke in the lungs longer to compensate for lower amounts of nicotine or tar. The current findings seem to support this notion.

"The major concern that the health community has is that people who smoke may defer quitting because they are misled into believing that ultralight or light cigarettes are less hazardous," Thun says. "In our study, the lung cancer risk was identical in people who smoke those brands."

Incredible Finding: Why It's So Easy for Some to Quit Smoking

Robert Baker, PhD, director, Ochsner Center for the Elimination of Smoking, and director, behavioral medicine unit, Ochsner Clinic Foundation Hospital, New Orleans.

Marc K. Siegel, MD, internist, New York University Medical Center, and clinical associate professor, New York University School of Medicine, New York City.

Health Psychology.

Why is it that some people can stop smoking by going cold turkey while other people struggle to quit again and again? Researchers from the Tobacco Use Research Center at the University of Pennsylvania say the reason is at least partly genetic.

Two genes in particular seem to help smokers quit successfully, and this combination of genes also makes them less likely to start smoking again.

"This study provides the first evidence that genes that alter dopamine function may influence smoking cessation and relapse during treatment," says study author Caryn Lerman, who is also associate director for Cancer Control and Population Science at the University of Pennsylvania.

Dopamine is a neurotransmitter that acts as a messenger between nerve cells in the brain.

THE STUDY

Lerman and her colleagues studied 418 people who were enrolled in a clinical trial to test the effectiveness of the antidepressant *bupropion* for smoking cessation. The study participants either received bupropion or a placebo for 10 weeks and behavioral counseling.

Blood samples were taken from the participants for genetic analysis. Smoking status was assessed at the end of the 10 weeks and then again after six months.

People who were more successful at staying off cigarettes and avoiding a relapse had particular variants of a dopamine transporter gene (SLC6A3) as well as a dopamine receptor gene (DRD2).

"One of the great mysteries in smoking cessation is why some people find it so easy and why it's so hard for others," says Robert Baker, director of the Ochsner Center for the Elimination of Smoking in New Orleans.

"I hear about people who smoked for 40 years and then just put them down one day. Others haven't smoked as long and seem to have a much harder time. I think genetic factors do play a role," he says.

Dr. Marc K. Siegel, an internist at New York University Medical Center, agrees with Baker. "It's not surprising to hear that someone's genetic makeup influences their response to quitting smoking. Some patients respond to Zyban [a form of bupropion], some to the [nicotine replacement therapy] patch."

FINDING MAY PROVIDE CUSTOMIZED HELP

What's exciting about this research, Siegel believes, is the possibility that one day doctors could specifically target smoking cessation treatment to each patient on the basis of his/her genetic makeup.

However, such a therapy is probably a long time away. "If you're waiting for a cure before you quit smoking," advises Baker, "you may not live that long."

Despite some compelling reasons to quit—including an increased risk of many cancers, heart disease and a one in five chance of developing emphysema or chronic bronchitis, according to the American Cancer Society—many people still smoke.

The good news is that plenty of people—those who have these genes and those who don't—have quit smoking. According to statistics from the American Cancer Society more than 44 million people in the United States have stopped smoking.

"You may have a more difficult time if you don't have these genes," says Baker, "but you can still get off cigarettes. I'm sure there are thousands upon thousands who have done just that."

info For more information on quitting smoking, visit the American Lung Association at *www.lungusa.org.*

Can't Sleep? It's All in Your Head—Really!

Sid Gilman, MD, chairman, and William Herdman, professor, department of neurology, University of Michigan School of Medicine, Ann Arbor.
Neurology.

If you've got a sleeping problem, it may be all in your head. Two recent studies have linked different sleep disorders to disturbances in brain chemistry.

This association doesn't necessarily indicate a cause-and-effect relationship, but it may reveal some of the roots of sleep disorders, according to researchers.

THE STUDIES' SUBJECTS

Both of the studies looked at the same 13 people who had a relatively rare disorder known as *multiple system atrophy* (MSA), a fatal disease that is almost always accompanied by sleep disorders.

All the patients also had rapid eye movement (REM) behavior disorder and obstructive sleep apnea.

People who have sleep apnea literally stop breathing repeatedly during their sleep, often for a minute or longer and as many as hundreds of times during a single night. These people may snore and have excessive daytime sleepiness, which can be a frequent cause of traffic accidents.

Sleep apnea has also been associated with high blood pressure, heart disease and with a higher incidence of stroke.

In REM behavior disorder, patients thrash about in their sleep, moan, speak, act out their dreams, get out of bed and even pummel their bed partners. This activity occurs during the REM phase of sleep.

METHODOLOGY OF THE STUDIES

The researchers used sophisticated sleep monitors and video recorders to observe the subjects in slumber.

The two studies explored the links between these sleeping disorders and the neurotransmitters *dopamine* and *acetylcholine.*

In the first study, the researchers wanted to see if dopamine was related to REM sleep behavior disorder.

"We already knew that in Parkinson's disease there's a very high incidence of REM sleep behavior disorder," explains Dr. Sid Gilman, author of the study as well as chairman of the department of neurology at the University of Michigan School of Medicine located in Ann Arbor.

Since Parkinson's is associated with a deficiency in dopamine, Gilman had a suspicion that it would also be related to the severity of REM sleep behavior disorder.

"We thought we'd see a correlation, which is exactly what we saw. It's a correlation only, but it certainly suggests that the amount of dopamine loss in the brain is related to this disorder," he says.

This finding has led Gilman to wonder if REM sleep behavior disorder could be a very early symptom of Parkinson's.

The second study looked for a relationship between the severity of obstructive sleep apnea and the degree of decrease of the brain molecule acetylcholine.

"Here once again, we found a good correlation," Gilman says. "It's not allowing us to conclude anything, but it's certainly suggesting that there might be a causative relationship between obstructive sleep apnea and this neurotransmitter."

STUDIES RAISE QUESTIONS

The findings raise a number of questions, not the least of which is whether obstructive sleep apnea in healthy people is due to the same type of chemical disturbance.

"It is an interesting area because it leads to the question about the basic science that is underlying sleep," Gilman says. "It's a somewhat unexpected finding. It could be central to so many things."

info For more information on sleep disorders try the American Sleep Apnea Association's Web site at *www.sleepapnea.org* or the National Sleep Foundation's Web site at *www.sleepfoundation.org.*

Sleep Problems Still Haunt Ex-Drinkers

Shawn Currie, PhD, adjunct assistant professor, psychiatry and psychology, University of Calgary, Alberta, Canada.
Kirk J. Brower, MD, associate professor, psychiatry, University of Michigan Medical School, and executive director, Chelsea Arbor Addiction Treatment Center, Ann Arbor, MI.
Alcoholism: Clinical & Experimental Research.

Sleep problems among reformed drinkers can linger for months or even years, a recent study has found.

Problems getting to sleep are more common than staying asleep, though both occur, according to the researchers.

University of Calgary psychologist Shawn Currie and his team studied 63 recovering alcoholics, all of whom were sober for at least one month but for less than five years. The researchers evaluated their sleep not in a sleep lab for one night—the standard approach—but rather at home for a week.

"We looked at sleep problems in a different way," Currie says. "Most of the research prior to this study has people spend one night in a sleep lab. We used portable sleep monitors—they look like a wristwatch—and we did it for seven nights."

"We found out that they definitely had sleep problems," says Currie. The study participants tended to be short sleepers, sleeping less than six hours per night.

PRIOR SLEEP PROBLEMS

More than half of the subjects reported that sleep problems preceded their alcohol dependence. They reported more problems getting to sleep, overall, than staying asleep. In the general population, just 10% to 15% of people have chronic insomnia, Currie says.

Why recovering alcoholics suffer lingering sleep problems isn't clear. Alcohol induces rapid sleep onset and deeper sleep the first half of the night, but causes sleep to become very fragmented the second half of the evening as blood alcohol levels fall. Chronic alcohol use may change brain chemistry in a way that disrupts the normal way sleep is regulated.

Currie says that there may or may not be a cause-and-effect relationship between the high rate of sleep problems and the alcohol dependence. He believes the topic needs further study.

SLEEP CAN IMPROVE

As prevalent as the problems were, Currie adds, the news isn't all bad. Many recovering alcoholics sleep soundly after they quit drinking. Sleep seems to improve after alcoholics have abstained for three to six months, other research shows, but disrupted sleep can sometimes continue even longer.

The new research "confirms some previous findings," says Dr. Kirk J. Brower, an associate professor of psychiatry at the University of Michigan Medical School in Ann Arbor and executive director of Chelsea Arbor Addiction Treatment Center, affiliated with the University. "We tell our patients that sleep is an important part of their recovery" as well as a way to prevent relapse.

Brower's clinic teaches good sleep habits: No naps, avoid caffeine late in the day, and keep regular bedtimes and wake-up times.

For those people whose sleep problems persist, Currie recommends non-pharmaceutical approaches, such as learning mental relaxation. Many recovering alcoholics get sleeping pills from their physicians, Currie says, but medication is not a good long-term solution, and may be a problem for people with addictive tendencies.

info Learn more about alcohol abuse from the National Institute on Alcohol Abuse and Alcoholism Web site at *www.niaaa.nih.gov.*

Good News! No Hepatitis A Booster Shots Needed

The Lancet.

Most people who have received an immunization against hepatitis A don't need booster shots to shore up the vaccine, British scientists have learned.

Protection from the disease continues even after protective antibodies can no longer be detected. A complete course of the vaccination, usually two to three doses, protects against hepatitis A for more than 10 years—possibly as many as 25 years—at least among people who have healthy immune systems, the researchers say. That makes booster shots unnecessary for those healthy people, they add.

However, the researchers stop short of saying booster shots are never necessary for anyone. Whether booster shots can be eliminated in people who have immune system problems or in people who initially received only a single dose of the vaccine is not yet known, they say.

■ ■ ■ ■

Preventing Hepatitis A

Hepatitis A is a liver disease caused by a virus that is often transmitted through sexual contact, sharing tainted drug needles or contact with the stool of a person carrying the virus. The virus is also spread by contaminated food and water.

Symptoms might include fever, fatigue, loss of appetite, nausea, abdominal discomfort, dark urine and jaundice (yellowing of the skin and eyes), according to health officials in the United States.

About 1.4 million cases of hepatitis A are reported each year, though experts suspect 10 times that many people worldwide actually contract the disease. The most susceptible are people who live in or travel to less developed parts of the world.

The Centers for Disease Control and Prevention (CDC) recommends the following people receive the hepatitis A vaccine…

●**Travelers to areas with increased rates of hepatitis A.**

●**Men who have sex with men.**

●**People who use injecting and non-injecting drugs.**

●**People who have blood clotting disorders** such as hemophilia.

●**People with chronic liver disease.**

The agency also recommends the vaccine for children older than two years who live in areas with high rates of hepatitis A.

In addition to the vaccine, you can avoid infection with hepatitis A by…

●**Getting injections of a protein called immune globulin** before and within two weeks after contact with the hepatitis A virus.

●**Washing your hands well with soap and water** after using the bathroom and changing a baby's diaper, as well as before preparing and eating food.

info You can learn more about hepatitis A from the Centers for Disease Control and Prevention's National Center for Infectious Diseases at *www.cdc.gov/ncidod.*

Osteoporosis Is Not For Women Only

Pamela Taxel, MD, assistant professor, medicine, University of Connecticut Health Center, Farmington.

Clifford J. Rosen, MD, director, Maine Center for Osteoporosis Research and Education, St. Joseph's Hospital, Bangor, ME.

New England Journal of Medicine.

Women have long been alert to the dangers of osteoporosis as they age, but few men worry about weakening bones. They should.

As many as 2 million American men have the bone-thinning disease, according to the National Institutes of Health. Men older than 50 years are at greater risk of osteoporosis-related fractures than they are of prostate cancer, the National Osteoporosis Foundation says.

"The importance of the bone health of men is starting to get on the radar screen," says Dr. Pamela Taxel, an endocrinologist at the University of Connecticut Health Center, who specializes in bones.

MORTALITY RISK

The National Osteoporosis Foundation reports that, among at-risk men older than 50, one in eight will experience an osteoporosis-related fracture. Mortality in men one year after a hip fracture is twice that of women.

These numbers, combined with the aging of the US population, spurred the National Institutes of Health's Institute of Arthritis, Musculoskeletal and Skin Diseases to begin a $24 million, seven-year, seven-site study of 5,700 men older than 65 to identify the prevalence and risk factors for osteoporosis.

Men are less susceptible than women to osteoporosis—women with the disease outnumber men 4 to 1—because most men have bigger bones than most women. Their bone loss begins later in life and progresses more slowly. And they don't have accelerated bone loss due to the rapid hormonal changes that women face during menopause, adds Dr. Clifford J. Rosen, director of the Maine Center for Osteoporosis Research and Education.

But as men move into their 70s and beyond, their bone loss increases to the same level as women's, says Rosen.

Scientists are exploring the gender-specific genetic characteristics that might make some men vulnerable to the disease. They are also studying the protein *IGF profactor-1,* which researchers believe could contribute to osteoporosis in men, Rosen says.

Of growing interest to researchers is the effect of men's estrogen levels on their bone health, says Taxel, which could lead to new treatments for men. "Not only testosterone but also estrogen may be important in men's bone health," she says.

There are no guidelines recommending that all men have bone-density screening tests. But Taxel believes that testing would be medically prudent.

Taxel says that men should have bone-density screening tests if they are older than 55 and have lost two inches of height. So should men who've had a bone fracture that was caused by a simple fall—a "fragility fracture"—not a major trauma, such as a car crash.

Other known risk factors for men, most of which parallel the risks for women, include a family history of the disease, kidney stones, alcoholism, smoking and a history of taking steroid medications.

Men who have problems with the production of male hormones and those on medication for prostate cancer that suppresses hormone production should also be tested.

DRUG THERAPY

Osteoporosis drugs approved for women have similar benefits for men. These include Actonel and Fosamax, a brand name for *alendronate sodium,* which increases bone density and lowers the risk of fracture.

A newer drug called *teriparatide,* manufactured by Eli Lilly and Co. and sold as Forteo, also shows promise. It increases the action of bone-building cells called osteoblasts, which in turn increases bone density. The drug must be injected daily, so it's only used for very serious cases, Taxel says.

Men with osteoporosis are also urged to increase calcium and vitamin D intake and exercise regularly, Rosen says.

info The National Osteoporosis Foundation has more information on the disease on-line at *www.nof.org.*

New Hope for People with Urinary Incontinence

Neil M. Resnick, MD, professor, medicine, University of Pittsburgh, PA.

Patricia S. Goode, MD, associate professor, medicine, University of Alabama, Birmingham.

Journal of the American Medical Association.

Approximately 13 million Americans, most of them women, suffer from urinary incontinence, and now a study is offering all of them new hope for dealing with the condition.

Several nonsurgical treatments are effective, and even self-administered behavioral therapy can cut the frequency of episodes in half, researchers have found. The new research should help dispel the common belief that surgery is the only way to ease the condition, according to Dr. Neil M. Resnick, professor of medicine at the University of Pittsburgh.

THE STUDY

Dr. Patricia S. Goode and her colleagues at the Department of Veterans Affairs Medical Center in Birmingham, Alabama, tested several treatments on 200 women, aged 40 to 78 years, who had incontinence.

Some women were assigned to behavioral training, which consisted of biofeedback-assisted exercises to train bladder muscles, bladder-control strategies and self-monitoring with bladder diaries. A second group had the same behavioral training, with the addition of pelvic floor electric stimulation, which is used to activate muscles involved in bladder control. A third group was told to follow self-help booklet instructions.

At the start of the study, the frequency of incontinent episodes was the same in all of the groups. After eight weeks, the incidence of episodes was reduced by 68.6% in women who had behavioral training and by 71.9% in women who also got electrical stimulation. Women who used the self-help booklet had a 52.2% reduction in episodes.

Although electrical stimulation did not give statistically significant improvement over behavioral training alone, "patient self-reports indicated that the women in the [electrical stimulation] group perceived significantly better outcomes," the researchers write.

"The take-home message is that nonsurgical treatments for incontinence are very effective," says Goode, an associate professor of medicine at the University of Alabama. "People who tried self-help at home reduced the incidence of episodes by 50%. Those who came to a clinic for treatment increased that to 70%."

Many family physicians overlook urinary incontinence in their patients because most patients don't want to talk about it and because they believe surgery is the only answer. But, Resnick says, doctors should ask their patients, especially older women, if they are having trouble.

Women should speak up, too, Goode adds. "A lot of women think this is normal after childbirth or menopause," she says. But women need to know that effective treatments are available to treat incontinence.

info For more on urinary incontinence, visit the National Institute of Diabetes & Digestive & Kidney Diseases at *http://kidney.niddk.nih.gov.*

Sperm Defects Increase Chances of Fertilization

American Journal of Human Genetics, online edition. Johns Hopkins Medical Institutions news release.

The sperm of older men appears to accumulate disease-causing genetic mutations that also seem to increase the sperm's chances of fertilizing an egg, says a study by researchers at Johns Hopkins Medical Institutions.

The researchers made this discovery while they were investigating the reason why a rare genetic disease, Apert syndrome, is more common in children born to older fathers.

Children who are born with Apert syndrome have webbed fingers as well as early fusion of the skull bones, which requires correction through surgery.

The Johns Hopkins scientists discovered that sperm mutation rates increased as men aged. But these mutation rates were not enough to fully account for the increased incidence of Apert syndrome in children who were born to older fathers.

That led the scientists to suspect that the disease-causing mutations in the sperm also offer some benefit to the sperm.

"For some reason, a sperm that has one of these mutations is more likely to be used to make a baby than normal sperm," says researcher Dr. Ethylin Jabs, director of the Center for Craniofacial Development and Disorders at Johns Hopkins.

This combination of an increased mutation rate and the fertilization advantage offered by the mutations may explain the nearly two dozen other genetic conditions that are associated with older fathers.

The Most Common Birth Defects

Birth defects are the leading cause of infant deaths in the United States, accounting for more than 20% of all infant deaths, according to the Centers for Disease Control and Prevention (CDC). Of the roughly 120,000 babies born each year in this country with a birth defect, 8,000 die during their first year of life.

There are thousands of birth defects. Some, like Down's syndrome—the leading cause of mental retardation—involve errant chromosomes or genes. Some occur when the fetus is exposed during development to chemicals that cause mutations. Maternal alcohol abuse, inadequate consumption of folic acid during pregnancy, smoking during pregnancy, infections and exposure to certain medications are just some of the known causes of birth defects. But, the cause of 70% of birth defects remains unknown, the CDC says.

It's possible to diagnose certain birth defects while a baby is still in the womb. And in some cases, the defects can be treated. For example, surgeons have successfully removed urinary-tract obstructions and lung tumors in fetuses, and have repaired hernias in the muscle that divides the chest and abdomen.

The March of Dimes, a birth defects support group, says more than 100 fetuses have undergone experimental prenatal surgery to repair spina bifida, a disorder in which the spinal cord doesn't properly fuse in early development.

Drug-Resistant Salmonella Discovered

Becky Goldburg, PhD, senior scientist, Environmental Defense, New York City.
The Lancet.

Doctors in Taiwan have identified a potentially lethal strain of salmonella. This new strain is resistant to two antibiotics that are widely used to treat serious bacterial infections.

The appearance of the resistant strain "is a serious threat to public health, and thus constant surveillance is warranted," according to physicians at the Chang Gung University College of Medicine.

ANTIBIOTIC RESISTANCE A SERIOUS CONCERN

The salmonella, which was isolated from a 58-year-old Taiwanese man, resists both Cipro and Rocephin, the Taiwanese doctors report. Although a resistance to Cipro is not uncommon, this is the first reported case that identifies a strain of salmonella that is resistant to Rocephin as well.

Previously, the same group of researchers reported that certain strains of salmonella can develop resistance to Cipro in less than two years. They found that although none of the samples they tested in 2000 were resistant to Cipro, 60% were resistant by the third quarter of 2001.

"These are the two powerful modern antibiotics that are used to treat serious cases of salmonella," says Becky Goldburg, a senior scientist at Environmental Defense, a New York–based group that has crusaded against the use of certain antibiotics in animal feed due to concerns about drug-resistant germs. "When the infection is resistant to [the antibiotics], it is untreatable."

Because the finding is just one instance of reported multiple resistance, "it is hard to know how common it might be," Goldburg says. But the fact that Cipro-resistant salmonella quickly became common in Taiwan is not a good sign, she adds.

MOST SALMONELLA INFECTIONS NOT DEADLY

Approximately 40,000 salmonella infections are reported in the United States each year. The bacteria, which is found in contaminated food and water, tends to be more common and more serious in the underdeveloped countries of the world.

Scientists have previously identified hundreds of strains of salmonella, and most are not particularly virulent, causing diarrhea and other intestinal problems that clear up in a few days without antibiotic treatment. But the resistant bacteria detected in Taiwan can cause potentially fatal infections, the researchers say.

Severe salmonella poisoning usually strikes infants, the elderly and people with weakened immunity.

A spokesperson for the Centers for Disease Control and Prevention (CDC) says the agency cannot comment on the Taiwan report because CDC scientists were not involved in the study.

info For more information on salmonella, visit the Food and Drug Administration's (FDA) Center for Food Safety and Applied Nutrition at *www.cfsan.fda.gov.*

Simple Ways to Keep Food-Borne Diseases At Bay

Jason Ellis, MS, extension specialist, Iowa State University's Food Safety Project, Ames, Iowa.

Andrea McNally, spokeswoman, US Department of Agriculture's Food Safety and Inspection Service, Washington, DC.

Food safety might not be on your mind when you're heading to the buffet, but US health officials estimate that 76 million Americans get sick, more than 300,000 are hospitalized and 5,000 people die from food-borne illnesses each year.

More than 250 food-borne diseases have been identified, and most are caused by a variety of bacteria, viruses and parasites.

Just one—salmonellosis, an infection with the salmonella bacteria—costs the United States more than $1 billion a year in medical expenses and lost wages, according to the Centers for Disease Control and Prevention (CDC).

That's why it is important to play it smart with your food.

SAFETY STEPS

Four steps—clean, cook, chill and separate —should be followed to prevent the spread of bacteria when working with or eating food, says Jason Ellis, an extension specialist with Iowa State University's Food Safety Project.

Always thoroughly clean the foods that you intend to eat raw, such as fruits and vegetables. Clean yourself as well—wash your hands with warm water and soap for at least 20 seconds before eating, before preparing a meal and after handling raw meat or poultry.

And when you've used a cutting board to cut meat, clean it (and the knife) before you cut anything else or use a different board and utensils. This way, bacteria from your meat doesn't end up in your raw salad, says Andrea McNally, a spokeswoman for the US Department of Agriculture's Food Safety and Inspection Service.

It is also necessary to cook your food thoroughly. Use a meat thermometer so you can make sure enough heat has been applied to kill germs and bacteria.

There's a food danger zone between 40° and 140° Fahrenheit, Ellis says. That's why you should cook food thoroughly (at a temperature above 140°F) and chill leftovers as soon as you're done eating (at a temperature below 40°F).

That warning to keep foods cold also holds true for foods that haven't been cooked yet. Get them home from the grocery store as soon as possible.

"Pick up your cold foods last at the store and be sure you go straight home and get them in a refrigerator," Ellis says.

If food has been left out for too long, reheating it won't necessarily make it safe, the US Food and Drug Administration says. Heating and reheating will kill food-borne bacteria, but some bacteria produce toxins that aren't destroyed by high cooking temperatures.

One such bacteria is *staphylococcus*. This bacteria produces a toxin in cooked foods left out at room temperature for more than two hours.

If in doubt as to whether any food is still safe to eat, you should err on the side of caution and throw it out.

And always follow the "sell-by" or expiration dates on fresh foods. Ellis says, "It's much cheaper to buy more food than to take the risk of making a family member sick from a food-borne illness."

When you are preparing lunches for work or school, know whether you or your family members have access to a refrigerator. If so, you can pack all manner of foods or leftovers. If there's no access to a refrigerator, you'll have to be more creative.

"Peanut butter and jelly sandwiches are a very good choice," Ellis says. "They can be stored at room temperature without the danger of illness."

Another tip is to make your sandwiches the night before and freeze them. They thaw over the course of the morning and are ready to be eaten at lunchtime.

■ ■ ■ ■

The Most Common Food-Borne Diseases

The most common food-borne infections are those caused by the bacteria *campylobacter, salmonella* and *E. coli O157:H7,* and by a group of viruses called *calicivirus,* which is also known as the Norwalk and Norwalk-like viruses.

•*Campylobacter* causes a fever, diarrhea, and abdominal cramps. Because the bacteria that cause this illness live in the intestines of healthy birds, most raw poultry meat has campylobacter on it. Eating undercooked chicken or food that has been contaminated with the juices from raw chicken is the most frequent source of this infection.

•*Salmonella* causes *salmonellosis.* Symptoms typically include a fever, diarrhea and abdominal cramps. In people who have poor underlying health conditions or weakened immune systems, it can invade the bloodstream and cause life-threatening infections. Like campylobacter, it is also widespread in the intestines of birds, reptiles and mammals. It can spread to humans via a variety of different foods of animal origin

•*E. coli O157:H7* often causes severe and bloody diarrhea and painful abdominal cramps, without much of a fever. In 3% to 5% of cases, *hemolytic uremic syndrome* (HUS) can occur several weeks after the initial symptoms. This severe complication includes temporary anemia, profuse bleeding and kidney failure. E. coli is usually found in cattle. Human illness typically follows the consumption of food or water that has been contaminated with microscopic amounts of cow feces.

•*Calicivirus,* or Norwalk-like virus is an extremely common cause of food-borne illness, though it is rarely diagnosed, because the laboratory test that identifies it is not widely available. Calicivirus causes an acute gastrointestinal illness, usually with more vomiting than diarrhea. This illness usually resolves within two days. Unlike many food-borne pathogens that have animal sources, it is believed that Norwalk-like viruses spread primarily from one infected person to another. If they have the virus on their hands, infected kitchen workers can contaminate a salad or sandwich as they prepare it.

Some other food-borne illnesses include the rare but deadly disease botulism, which occurs when the bacterium *Clostridium botulinum* grows and produces a powerful paralytic toxin in foods.

People can also become ill if a pesticide is inadvertently added to a food, or if naturally poisonous substances are used to prepare a meal. Every year, people become ill after mistaking poisonous mushrooms for a safe species, or after eating poisonous reef fishes.

Hard to Swallow: Farm-Raised Salmon Pose Health Risk

David O. Carpenter, MD, professor, environmental health and toxicology, and director, Institute for Health and the Environment, State University of New York at Albany.
Science.

The health benefits of eating salmon are well known, but farm-raised salmon may actually be hazardous to your health.

Chemical contaminants in farm-raised salmon are at unacceptably high levels and may increase the risk of cancer dramatically, according to a report.

The key contaminant, *polychlorinated biphenyl* (PCBs) has been banned in the United States since the late 1970s. PCBs have been linked to cancer and impaired brain development in fetuses.

THE STUDY

In the study, which is the largest to date, co-researcher Dr. David O. Carpenter, a professor of environmental health and toxicology and director of the Institute for Health and the Environment at the State University of New York at Albany, tested more than two metric tons of farmed and wild salmon from around the world.

The researchers discovered that farm-raised salmon had significantly higher PCB levels than wild Pacific salmon. "Levels of 14 different chemical contaminates and pesticides are higher in farmed salmon than in wild salmon," explains Carpenter. High PCB levels in farmed salmon come from the fish meal and fish oil they are fed.

CONFLICTING STANDARDS

Although these levels of PCB are far below those called dangerous by the US Food and Drug Administration (FDA), they are considered unsafe by US Environmental Protection Agency (EPA) standards. FDA standards have not been changed since 1984.

Carpenter notes the FDA's PCB limit is not health-based (the FDA is a regulatory advisory agency), while the EPA limit is based only on health effects.

"I hope the FDA and the EPA will come together and review the standards, because the present circumstance is confusing to the consumer."

RECOMMENDATIONS

"To avoid an excessive risk of cancer, people should reduce their consumption of farm-raised salmon," Carpenter says. On average, people should limit their consumption of farmed salmon to once a month, he advises.

info To learn more about PCB contamination in fish, visit the EPA's Web site at *www.epa.gov/waterscience/fish/pcb99.html.*

New Lights Zap Germs

The Lancet.
The Lancet news release.

Installing special ultraviolet lights in office heating, ventilation and air conditioning systems can cut the number of respiratory infections that may be spread in the workplace. A Canadian study sought to address the mysterious question of why.

THE STUDY

The study included 771 volunteers in Montreal office buildings. The drip pans and cooling coils that are within office ventilation systems were exposed to *ultraviolet germicidal irradiation* (UVGI). The UVGI was alternately turned off for 12 weeks and on for four weeks, and the cycle was repeated three times.

The study found that UVGI reduced by 99% the concentrations of microscopic organisms and toxins secreted by bacteria on irradiated surfaces within the ventilation systems. The volunteers reported no adverse effects and the use of UVGI was associated with significantly fewer workplace symptoms overall.

The authors conclude that the installation of UVGI in most North American offices could resolve work-related symptoms in approximately 4 million employees.

In addition, they suggest that the expense of UVGI installation could prove cost effective in the long run compared with the cost of employee absence due to building-related illness.

■ ■ ■ ■

Sick Building Syndrome

Employees in modern office buildings frequently have unexplained work-related symptoms or combinations of symptoms. "Sick building syndrome" is the term for ailments that are believed to be associated with indoor air quality, but which can't be linked to a specific cause.

In 1984, a committee for the World Health Organization (WHO) said that as many as 30%

of new and remodeled buildings around the world may be implicated in complaints about indoor air quality.

Although the situation in the building is usually temporary, some structures have chronic problems.

Some of the various signs of sick building syndrome may include...

●**Occupants complain of acute discomfort.** They report headaches; eye, nose or throat irritation; a dry cough; dry or itchy skin; dizziness and nausea; difficulty in concentrating; fatigue; and sensitivity to odors.

●**The reason people are experiencing these symptoms is not known.**

●**Most complainants report relief soon after leaving the building.**

Sometimes, a specific disease-causing agent is identified in a building outbreak. These cases are called "building-related illnesses."

■ ■ ■ ■

How to Know if a Building Is Making You Ill

The Environmental Protection Agency (EPA) identifies the following signs of building-related illnesses...

●**Building occupants complain of symptoms such as cough;** chest tightness; fever, chills; and muscle aches.

●**The symptoms can be defined clinically** and have clearly identifiable causes.

●**Complainants may require prolonged recovery times after leaving the building.**

One of the most virulent forms of building-related contamination is Legionnaire's disease, which infects an estimated 8,000 to 18,000 people each year in the United States alone. Legionnaire's disease is fatal for between 5% and 30% of those who contract the illness, according to the Centers for Disease Control and Prevention (CDC).

info You can learn more about sick building syndrome and building-related illness from the National Safety Council at *www.nsc. org/library/facts/sickbldg.htm.*

Dust Mite Bedding— A Waste of Money

Adnan Custovic, MD, professor, Wythenshawe Hospital, Manchester, England.

Darryl Zeldin, MD, senior scientist, National Institute of Environmental Health Sciences, Research Triangle Park, NC.

New England Journal of Medicine.

If you have invested in impenetrable bedcovers to free yourself from your bed's dust mites, don't be surprised if you find yourself still wheezing and sneezing.

Research shows the covers do reduce exposure to dust mite allergens, but they do not reduce it enough to prevent allergy and asthma flare-ups in people who are sensitive to the microscopic menaces.

Dr. Adnan Custovic, an allergist at Wythenshawe Hospital in Manchester, England, and his colleagues tried to find out whether bedding covers could reduce breathing trouble in adult asthmatics.

"Covering your mattress, pillows and quilts won't work," says Custovic.

In their study, the bedcovers—which are designed to prevent dust mite particles from reaching people who are sleeping—did reduce exposure to allergy-causing proteins. But doing so wasn't enough to reduce symptoms in the long run.

BETTER THAN BEDCOVERS ALONE

Dust mites are a leading cause of allergies and asthma in the United States. Dr. Darryl Zeldin, a senior scientist and a dust mite expert at the National Institute of Environmental Health Sciences, and his colleagues recently found that 85% of American homes had detectable levels of the pests in the bedding. Half of the homes had levels that topped 2 micrograms (mcg) per gram of dust—an amount that is considered enough to make a person become sensitive to the allergen. One in four homes had enough mites in bedding to trigger asthma.

Zeldin says the findings from Custovic's study shouldn't discourage people with allergies or asthma from using bedcovers.

Instead, you should include the bedcovers as part of an overall allergy prevention program that also includes ridding your home of cockroaches or pet dander (with traps and frequent vacuuming), and washing bedding frequently in hot water, which has been shown to remove dust mite allergens.

Still, Zeldin believes that the new research underscores gaps in what scientists understand about allergies and allergens. "It may be that you get rid of one allergen and you just respond to another," he says.

■ ■ ■ ■

Reducing Allergens in Your Home

The Asthma and Allergy Foundation of America has published some additional suggestions for keeping dust and dust mites at a minimum in your home…

●**Avoid having wall-to-wall carpeting,** blinds, wool blankets, upholstered furniture and down-filled covers and pillows in your bedroom.

●**Keep pets out of the bedroom** as well.

●**Windows should have roll-type shades** instead of curtains; if you do have curtains, be sure to wash them often.

●**It is ideal for someone without a dust mite allergy to do the cleaning** of the bedroom. If this is not possible, wear a filtering mask when dusting or vacuuming.

●**Special filters for vacuum cleaners** can help to keep mites and mite waste from circulating back into the air. These filters can be purchased from an allergy supply company or in some specialty vacuum stores.

●**Wash rugs in hot water** whenever possible. Cold water leaves up to 10% of mites behind. Dry cleaning kills all mites and is also good for removing dust from fabrics.

info The Asthma and Allergy Foundation of America has more information about protecting you and your family from allergens at *www.aafa.org*.

Tight Neckwear May Be 'Tied' to Glaucoma

Robert Ritch, MD, professor of clinical ophthalmology, and chief, Glaucoma Service, The New York Eye and Ear Infirmary, New York City.

George Shafranov, MD, assistant professor and director of the glaucoma section, Yale University, New Haven, CT.

British Journal of Ophthalmology.

Ties that bind the neck may raise the risk of the eye disease glaucoma. So says a controversial study that found snug neckwear can increase *intraocular pressure* (IOP) in the eyes, possibly leading to glaucoma.

"If men wear tight neckties when their IOP is measured, it can raise their IOP," says Dr. Robert Ritch, lead author of the study and a professor of clinical ophthalmology at The New York Eye and Ear Infirmary.

DOUBLE TROUBLE

That double Windsor may be double trouble. If a person has moderate or severe glaucoma damage, the increase in IOP caused by a tight tie may worsen the damage. What's more, patients without glaucoma whose tight tie falsely increases IOP might end up being treated for glaucoma when they don't need to be. Although there are no reported cases of glaucoma being caused by a tight necktie, Ritch says it's theoretically possible.

Ritch became aware of the phenomenon during his regular practice. "I just noticed that some patients had tight neckties, and I just loosened their neckties and their IOP would go down several points," he says.

To quantify his observation, Ritch and his colleagues looked at 20 healthy men and 20 men with open angle glaucoma, the most common form of the disease.

The researchers measured IOP first while the men weren't wearing neckties, then three minutes after they put on a tight necktie, and again three minutes after the tie was loosened.

Ritch's team found that in 70% of the healthy men, a tight necktie increased mean IOP, as it did in 60% of those with glaucoma. Increases in IOP while wearing a tight necktie ranged from more than 2 to more than 4 mmHg (millimeters of mercury), compared with IOP readings when no ties were worn and after ties were loosened.

Ritch speculates that when a necktie exerts too much pressure on the jugular vein located in the neck, pressure is increased in the entire venous system, including in the eyes.

LOOSEN UP!

According to the Glaucoma Research Foundation (GRF), open angle glaucoma is the most common type of glaucoma and affects about 3 million Americans. Open angle glaucoma develops over time as the drainage canals of the eyes become clogged.

According to the GRF, most people have no symptoms of glaucoma and no early warning signs of the disease.

If open angle glaucoma fails to be diagnosed and treated, it can cause a gradual loss of vision. This type of glaucoma develops slowly, and sometimes without noticeable sight loss for many years. However, it usually responds well to medication, especially if caught early and treated.

George Shafranov, an assistant professor and director of the glaucoma section at Yale University in New Haven, Connecticut, says tight neckties "certainly don't cause glaucoma. Ties do increase IOP if the tie is really pressing on the neck and may make some ophthalmologists believe that glaucoma is present."

Neckties can affect the measurements of IOP, Shafranov notes. And a tight necktie is something physicians should be aware of when measuring IOP, in addition to other factors that can increase the pressure during an examination.

"If you have glaucoma, do not wear your necktie so tight that it can constrict your neck," Ritch advises.

"And if you are going to have your IOP measured during an eye exam, whether you do or don't have glaucoma, loosen your tie," he adds.

info To learn more about glaucoma, visit the Glaucoma Research Foundation at *www.glaucoma.org*.

Most Common Cause of Multiple Sclerosis

George C. Ebers, MD, professor and head of the department of clinical neurology, University of Oxford, England.
Stephen Reingold, PhD, vice president for research programs, National Multiple Sclerosis Society, New York City.
Proceedings of the National Academy of Sciences.

Genes contribute to the onset of multiple sclerosis (MS), according to a large study of Canadian twins, confirming much of what scientists already know.

Many studies of twins, which are considered the gold standard for trying to distinguish genetic influences from the environmental ones (because of the identical set of genes that twins have), have focused on MS, but most have been small studies.

THE STUDY

The main distinguishing feature of the new study is its size. Over 20 years, the researchers identified and analyzed more than 80% of all Canadian twins with MS. This amounted to a total of 370 pairs, 120 of them male pairs and 250 female pairs.

Most of the findings from this study are in accordance with previous data. For example, the researchers found that the identical twin of an MS patient was more likely to develop the disease than a nonidentical twin. Slightly more than 25% of identical twins with MS had a twin with the disease. Among fraternal twins, that rate was only 5.4%; among regular siblings, it was even lower (2.9%).

FEMALES MORE SUSCEPTIBLE

This concordance (when both twins had MS) was most pronounced in females. Thirty-four percent of female identical twins with MS had a twin with the disease, which was approximately 10 times the rate among female fraternal twins (3.8%).

For male identical twins, the rate at which both had MS was only 6.5%. Again, this supports previous findings.

No one is sure why females are more susceptible to the disease, but Dr. George Ebers, the lead author of the study and professor and head of the department of clinical neurology at the University of Oxford in England, suspects that the risk may come from a gene the mother passes on.

Finally, the authors determined that "twinning" itself did not have a relationship to MS. In other words, being a twin does not mean you're at a higher risk of developing the disease.

Whatever the genetic factors at play, they clearly are only part of the story.

"Even in identical twins, which are largely genetically the same, the concordance rate is only 25% to 30%," says Stephen Reingold, vice president for research programs at the National Multiple Sclerosis Society (NMSS). "That means other things are going on."

Further studies are necessary to determine the other factors.

■ ■ ■ ■

About Multiple Sclerosis

Multiple sclerosis (MS) is one of the most common neurological disorders among young adults. According to the National Multiple Sclerosis Society, approximately 400,000 Americans have MS and the disease may affect 2.5 million people worldwide.

The diagnosis of MS is most often made when the person is between 20 and 50 years old, and women are more likely to be affected than men.

The symptoms of MS are caused by the destruction of myelin, fatty tissue that protects nerve fibers and helps them conduct electrical impulses. Those symptoms can vary from person to person and from time to time in the same person.

For example, one person might experience abnormal fatigue, while another might have severe vision problems. One person who has MS could experience a loss of balance and muscle coordination; another might have slurred speech, tremors, stiffness and bladder problems, the Society says.

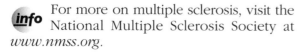 For more on multiple sclerosis, visit the National Multiple Sclerosis Society at *www.nmss.org.*

Kids, Go Out and Play— It May Help Prevent MS

British Medical Journal.

There is a positive side to all those years many of us ran around without protective clothing or sunblock—people who receive more sun exposure during their childhood and adolescence may have a reduced risk of developing multiple sclerosis (MS), according to a study.

The study notes that MS is more common at higher latitudes. These locations generally have lower ultraviolet radiation levels.

THE STUDY

Researchers surveyed 136 people who had MS and 272 control subjects who didn't have the disease. They all lived in Tasmania, which is located at a high latitude and has a high prevalence of MS.

The participants in the study were asked about their past sun exposure, sun-protection measures, use of vitamin D supplements, medical history and other factors believed to be associated with MS. Their skin damage and skin color were also assessed.

The researchers discovered that higher sun exposure at ages 6 to 15 years old (an average of two to three hours a day in summer and during weekends and holidays) and greater skin damage were associated with a decreased risk of MS.

The study also found that higher sun exposure in winter seemed more important than higher sun exposure in summer.

The association between sun exposure and a decreased risk of MS persisted after the researchers adjusted for fair skin and for sun exposure after the onset of MS.

Insufficient amounts of either vitamin D or ultraviolet radiation, or both, may influence development of MS, the study authors suggest.

EXPERTS URGE CAUTION

Talk with your doctor about the dangers of sun exposure in relation to the potential benefit of lowering your risk of developing MS.

Multiple Sclerosis Theories: Genes vs. Environment

Although the origin of MS is still unknown, the University of California at San Francisco offers some theories on the causes of the crippling disease…

The environmental theory: This theory suggests that regional differences are implicated in MS.

The disease is diagnosed more often in temperate than in tropical or subtropical climates, and there are more cases of MS in northern climates. For example, the prevalence of MS in North Dakota is approximately twice that of Florida.

People who are born in a high-risk region seem to acquire a lower risk if they relocate to a low-risk region before age 15 years.

The opposite also holds true for those people who were born in low-risk areas who then move to high-risk areas—they seem to acquire a greater risk of getting MS.

The genetic theory: This theory suggests that the risk of getting MS is influenced by genetic factors.

MS is common in Caucasians but rarely is seen in Native Americans, African-Americans native to Africa and Asians living in high-risk areas in the United States.

If it is true that an environmental factor contributes to MS, perhaps only those who are genetically susceptible actually go on to develop the illness.

Researchers have found that certain genes occur more frequently in people who have MS than those who do not have the disease.

In addition, several studies of families in which more than one member has MS indicate other family members are at an increased risk of developing MS compared with the general population.

The risk of developing MS in the general population is approximately 0.15%. However, the risk to members of families who have a father, mother, sister or brother with MS is between 1.0% and 4.0%.

info You can learn more about multiple sclerosis from the National Institute of Neurological Disorders and Stroke at *www. ninds.nih.gov.*

Do You Know How to Put on a Bike Helmet?

Gregory Parkinson, MD, community pediatrician, Falmouth Pediatric Associates, Falmouth, MA.
Ken Giles, spokesman, US Consumer Product Safety Commission, Bethesda, MD.
Pediatrics.

Even if you and your family members all wear bicycle helmets regularly, chances are the helmets fit you incorrectly. In fact, a study says that 96% of the people who wear them have them on wrong.

Dr. Gregory Parkinson admits it took him approximately 12 years to learn how to put on his bicycle helmet properly. Now Parkinson is on a mission to show kids and their parents how to master this task. In his study, Parkinson found an overwhelming majority of children, adolescents and parents cannot properly fit a bicycle helmet.

Experts agree that wearing a helmet while riding a bike, scooter, skateboard or in-line skates is a smart idea. According to the US Consumer Product Safety Commission (CPSC), about 900 people—including more than 200 children—are killed every year in bicycle-related accidents, and about 60% of these fatalities involve head injuries. According to the study, in 1997 about 4,000 head injuries resulted from in-line skating. And in 1999, an estimated 59,000 skateboard injuries occurred, about 7% of them involving the head.

The CPSC says that wearing a helmet when riding a bicycle can reduce the risk of a head injury from an accident by up to 85%—but only if the helmet is worn properly.

To find out how many people were wearing helmets correctly, Parkinson launched a study in his own private practice in Falmouth, Massachusetts, recruiting 395 families with a total of 479 children. At their regular pediatric visit, the participants were questioned and then demonstrated how they fit a helmet.

Eighty-eight percent of the kids in the study owned a bicycle helmet, but only 4% percent passed the test. None of the parents passed.

The main problems were the helmet resting too high up on the forehead, the wrong strap positions and excessive movement of the helmet—moving too loosely from the front to the back of the head.

GET IT RIGHT FOR SAFETY!

To get his own helmet adjusted correctly, Parkinson consulted the guidelines put out by the Harvard Research Center in Seattle.

Using those guidelines, he developed his new mantra: Be a Bike Helmet MVP.

M: Move it down the forehead (less than two fingers' width above the brow).

V: The straps should create a "V" around the ear.

P: Pull the chinstraps snugly.

"If you can do those three things in that order, it substantially improves safety," Parkinson says. The key is to do them in order.

"If they're going to be effective, the helmets have to cover the skull as completely as possible," Giles says.

"Some people wear them sunbonnet style—kind of pushed up and on the back of head—and that's just not effective. The helmet has to be flat on the head. The straps should make a 'V' around the ears and the straps should be snug," he explains.

Parkinson suggests that once the straps are adjusted properly, parents should sew or tie them in place. They won't have to be adjusted more than once a year, even for kids, he says.

info To see the correct way to fit a helmet, do what Dr. Parkinson did and visit the Consumer Product Safety Commission at *www.cpsc.gov/kids/kidsafety/correct.html.*

■ ■ ■ ■

Staying Safe on Your Bicycle

About 67,000 head injuries occur every year from bicycle accidents.

The University of Michigan (U-M) Health System offers some tips on helmet use and on bicycle safety in general…

THE HELMET

- **It should fit snugly.**
- **Chin straps should be sturdy.**
- **It should sit on the head evenly,** not too far forward or backwards. Light-colored helmets are best because they're more visible to drivers.
- **Always replace a helmet after a crash.**
- **Make sure that the helmet has a sticker saying it is safety certified.** Riders should always wear their helmets, even on short trips. Parents need to encourage their children to wear helmets and should set an example by wearing helmets themselves.

BICYCLE SAFETY

- **Wear close-fitting,** light-colored or reflective clothing.
- **Walk bikes across busy intersections.**
- **Never ride against traffic.**
- **Never wear headphones while riding.**
- **Always stop before entering a street.** Look left, look right and then left again before you proceed.

Loss of Consciousness Not the Only Sign Of Concussion

Study, presented to the American Orthopaedic Society for Sports Medicine.
American Orthopaedic Society for Sports Medicine news release.

One of the clearest signs of a probable concussion is loss of consciousness. But if that's the only sign doctors and coaches look for, they may send seriously injured players back into competition, researchers have found.

Athletes who get a severe concussion don't always lose consciousness, but they may experience amnesia or confusion, according to a study by doctors at the University of Pittsburgh Medical Center.

"Athletes may sustain a severe concussion without losing consciousness. Amnesia and confusion on the field after injury may be as important, if not more important, in making a return-to-play decision," study lead author Mark R. Lovell, director of the sports concussion program, says in a news release.

He and his colleagues evaluated 181 high school and college athletes with sports-related concussions. Thirty of the students had lost consciousness, while 151 had not.

They recommend not allowing any athlete thought to have a concussion back into an athletic contest until he or she has been thoroughly evaluated by a physician and undergone neuropsychological testing. "This is especially important with athletes 18 years of age and younger because their brains are still developing," Lovell says.

In another study presented at a meeting of the American Orthopaedic Society for Sports Medicine, researchers tested a simple method to measure concussion severity. The Immediate Post-concussion Assessment and Cognitive Test (ImPACT) evaluates different areas of the brain that are sensitive to concussion.

ImPACT measures reaction time, processing speed, cognitive ability and memory. The test is used by many national and international sports organizations, as well as hundreds of American colleges, universities and high schools.

In a study of 231 high school and college athletes who had a concussion and 50 control subjects without a concussion, the researchers found ImPACT accurately identified the concussed athletes. They also determined that up to 10 days are required to recover from concussion, even though many athletes report improved symptoms by the fifth day.

■ ■ ■ ■

Concussion Linked with Depression, Alzheimer's

There are about 300,000 sports-related concussions each year in the United States. At least 62,000 of those are suffered during high school contact sports. Approximately 34% of college football players have sustained a concussion, and an estimated 20% have had multiple concussions.

A study of retired National Football League players found that 61% had sustained at least one concussion during their pro career, according to the American Association of Neurological Surgeons. Nearly 24% had sustained three or more concussions while in the league, while 12% said they endured five or more of the head injuries.

But the injuries rarely kept athletes off the playing field. About 70% said they continued to participate in the sport on the day they had their concussion.

One study has linked the repeat concussions in pro football players to an increased risk of depression. Players who'd had three or more concussions in their pro careers were nearly three times as likely to suffer clinical depression than those who'd suffered no concussions, the study found.

Scientists have also learned that mild but recurring head injuries, such as repetitive concussions, increase a person's chances of developing Alzheimer's disease later in life.

Seizure Surgery Stops Epilepsy for Some

Susan S. Spencer, MD, neurologist, Yale University School of Medicine, New Haven, CT.

Edwin Trevathan, MD, MPH, director, Pediatric Epilepsy Center, Washington University, St. Louis, MO.
Neurology.

Surgery that removes a small part of the brain often stops or significantly reduces seizures among people who have epilepsy after their medications fail to do so, researchers have found.

Scientists from the Yale University School of Medicine in New Haven, Connecticut, discovered the chances of remaining seizure-free were 83% for three years after surgery, 72% for five years and 56% for 10 years.

THE STUDY

Of the 175 patients tracked for an average of more than eight years, 110 (63%) never suffered another seizure. And of the 65 patients who did have another seizure, more than half experienced one or fewer per year, a promising sign, as longer periods without seizures mean less-severe relapses, the researchers say.

"We were very encouraged by these results," says study author Dr. Susan S. Spencer, a neurologist at Yale. "It turns out that surgery has excellent results for the very long-term treatment of a group of people who have not been able to control their seizures with medications."

Usually, the part of the brain removed in epilepsy surgery can be taken out without any adverse consequences because it is not performing any critical functions, Spencer says.

Only people whose seizures start in a localized area of the brain—called "partial epilepsy"—can be treated surgically, however. Generalized seizures are a result of abnormal neuronal activity in many parts of the brain.

Approximately 60% of epileptics have partial epilepsy, and surgery could be used much more often for those partial epileptics whose seizures don't respond to medications, says Dr. Edwin Trevathan, director of the Pediatric Epilepsy Center at Washington University in St. Louis.

"Epilepsy surgery is definitely underutilized, and I think the reason is because people have the perception that it's quite risky and that the next new medicine is going to work," says Trevathan.

DON'T WAIT

Trevathan says that surgery should be considered sooner for patients who have seizures that don't respond to medications. If two drugs fail to stop seizures, Trevathan says, surgery is much more likely to stop seizures than adding another drug to the regimen.

Few people in the Yale study had surgery within the first 10 years of their epilepsy, he says. So the research did not prove that early surgical intervention is better than delaying surgical treatment.

"But as a general rule, the longer surgery is delayed, the more years of frequent seizures, further impairing patients' quality of life and increasing the risk of seizure-associated injuries and even death," he says.

The study did establish a link between the amount of time patients had epilepsy before surgery and the likelihood of additional seizures, or relapse.

Those patients who remained seizure-free had epilepsy an average of 16 years before surgery; those who relapsed had the disease an average of 20 years before surgery, the study found.

"We're trying to encourage physicians and patients alike to consider surgery as an early option rather than waiting 20 years before seeking this effective therapy," Trevathan says.

"Based on what we know, it is clear that there are thousands of individuals with uncontrolled epilepsy in the United States alone who have not been considered for this kind of [surgical] treatment that may permanently cure them," Spencer says.

According to the American Academy of Neurology, more than 2.3 million Americans—and 50 million people worldwide—have epilepsy. The disorder is the most common serious neurological problem among children.

info For more on surgery to treat epilepsy, visit the Epilepsy Foundation at *www. epilepsyfoundation.org*. Click on "Medical Aspects" under "Answer Place."

Cochlear Implants Linked to Meningitis

Jennita Reefhuis, PhD, researcher, National Center on Birth Defects, US Centers for Disease Control and Prevention, Atlanta, GA.
George A. Gates, MD, professor, otolaryngology/head and neck surgery, University of Washington, Seattle.
New England Journal of Medicine.

Government scientists have confirmed reports linking cochlear implants to an increased risk of meningitis.

The good news: Researchers regard the risk as small and manageable.

"The rate of meningitis for children who received cochlear implants is higher than it is among the general population," says study author Jennita Reefhuis, a researcher with the Centers for Disease Control and Prevention (CDC). "However, it is not known how much of the risk is due to the cochlear implant and how much is due to other factors."

Reefhuis notes that meningitis is more common among deaf children—even without cochlear implants—than among the general population.

Cochlear implants are surgically placed in the inner ear. They contain electrodes that activate nerve fibers to allow sound signals to be transmitted to the brain. These implants can help children and adults who have hearing loss perceive sounds and learn to speak. In the United States, almost 10,000 children and 13,000 adults with severe to profound hearing loss have received cochlear implants.

THE STUDY

The study looked at 4,264 children younger than six years who received a cochlear implant over a five-year period.

Researchers identified 29 cases of bacterial meningitis in 26 children (three children had two bouts of the disease). Of these children, 15 had meningitis caused by the *streptococcus pneumoniae* bacterium. In the general population, less than one case in a group this size would have been seen, according to the report.

Nine of the 29 cases that were identified occurred within a month following the implant. The other 20 cases occurred up to 36 months after surgery. In children with a cochlear implant, the risk of meningitis is 4.5 times higher when a device called a "positioner" is used, Reefhuis says. She notes that because of this increased risk, the positioner is no longer being produced.

Reefhuis says physicians should make sure that patients who are candidates for a cochlear implant are up-to-date on their vaccinations. Patients who have cochlear implants should follow the recommendations for pneumococcal vaccinations that apply to members of other high-risk groups.

Physicians should assess their patients for risk factors for meningitis. After surgery, they should watch for any signs of meningitis, including sore neck and the inability to lift the head, high fever, lethargy and possibly nausea and vomiting, Reefhuis says.

Anyone who is considering a cochlear implant should discuss the advantages and risks of having the implant with their health-care provider, Reefhuis advises.

INFECTION RISK SHOULDN'T AFFECT DECISION

George A. Gates, an ear specialist at the University of Washington in Seattle, comments that the risk of contracting meningitis is so small that it shouldn't influence the decision to have a cochlear implant. "The risk for meningitis is not much greater than for people who don't have a cochlear implant," he says.

"Cochlear implants have been the greatest thing since sliced bread for people with severe to profound hearing loss and for whom hearing aids don't improve their understanding," Gates adds. "It is hard to imagine how isolated you can be with hearing loss. It has a very powerful effect on the quality of life."

info To learn more about the connection between the implants and meningitis, visit the US Food and Drug Administration *www.fda.gov/cdrh/safety/cochlear.html.*

10

Heart Disease

Here's a Sweet Way to Fight Heart Attacks

Giving heart cells a dose of sugar in the important first few hours after a heart attack improves the chances of survival for most patients, according to the results of a Dutch study.

THE STUDY

An infusion of a solution that combined glucose, insulin and potassium decreased the death rate by nearly 75% for heart attack patients who did not also have heart failure, the report says. (Only 10% of heart attack patients actually have heart failure, a serious condition in which the heart progressively loses its ability to pump blood.)

In the Dutch study, only 1.2% of the heart attack patients without heart failure who were given the infusion died, compared with 4.2% of patients who did not receive the infusion.

The infusion did not help the patients who had heart failure.

Sick heart cells need energy. In an ailing heart, "oxygen is not available, so free fatty acids are burned without oxygen, and the results are toxic to the myocardium [heart muscle]," explains Dr. Iwan C.C. van der Horst, a cardiologist who led the study. "The infusion of glucose allows cells to use glucose as the source of energy. This prevents the toxic products, and glucose produces more energy."

The insulin and potassium also have positive effects, including widening arteries to increase blood flow, van der Horst says.

LARGER STUDIES NEEDED

Results of the study have been presented at several international cardiology meetings, and the Dutch work has been praised as "a landmark study for the treatment of myocardial

Iwan C.C. van der Horst, MD, cardiologist, Hospital de Weezenlanden, Zwollen, the Netherlands.

Richard C. Becker, MD, professor, medicine, University of Massachusetts Medical School, Worcester, and spokesman, American Heart Association.

Journal of the American College of Cardiology.

infarction [heart attack]" by Dr. Carl S. Apstein of Boston University School of Medicine.

But now, he says, larger studies are necessary to prove the point.

No such studies are in sight, says Dr. Richard C. Becker, a professor of medicine at the University of Massachusetts Medical School and a spokesman for the American Heart Association, even though the scientific rationale for the treatment is compelling.

"Since the 1960s, there have been a number of small-scale trials of this kind of therapy. The results have been promising," Becker says.

The pharmaceutical industry, which is a possible source of money for a large-scale trial, "is not getting excited," because the components of the infusion are cheap and common, according to Becker.

info An overview of heart attack treatments is available on the American Heart Association Web site at *www.americanheart.org*.

■ ■ ■ ■

Heart Attack Risk Factors

R isk factors for heart attack can be broken down into two groups, according to the National Institutes of Health.

Following is a list of those risk factors that can be controlled…

- **Smoking.**
- **High blood pressure.**
- **High cholesterol.**
- **Obesity.**
- **Physical inactivity.**

Among those risk factors that cannot be controlled are…

- **Age.**
- **Family history of early heart disease.**
- **Pre-existing coronary diseases,** including a previous heart attack or angina, or prior angioplasty or bypass surgery.

Aspirin Cuts the Risk of a First Heart Attack by 32%!

Patricia Hebert, PhD, associate professor, cardiology, Yale University, New Haven, CT.
David Katz, MD, MPH, associate clinical professor, public health, Yale University, New Haven, CT.
Archives of Internal Medicine.

D octors have known of aspirin's ability to prevent second heart attacks and stroke for a long time, but a recent analysis finds that aspirin users have a significantly lower risk of a first heart attack.

Study co-author Patricia Hebert, an associate professor of cardiology at Yale University, and her team collected data from five studies that included 55,580 people, 11,466 of whom were women.

"Aspirin reduces the risk of a *first* attack in healthy people by 32%," says Hebert. The researchers also found aspirin cut the risk of all major cardiac events by 15%.

RISK PROFILE

Doctors need to look at your 10-year risk of having a first heart attack, and if that risk is 10% or higher, then you should be taking aspirin every day, Hebert says. These are the recommendations of both the US Preventive Services Task Force and the American Heart Association.

"If your risk of a first heart attack is 10% or more, then the chances are that the benefits of aspirin therapy will outweigh the risks."

Risks of aspirin therapy can include gastrointestinal bleeding and a slight risk of hemorrhagic stroke.

Hebert says your risk profile is based on a number of factors, including age, sex, weight, family history, diabetes, smoking and blood pressure and cholesterol levels.

DAILY ASPIRIN SUGGESTED

"Daily aspirin therapy is underused to prevent a first heart attack," Hebert says.

People should talk with their doctors about what their risk for a heart attack is to see if they should be taking aspirin daily, she advises. The optimum daily dose of aspirin is approximately 75 milligrams (mg), according to Hebert. Patients who have similar risk profiles for a heart attack also might want to take cholesterol-lowering drugs, called statins.

"If more people took aspirin every day, it is estimated that 150,000 cardiovascular deaths could be prevented each year," Hebert says.

HEALTHY LIVING

'There are approaches to preventing heart disease that have no risks associated with them, he adds, including not smoking, being active and eating a healthy diet, says Dr. David Katz, an associate clinical professor of public health at Yale University.

"It comes down to making a choice," Katz adds. "People who are willing to commit to the harder work of living a health-promoting lifestyle may never need aspirin in order to prevent heart disease. And for those who can not make that commitment, or who have risk factors because of a genetic component, they will find aspirin a very useful strategy for preventing heart disease, because it is very effective and not very toxic."

■ ■ ■ ■

What Happens During A Heart Attack

A heart attack occurs when the blood supply to part of the heart muscle—the myocardium—is severely reduced or stopped. This happens when one or more of the coronary arteries that is supplying blood to the heart muscle is blocked. This blockage is usually caused by the buildup of plaque inside the arteries, a process called atherosclerosis. The plaque can eventually burst, tear or rupture, creating a "snag" where a blood clot forms and blocks the artery.

If the blood supply is cut off for more than a few minutes, muscle cells suffer permanent injury and die.

According to the American Heart Association there are 1.2 million new and recurrent cases of heart attack per year. About 42% of all heart attacks are fatal.

Aspirin Alone Not Enough To Conquer Clots

Presentation, American Heart Association annual conference, Orlando.
The Johns Hopkins Medical Institutions news release.

A spirin by itself is not strong enough to prevent blood clots from developing in some people with heart problems. So say researchers from The Johns Hopkins Medical Institutions, who analyzed the blood of heart patients to see how well aspirin prevented clotting.

THE STUDY

The study researchers collected blood samples from 33 patients hospitalized for chest pain—18 with cardiac chest pain and 15 with noncardiac chest pain. All the patients were taking 81 to 325 milligrams (mg) of aspirin per day.

The blood samples were treated with low doses of epinephrine and ADP, medications that allow blood cells called platelets to clump together. Despite treatment with aspirin, platelets clumped together 5% to 10% more in the samples that were taken from patients who had heart disease than in the blood of the people without heart disease.

The more that blood platelets clump together, the greater the risk of clot formation and heart attack.

"Even though these patients were receiving aspirin therapy, they still had very active platelets," says lead author Dr. Marlene S. Williams, an assistant professor of medicine.

Williams plans to investigate the effectiveness of adding other anti-clotting agents to aspirin therapy. She also recommends that patients taking daily aspirin therapy continue to do so.

■ ■ ■ ■

Why Aspirin?

A spirin therapy prevents heart problems by thinning the blood and reducing the size of clots, which can cause heart attacks and strokes.

According to the US Food and Drug Administration, low-dose treatment with aspirin has been shown to…

•**Prevent a heart attack in those who have had a previous heart attack** or who experience angina (chest pain).

•**Reduce the risk of death or complications from a heart attack** if it is taken at the first signs of a heart attack.

•**Prevent recurrent blockage** for those who have had heart bypass surgery or other procedures to clear blocked arteries, such as balloon angioplasty or carotid endarterectomy.

•**Prevent stroke in those who have had a previous stroke** or who have had a warning sign called a *transient ischemic attack* (TIA or mini-stroke).

In addition, studies show that aspirin helps prevent heart attacks and strokes in people at high risk for these conditions.

Although aspirin has been used for more than 100 years, it's not free of risk. It can cause stomach upset, as well as serious gastric bleeding in people who take it over long periods of time. This effect is exacerbated by alcohol use, so experts advise against drinking alcohol while taking aspirin regularly.

High doses of aspirin have also been linked to ringing ears and hearing loss, problems which typically resolve when the drug is stopped or scaled back. In addition, a small percentage of people are allergic to aspirin.

The Best Hospitals for Heart Attack Survival

Henning R. Andersen, assistant professor of cardiology, Aarhus University Hospital, Copenhagen, Denmark.

John G. Canto, director, coronary care unit and chest pain center, and assistant professor of medicine, University of Alabama, Birmingham.

New England Journal of Medicine.

People who have heart attacks do better if they are sent quickly to major medical centers for artery-opening angioplasty operations than if they stay in community hospitals where they get the clot-dissolving treatment, according to a Danish study. Angioplasties were found to be much better at preventing a second heart attack than the clot-dissolving treatment.

However, the short-term benefits of quick angioplasty might not be overwhelming. In the Danish study, the death rate for the patients who had angioplasty and for those who had clot-dissolving treatment was not very different—6.6% for angioplasty, 7.8% for clot-dissolving treatment.

The big gain was in prevention. Only 1.6% of the angioplasty patients had a second heart attack, compared with 6.3% of those getting clot-dissolving treatment.

WILL RESULTS TRANSLATE?

So can the results of the trial, and others with similar results, be applied here in America, where it takes the majority of heart attack patients a long time to reach major medical centers that do angioplasty?

Some American experts say "yes."

The Danish trial shows that "now is the time to discard the practice of transporting patients with acute myocardial infarction [heart attack] to the nearest hospital, and to transport them preferentially to centers of excellence," says Dr. Alice K. Jacobs of Boston University Medical Center.

Among the physicians who are not so sure these study results are applicable in the United States is the lead author of the report, Henning R. Andersen, assistant professor of cardiology at the Aarhus University Hospital in Copenhagen. For one thing, the medical systems of the two countries are very different, he says.

"In my country, we don't have private hospitals," he says. "Everything is paid for by the government. In the US, a hospital may be reluctant to transfer a patient because of the income their stay will generate."

OTHER DIFFERENCES

In addition, there are other differences, adds John G. Canto, director of the coronary care unit and chest pain center at the University of Alabama at Birmingham.

"Denmark is amazing," Canto says. "From the time patients present for the initial hospitalization to when they get the artery open is shorter than when patients present here. They can open an artery much faster than we can in the United States."

And geography is another factor, explains Canto. Jacobs works in Boston, where a high-skilled medical center is only minutes away. The same is true of Birmingham, where "we have 16 hospitals, and 12 can do that intervention," Canto says. "But if you are in a rural part of Alabama, I don't know whether the two hours you would have to drive would be worth it."

Angioplasty is the better treatment, Canto adds. "But if the question is whether the Danish results can be extrapolated to the United States, my answer is that we don't know."

Canto's advice: When someone appears to be having a heart attack, take him to the nearest hospital, whether or not it is equipped to do angioplasty.

"Once you get the patient to a hospital, it can be decided whether he or she should be transported to a medical center where they do primary angioplasty," Canto says.

New Clue to Sudden Coronary Death

Frank D. Kolodgie, PhD, research scientist, Armed Forces Institute of Pathology, Washington, DC. *New England Journal of Medicine.*

Coronary artery disease most often results from a condition known as *atherosclerosis,* which happens when a waxy substance called a *plaque* forms inside the arteries that supply blood to your heart.

Plaque is made of cholesterol, fatty compounds, calcium and a blood-clotting material called fibrin.

TWO TYPES OF PLAQUE

There are two kinds of plaques: Hard plaque and soft plaque.

Hard plaque is the most common. If hard plaques build up in the arteries that supply blood to your heart, the blood flow can slow down or even stop entirely. This decreases the amount of oxygen that gets to the heart, which can lead to a heart attack.

But doctors have now discovered that most heart attacks are caused by soft plaques, or inflamed parts of an artery that can burst.

Pathologists studying tissue from people who died suddenly of coronary disease have discovered that when plaques rupture, the debris can block the blood vessel and cut off blood flow to part of the heart or brain.

THE STUDY

An analysis of plaques from 24 people who died suddenly of coronary disease shows fatal ruptures can occur when tiny blood vessels that have grown into a plaque burst, according to researchers at the Armed Forces Institute of Pathology.

The study shows that hemorrhages of the blood vessels that invade plaques can cause the plaques to rupture, says the author of the study, Frank D. Kolodgie, a research scientist at the Institute. That finding makes *angiogenesis,* the process of blood vessel growth, a possible target of treatment.

"If you can prevent angiogenesis, you may be able to stabilize those plaques so they are less prone to rupture," Kolodgie says.

When he and his colleagues tested plaques from the coronary patients, they looked for a molecule called *glycophorin A* and for excess amounts of iron, both of which are signals of a hemorrhage. Both were found in plaques that were the most unstable and most likely to rupture.

To verify the finding, the researchers force-fed rabbits with high-fat foods to stimulate the formation of plaques in their arteries. An analysis of the rabbit plaques found results that were similar to the human samples.

info Learn to reduce your risk of coronary artery disease from the American Academy of Family Physicians at *http://familydoctor.org/239.xml.*

Survive a Heart Attack With Hormones

David Haines, MD, director, heart rhythm center, William Beaumont Hospital, Royal Oak, MI.

Volker Wenzel, MD, associate professor, anesthesiology and critical care medicine, Leopold-Franzens University, Innsbruck, Austria.

New England Journal of Medicine.

Minneapolis Heart Institute Foundation, coronary heart disease fact sheet.

A hormone may improve the chances for people who have the worst odds of surviving after cardiac arrest.

A European study found that *vasopressin* raised the odds of surviving cardiac arrest in the worst cases up to 50% compared with the standard treatment, in which the hormone *epinephrine* is administered.

The realities of cardiac arrest are very different from television and the movies—where it is often successfully treated with a shock or two from a defibrillator.

Approximately 600,000 people die from sudden cardiac arrest every year in North America and Europe, the study says. According to the American Heart Association (AHA), 95% of people who have cardiac arrest die before they even get to the hospital.

"Sudden death statistics are just abysmal," confirms Dr. David Haines, who is director of the heart rhythm center at William Beaumont Hospital in Royal Oak, Michigan. He was encouraged by the findings.

"This is really the first therapy that has been shown effective above and beyond CPR [cardiopulmonary resuscitation]. This offers a real window of hope for some people," he says.

THE STUDY

For the study, nearly 1,200 people in cardiac arrest were randomly selected to receive vasopressin (also known as antidiuretic hormone) or epinephrine (adrenalin), which has been the standard treatment for almost 100 years.

The patients were from 33 hospitals in Austria, Germany and Switzerland. Each person was given two injections each of vasopressin or epinephrine. If both of these treatments failed, then an additional injection of epinephrine was given.

Cardiac arrest can take several forms. One is *ventricular fibrillation,* a potentially fatal heart rhythm. Another is *asystole* in which there is no heart activity at all.

In the study, the group that was given vasopressin fared only slightly better than the group that was given epinephrine if they had ventricular fibrillation.

However, people with asystole fared much better when they were treated with vasopressin. Twenty-nine percent of the patients survived to hospital admission, compared with only 20% of the epinephrine group.

More than 700 people required the additional injection of epinephrine, and the combination of the vasopressin and the epinephrine appeared to be more effective than either of the drugs alone.

Almost 26% of those who received vasopressin and epinephrine survived to hospital admission, while only 16.4% of the epinephrine-only group did.

"Vasopressin is most helpful when shock or cardiac arrest is prolonged," says Dr. Volker Wenzel, an associate professor of anesthesiology and critical care medicine at the Leopold-Franzens University in Innsbruck, Austria, and author of the study.

"It is nice to see that the patients with the worst prognosis now have a better chance to survive," he adds.

info To learn more about cardiac arrest, visit the Duke University Health System at *www.dukehealth.org.*

■ ■ ■ ■

Coronary Heart Disease Symptoms

Although many of the symptoms of coronary heart disease are subtle or silent, there are some signs that a person may have the illness. *The Minneapolis Heart Institute Foundation lists the following signs that a person may have heart disease...*

●**Pressure, discomfort or squeezing** in the center of the chest. This is the most common symptom for coronary heart disease and is the result of an insufficient supply of oxygen to the heart muscle.

●**Shortness of breath** when performing light to moderate activities.

●**Radiating pain** that travels to your shoulders, neck, arms or jaw. This pain may occur alone or with chest pain.

●**Sweating** with or without chest pain.

●**Feeling faint,** lightheaded or suddenly becoming dizzy and weak without the loss of consciousness.

●**Fatigue can be a symptom of heart failure** because the heart is not pumping a sufficient amount of blood.

Additionally, the Minneapolis Heart Institute Foundation lists several significant differences in the ways women and men present with coronary heart disease symptoms.

WOMEN

●**Tightness in the chest,** sometimes with radiating pain.

●**Shortness of breath.**

●**Fatigue** that is overwhelming and unusual.

●**Dizziness** and unexplained lightheadedness, sometimes with blackouts.

●**Swelling,** particularly of the ankles and lower legs.

●**Rapid heartbeats.**

●**Nauseous feeling** or upset stomach.

MEN

●**Sudden pressure,** fullness or squeezing pain in the center of the chest.

●**Radiating pain** from the center of the chest to the arms and neck.

●**Lightheadedness,** fainting, sweating, and shortness of breath.

●**Sudden rapid heartbeats.**

Inflammation Swells Risk Of Cardiovascular Disease

C. Michael Stein, MD, associate professor, medicine, Vanderbilt University School of Medicine, Nashville, TN.

Mary J. Roman, MD, professor, medicine, Weill Medical College of Cornell University, New York City.

New England Journal of Medicine.

There is growing evidence that chronic inflammation plays a major role in cardiovascular disease, researchers say.

And two new studies that focused on the accumulation of fatty deposits in the arteries of people who have lupus support this theory.

Systemic lupus erythematosus (SLE) is a condition in which the immune system mistakenly attacks part of the body, causing inflammation of connective tissue, such as tendons and cartilage. Patients have periodic bouts of symptoms which can include fever and fatigue. It affects approximately 1.5 million Americans, 90% of them women.

Doctors have known that there is an increased incidence of cardiovascular disease in SLE patients, and now researchers at Vanderbilt University School of Medicine and Weill Medical College of Cornell University report that the buildup of fatty deposits in the arteries (atherosclerosis), starts earlier and progresses faster in SLE patients.

The finding points directly to inflammation as a factor in atherosclerosis, Roman says.

THE STUDY

The two groups used different techniques to obtain images of arteries in the SLE patients —*electron-beam computed tomography* at Vanderbilt, *ultrasonography* and *echocardiography* at Cornell. Both produced strikingly similar results.

The Vanderbilt study of 65 SLE patients and 69 people without the condition found that "the prevalence of coronary artery atherosclerosis is elevated and the age at onset is reduced" in SLE subjects.

After comparing 197 SLE patients with 197 people without the condition, the Cornell researchers found that "atherosclerosis occurs prematurely in patients with SLE and is independent of traditional risk factors."

Dr. C. Michael Stein, an associate professor of medicine and the leader of the Vanderbilt group, says, "We started the study based on the inflammatory hypothesis. We're not sure which aspect of inflammation is involved, but this kind of study may help us understand the relationship of atherosclerosis to inflammation in the general population."

"The next big step is to try to figure out what is the best way to retard the progression of atherosclerosis," says Dr. Mary J. Roman, a professor of medicine and leader of the research group at Cornell.

info Get a primer on SLE from the National Institute of Arthritis and Musculoskeletal and Skin Diseases at *www.niams.nih.gov.* Click on "Health Information."

'Top' Predictor of Heart Disease

Eliseo Guallar, MD, assistant professor, epidemiology, The Johns Hopkins School of Public Health, Baltimore.

Daniel Jones, MD, dean, School of Medicine, University of Mississippi Medical Center, Jackson.

Annals of Internal Medicine.

When a medical professional takes your blood pressure and gives you two numbers, such as 120 over 80, it can be confusing. What are these numbers and what do they mean? Should you care about one number or both? What about the difference between the two?

Relax. Research confirms that the first number (systolic) is more important than the second (diastolic). The difference between them —the little-known *pulse pressure*—does not mean much at all.

"We believe that the number to watch more closely is the higher blood pressure number," says Dr. Eliseo Guallar, a researcher at The Johns Hopkins School of Public Health and co-author of the study, as it's a better indication that a seemingly heart-healthy person will die of heart disease.

The systolic number measures the pressure when the heart pumps blood out, and the diastolic number measures the pressure between the pumps. The pressure doesn't drop down to zero between heartbeats, but it does descend a bit.

High blood pressure is a sign that the heart is working extra hard to push blood through the body.

"Too much pressure is bad because it makes your heart overwork, making it more prone to arrhythmias and heart failure," Guallar says. "And as you are pumping blood with more force, you're damaging your arteries."

Arteries that are stressed out, in turn, can lead to heart disease, stroke, vascular diseases and kidney disease.

IMPORTANT NUMBER IS ON TOP

Doctors have realized the importance of systolic pressure after placing too much emphasis on diastolic pressure, says Dr. Daniel Jones, dean of the School of Medicine at the University of Mississippi Medical Center and spokesman for the American Heart Association.

Recently, however, some researchers have speculated that the pulse pressure could also be a sign of heart trouble.

Guallar and his team examined the medical records of 7,830 Americans—both men and women—who were followed up for 15 years. They were aged 30 to 74 years and seemed to have no sign of heart disease.

Those with higher systolic pressure levels were more likely to die of heart disease. Diastolic pressure may play a role in death rates in older patients, as may unusually low blood pressure. But pulse pressure didn't seem to be directly connected to mortality.

Doctors say any systolic pressure above 120 is cause for concern. Ways to lower your blood pressure include eating healthy foods, reducing the amount of sodium in your diet, losing weight, exercising more often, limiting your alcohol intake and quitting smoking.

Experts Urge Tighter Cholesterol Control

Scott Grundy, MD, director, Center for Human Nutrition, University of Texas Southwestern Medical Center, Dallas.
Sidney Smith, MD, chief, cardiology, University of North Carolina, Chapel Hill.
Circulation.

Just as it did in 2003 with blood pressure, the United States government has changed the standards for what it considers safe levels of cholesterol. The new guidelines reflect experts' beliefs that more Americans are at risk than they thought—at least statistically.

The new guidelines are based on the results of trials conducted in the last few years, according to Dr. Scott Grundy, director of the Center for Human Nutrition at the University of Texas Southwestern Medical Center and chairman of the panel that made the health recommendation.

"Evidence from many trials on lowering cholesterol has been accumulating rapidly," Grundy says. "Our last report was in 2001. Since that time there have been five major trials, so we felt the field needed new guidelines."

As a result, a panel of medical experts has created an entirely new category of patients who should be considered at very high risk of a heart attack. This category includes those people who have heart disease, plus diabetes and high blood pressure, are smokers or also have "metabolic syndrome," a constellation of symptoms, including high levels of triglycerides (another fatty substance) and low levels of HDL (high-density lipoprotein), the "good" cholesterol.

For these people, experts are now recommending that they lower their LDL (low-density lipoprotein), or "bad" cholesterol, to below 70 milligrams per deciliter (mg/dL). Previous guidelines said their LDL should be 100, at most.

The panel also recommended that people at moderately high risk try to cut their LDL level to no more than 100 mg/dL, a reduction from the previous limit of 130. This risk group includes people who have had a heart attack.

The study was sponsored by the National Cholesterol Education Program (NCEP), a joint effort of the American Heart Association, the American College of Cardiology and the National Heart, Lung and Blood Institute.

"It is very important to emphasize that the recommendations for more aggressive treatment of cholesterol in no way suggests that behavior modifications and diet are not important," says Dr. Sidney Smith, chief of cardiology at the University of North Carolina at Chapel Hill, a member of the panel as well as a spokesman for the American Heart Association. "We're not saying that all you have to do is take a pill," he adds

The decision on how aggressive treatment should be must be made on an individual basis, Grundy says. "High doses of drugs can cause side effects, so there is a potential downside to pushing cholesterol levels way down," he explains.

Age should not be a consideration, according to the guidelines. The study results indicate that it is never too late to benefit from reducing high levels of LDL, Grundy says.

info More information about lowering cholesterol can be found at the National Heart, Lung and Blood Institute at *www.nhlbi. nih.gov*.

Statins Pump Up Heart Health Even When Cholesterol's Normal

Circulation news release.
American Heart Association.

Cholesterol-lowering drugs called *statins* seem to benefit heart failure patients who have normal cholesterol levels, according to a study by Japanese and American researchers.

"This is the first prospective study to show that statins have beneficial effects in heart failure in the absence of coronary artery disease or high blood cholesterol levels," says senior author Dr. James K. Liao, an assistant professor of medicine at Harvard Medical School.

THE STUDY

Liao's study included 51 Japanese patients with moderate heart disease. They received either 5 milligrams (mg) of simvastatin for four weeks followed by 10 mg of the drug for 10 weeks, or a placebo.

Of the participants taking the statin, 39.1% showed improved heart function, 56.6% had no change and 4.3% experienced a decrease in heart function. Among those in the placebo group, 16% improved, 72% had no change and 12% got worse.

The left ventricular fraction, a measure of heart function, rose from 34% to 41% in the statin group but stayed the same in the placebo group.

"These improvements are significant, given that these patients had only moderate heart disease and were treated for only 14 weeks. This opens up a new treatment strategy for patients with heart failure, regardless of their cholesterol levels," Liao says.

MORE RESEARCH NECESSARY

But larger studies are needed before statins can be recommended to treat patients with this form of chronic heart failure, according to the researchers.

■ ■ ■ ■

The Benefits and Risks Of Statins

There are now five forms of statins available in the United States—lovastatin, simvastatin, pravastatin, fluvastatin and atorvastatin.

A sixth drug, cerivastatin, was withdrawn from the market by Bayer in August 2001 because of concerns that it was linked to potentially deadly muscle breakdown.

Still, heart experts say people who have high cholesterol shouldn't be scared away from statins.

"Statins, like all drugs, have side effects, but the benefits of using statins to manage patients' cholesterol far outweigh the risks of serious side effects from their use," says Dr. Douglas P.

Zipes, president of the American College of Cardiology.

Statin drugs have been shown to reduce LDL (low-density lipoprotein, or "bad") cholesterol by 20% to 60%, and to lower other blood fats called triglycerides. They also appear to raise HDL (high-density lipoprotein, or "good") cholesterol, which protects the heart and vessels.

Lowering high LDL levels in the short run can slash the risk of a heart attack and heart disease by as much as 40%. The earlier in life that a person develops high cholesterol, the greater their risk of having a heart-related illness later in life.

info You can learn more about cholesterol and statins from the US government's MedlinePlus Web site *www.nlm.nih.gov/med lineplus/cholesterol.html.*

Heart Scans 'Beat' Other Tests at Measuring Statins

Article and news release, *Journal of the American College of Cardiology.*

Heart scans may offer a clearer picture of the effectiveness of cholesterol-lowering statin drugs in people with coronary artery disease, a study says.

The pilot study discovered that using heart scans to monitor stress-induced coronary artery blood flow abnormalities may be a better way to evaluate how well statin therapy is working than measuring changes in blood cholesterol levels.

Coronary artery disease (CAD) is caused by a build-up of fatty deposits in the arteries, which can block the flow of blood and oxygen to the heart. Each year, more than 1 million Americans have heart attacks, and about 500,000 people die from heart disease.

THE STUDY

Over a six-month period, researchers compared changes in blood flow to the heart muscle with blood cholesterol profiles in people who had coronary artery disease who also took *pravastatin,* a cholesterol-lowering drug that has been shown to reduce heart attack and cardiac death.

Six weeks into treatment with pravastatin, the patients' cholesterol levels started to decline. But improvements in blood flow to the heart muscle as detected by heart scans became statistically significant only after six months of drug therapy.

The study found that some of the patients showed improvements in the blood flow to the heart along with expected substantial reductions in cholesterol. But, in others, the improvement in blood flow wasn't associated with major decreases in blood cholesterol levels.

And some patients in the study had improved cholesterol levels during the early period of treatment with no change—for better or worse—of the blood flow to the heart.

WHICH TEST IS BEST?

So which test is the better predictor of a patient's response to statins?

"It seems likely the heart scans...track the expected benefit of statin therapy better than cholesterol levels. However, further results from larger ongoing trials that are now taking place are required to evaluate this question," said researcher Dr. Ronald G. Schwartz of the University of Rochester Medical Center.

■ ■ ■ ■

Cholesterol and Heart Disease

When you have too much cholesterol in your blood, it builds up in the walls of your arteries. Over a period of time, this build-up narrows arteries and slows down or blocks blood flow to the heart.

The blood carries oxygen to the heart, and if enough blood and oxygen cannot reach your heart, you may have chest pain. If the blood supply to a portion of the heart is completely cut off by a blockage, the result is a heart attack.

High blood cholesterol by itself does not cause any symptoms, so many people are unaware that their cholesterol level is too high.

It is important to find out what your cholesterol numbers are because lowering cholesterol levels that are too high lessens the risk of developing heart disease and reduces the chance of a heart attack.

Manmade Cholesterol Unclogs Arteries In Just Weeks

E. Murat Tuzcu, MD, cardiologist and professor of medicine, Cleveland Clinic Foundation, OH.
Roger Blumenthal, MD, cardiologist, The Johns Hopkins School of Medicine, Baltimore.
Cleveland Clinic statement.
Journal of the American Medical Association.

A new weapon in the ongoing war on heart disease has been forged by some very healthy Italians.

A manmade form of cholesterol that mimics a protein in the Italians' blood took only weeks to reverse atherosclerosis in patients whose arteries had become clogged over decades.

REMARKABLE FINDING

If the success of this therapy continues, it could mean huge strides in the battle against heart disease—the leading cause of death in the United States. In the last decade, the gold standard of preventive medicine has been the use of statin drugs, which lower low-density lipoprotein (LDL, the "bad" cholesterol). In this study, however, the patients received an intravenous infusion of synthetic high-density lipoprotein (HDL, the "good" cholesterol).

"This is an extraordinary and unprecedented finding," says Dr. Steven Nissen, a Cleveland Clinic cardiologist who directed a study of the manmade cholesterol. "This is the first convincing demonstration that targeting HDL, good cholesterol, can benefit patients with heart disease."

HOW IT DEVELOPED

The development of the manmade cholesterol started 30 years ago, when researchers noticed that 40 people who were living in the village of Limone sul Garda in northern Italy were heart-healthy despite having very low levels of HDL, which should have left them vulnerable to disease. They lived long lives, and their arteries were remarkably clear.

"Normally, we would get very, very concerned because [we believed people with low HDLs would be] at high risk," says Dr. E. Murat Tuzcu, a cardiologist and professor of medicine at the Cleveland Clinic who took part in the study. "There was clearly something that was abnormal."

The researchers discovered that these people carried a variant in a blood protein called apolipoprotein A-1, which is a component of HDL. They named it ApoA-1 Milano, after the city of Milan, where the original work was conducted. Researchers at Esperion Therapeutics Inc., a biotech firm in Ann Arbor, Michigan, derived a synthetic version of this protein. Esperion then sponsored the study of the synthetic cholesterol.

THE STUDY

The study, which was led by the Cleveland Clinic team, was done at 10 centers across the United States. The trial was small—involving only 47 patients, aged 38 to 82 years, who had angina or had previously had a cardiovascular event such as a heart attack.

The patients underwent ultrasound at the start of the study to determine the amount of blockage in their arteries. They were then randomly assigned to one of three groups—high-dose or low-dose synthetic cholesterol or placebo. The injections were given every week for five weeks.

After six weeks, the researchers again conducted ultrasounds on the patients' arteries. Tuzcu says those who received the therapy saw their arteries clear by 4%. "That might not sound great, but actually it is," he says. "It is the first time in a human being that we can change or regress atherosclerosis in six weeks. Incredible!"

However, more and larger studies are needed, Tuzcu cautions.

Dr. Roger Blumenthal, a cardiologist at The Johns Hopkins School of Medicine as well as a spokesman for the American Heart Association, says most of the focus of existing medicines to treat heart disease has been on lowering LDL and triglycerides. But this study shows the benefits of trying to raise HDL levels, which "is another way to go about the problem of high cholesterol."

■ ■ ■ ■

Number of People Who Have High Cholesterol Rising

More than 100 million adults in America have at least borderline-high cholesterol, considered a reading of 200 milligrams per deciliter (mg/dL) of blood, according to the National Institutes of Health. Within this group, 37 million people have high cholesterol, which is defined as a reading of 240 mg/dL or higher.

Cholesterol levels are also alarmingly elevated among children and adolescents, with 10% of 12- to 19-year-olds having borderline-high levels, health officials say.

High cholesterol is a leading risk factor for heart attacks and strokes, but it's not impossible to reverse. A 10% drop in total cholesterol may reduce a person's risk of heart disease by as much as 30%, health officials say.

Does Red Wine Put a Cork in Cholesterol?

Alice H. Lichtenstein, DSc, director, Cardiovascular Nutrition Laboratory, Gershoff Professor of Nutrition, US Department of Agriculture's Human Nutrition Research Center, Tufts University, Boston, and vice chairwoman, nutrition committee, American Heart Association.

Presentation, American Chemical Society national meeting, New York City.

Red wine has long been linked to a reduction in heart disease, thanks largely to the healthy effects of a molecule called *resveratrol*.

Now, scientists say that they have found another group of chemicals that may share the responsibility for red wine's cholesterol-lowering effects.

. But don't plan a visit to the Napa Valley just yet, some experts say.

"It's always of interest to find naturally occurring compounds that decrease cholesterol levels, but one needs to keep it in context," says Alice H. Lichtenstein, Gershoff Professor of Nutrition at the US Department of Agriculture's Human Nutrition Research Center at Tufts University in Boston.

The evidence supporting the new chemicals' worth is inconclusive, she explains.

The new compounds, called *saponins,* have already been found in other foods, such as soy beans and peas, and are also thought to be in the skin of grapes, say the researchers, from the University of California, Davis.

THE STUDY

For the study, the researchers compared the saponin content of six types of California wines—four red and two white. They found red wine contains three to 10 times as much saponin as white wine. Red zinfandel topped the chart, followed by syrah, then pinot noir and cabernet sauvignon.

The scientists also discovered that the higher the alcohol content, the higher the saponin levels.

Resveratrol, an antioxidant, is believed to act by blocking cholesterol oxidation. Saponins are thought to work by preventing the absorption of cholesterol into the body.

WARNING

Even if saponins do contribute to lowering cholesterol levels, the American Heart Association points out that alcoholic beverages, including wine, can have negative health effects by increasing triglyceride levels, raising blood pressure and providing extra calories that can contribute to obesity.

So you might want to take this news about wine with a grain of salt.

"There are a number of naturally appearing compounds that can lower cholesterol levels, but one needs to take into consideration how much a person will probably get from normal consumption, and I don't have a good idea of the cholesterol response," Lichtenstein says.

■ ■ ■ ■

Red Wine May Slow Aging and Fight Cancer

Researchers are investigating the properties of red wine to determine if it can help stave off aging and fight cancer...

●**Antiaging.** Researchers at Harvard have found that a class of chemicals that includes resveratrol, an active ingredient in red wine— extended life by 70% in fruit flies, yeast and worms. So dramatic are the life-extension benefits, say the scientists, that they mimic the life-extending effects of calorie restriction, which many people would view as a lot less palatable than drinking red wine. Molecules like resveratrol regulate other proteins, which interfere with the natural process of cell death, the researchers say.

●**Cancer fighter.** Recent studies that have been conducted on red wine have examined its effects in fighting leukemia, skin, breast and prostate cancers in animals. However, studies of the association between red wine consumption and cancer in humans are in their initial stages. Although consumption of large amounts of alcoholic beverages may increase the risk of some cancers, there is growing evidence that the health benefits of red wine are related to its nonalcoholic components.

Astounding! High Cholesterol May Help People with Heart Failure

Andrew L. Clark, MD, Department of Academic Cardiology, University of Hull, Hull, England.

Robert Doughty, MD, research fellow, University of Auckland, New Zealand.

Journal of the American College of Cardiology.

A recent study turns common sense on its head by suggesting that high cholesterol levels may help, and not harm, people with heart failure.

High total blood cholesterol has been linked to an increased risk of coronary artery disease, especially when it is found in combination with other risk factors.

So the finding that higher cholesterol levels may be beneficial to some patients has researchers scratching their heads.

"On the face of it, this result seems quite surprising, given the strong association between cholesterol and vascular disease. However, we have been developing for some time the notion that heart failure is a metabolically stressful illness," says co-author Dr. Andrew L. Clark of Castle Hill Hospital and the University of Hull in England.

"A high cholesterol level can be seen as good in that it indicates a greater reserve to deal with metabolic stresses. And this is supported by some of the other studies...which show a greater survival with increasing body weight in heart failure and following heart surgery," Clark adds.

THE STUDY

Researchers from Castle Hill Hospital, along with colleagues in London and Berlin, studied 417 patients with chronic heart failure and found that, on average, patients with a total cholesterol level of 232 mg/dL had a 25% higher survival rate than heart failure patients with a total cholesterol level of 193 mg/dL. Experts say a total cholesterol figure under 200 mg/dL is desirable.

Although the results of this study contradict the usual advice—"lower cholesterol is better"—they reinforce the findings from several previous studies that linked lower cholesterol levels with poorer prognosis in heart failure patients.

ONE EXPLANATION

Clark offers one explanation for the paradoxical relationship.

An intriguing notion is that the reason for the immune system activity seen in heart failure patients is that as fluid builds up in the bowels, bacteria there can escape.

It may be that cholesterol mops up any of these renegade bacteria's toxins before they set off the immune system, he says. So he discourages the use of cholesterol-lowering statins for chronic heart failure patients.

"If [health professionals] are using cholesterol-lowering statins [for heart failure patients], they are doing that without evidence that what they are doing is correct. What we say to them is get those patients with chronic heart failure to clinical trials so it can be studied further," Clark says.

CAUSE AND EFFECT NOT PROVED

However, some experts caution that lower cholesterol is not necessarily the cause of the higher mortality in heart failure patients, but could be an indicator of other factors that are at fault.

Dr. Robert Doughty, a research fellow at the University of Auckland in New Zealand, who was not connected with the study but reviewed the data, emphasized that the results cannot unequivocally prove that low cholesterol was the cause of worse outcomes in the heart failure patients.

"We must be careful about this data," says Doughty. "Just because there's an association doesn't mean there is causality. This study is important, but there is more work that needs to be done," he adds.

Lifesaving News: Cures for Ailing Hearts

Augustus O. Grant, MD, PhD, president, American Heart Association, co-director, Heart Station, and professor of medicine, Duke University Medical Center, Durham, NC.

Edwin C. Weiss, MD, clinical assistant professor of medicine, New York University School of Medicine, New York City.

Heart damage is hard to mend, but recent findings show that science is making progress.

There are defibrillators that are easier to use than a VCR, and techniques that may help a damaged heart repair itself.

One of the most exciting areas of heart research is that of stem cell transplantation, says Dr. Augustus O. Grant, president of the American Heart Association.

Hearts that are damaged—by a heart attack, for example—lose some of their ability to pump blood. The traditional treatment doctors have used has been medications to try to counteract the damage, but that method doesn't rejuvenate the heart.

Now, however, researchers can inject stem cells derived from a person's bone marrow into a damaged heart and hope cells will revitalize the heart.

Researchers are also trying to reverse heart damage by taking stem cells from a person's vein and placing them on a donated heart valve. The stem cells grow on the valve, and soon it is covered by the person's own cells. That valve replaces a pulmonary valve that regulates the flow of blood from the heart to the lungs.

The procedure has been done in a small number of people, with promising results.

Another device that is helping people who have heart trouble is public-access defibrillators. They are currently available in airports, restaurants and bus and train stations, and they are saving many lives that might otherwise have been lost.

A defibrillator is an electronic device that administers an electric shock to the heart in an attempt to restore the normal rhythm in the event of a life-threatening arrhythmia.

A new type of stent, which is used to prop open arteries, is also getting positive reviews from researchers. The stent is coated with medication that reduces the inflammation and scarring that can cause arteries that have been opened with regular stents to close again.

And dual-chamber devices, which synchronize the two chambers of the heart so it beats properly, are "clearly showing an improvement in survival in patients and an improvement in quality of life," says Dr. Edwin C. Weiss, a clinical assistant professor of medicine at New York University School of Medicine in New York City.

IT'S NOT ALL GOOD NEWS

Despite scientific advances that are helping many patients, troubling news is also on the horizon, including rising rates of obesity, diabetes and metabolic syndrome, especially in children.

One in eight children has metabolic syndrome, a risk factor for developing diabetes and heart disease, researchers report.

"Doctors really need to be on target," Weiss comments. "We need to emphasize the importance of a healthy lifestyle. It may not be a new message, but it is the most important one."

Drug-Coated Stents Reduce Heart Attack Risk by 50%

Jeffrey Moses, MD, chief, interventional cardiology, Lenox Hill Hospital, New York City.

David Faxon, MD, chief of cardiology, University of Chicago, and past president, American Heart Association. *Circulation.*

Starting in the 1990s, bare metal stents have helped keep arteries open in angioplasty patients. But these devices can provoke inflammation and scarring, which can then cause the artery to close again.

The Cypher stent, which contains an antibiotic and an anti-inflammatory agent, could be the solution to this problem, according to a recent study.

The safety of the Cypher stent, which originally used an antibiotic called *siroliumus,* was called into question after a number of patient deaths occurred. However, researchers were able to make the changes that were necessary to give the stent system a safe-to-use status.

The stents now appear to be safe and effective even in a "real world" group of individuals who are more diverse and have more complicated medical problems than those who were included in the original clinical trials, and the results could clear the way for widespread use.

After one year, results from the Rapamycin-Eluting Stent Evaluated At Rotterdam Cardiology Hospital (RESEARCH) registry showed that patients who received the drug-eluting stents had approximately half the rate of heart attacks and other major problems as those who got the old-fashioned stents.

THE STUDY

This study looked at patients who represent the real world of medical care.

A total of 508 patients were treated with the Cypher stents, and 450 patients were treated with the conventional bare metal stents. Approximately half of the individuals in each group had experienced heart attacks or angina, and 16% had diabetes.

One year after implantation, only 9.7% of the patients who had received the drug-eluting stents had experienced a heart attack or other "major adverse cardiac event." This compared with 14.8% of the patients who had received the bare metal stents.

In the drug-eluting group, 3.7% had a re-narrowing of the vessel that required a repeat procedure, compared with 10.9% in the bare-metal stent group.

"I think there has been some limitation on the use [of the drug-eluting stents], and this may open doors," says Dr. Jeffrey Moses, chief of interventional cardiology at Lenox Hill Hospital in New York City. Moses was the principal investigator on the original trial, which paved the way for US Food and Drug Administration (FDA) approval of drug-coated stents in April 2003.

"If you look at all of the studies, which would include this and the randomized trials that have been conducted, there is no higher incidence of complications than one would expect from stents that don't have drugs in them," says Dr. David Faxon, chief of cardiology at the University of Chicago.

"[Using drug-eluting stents is] not riskier than what we currently do and it has better outcomes," he adds.

info To learn about the Cypher stent, visit the Food and Drug Administration Web site at *www.fda.gov.*

On-Pump Heart Bypass Beats Off-Pump Technique

Anthony De Souza, MD, consultant cardiac surgeon, Royal Brompton Hospital, London.

Gus J. Vlahakes, MD, division of cardiac surgery, Massachusetts General Hospital, Boston.

Nirav Patel, MD, cardiac surgeon, Lenox Hill Hospital, New York City.

New England Journal of Medicine.

Heart surgery that forgoes the use of a mechanical pump has become increasingly popular over the last decade and has compared favorably with traditional on-pump surgery. However, recent research has found that fewer grafted arteries remain open in patients who have the off-pump procedure.

"Our study is the only one that has shown a major difference between patients who undergo off-pump procedures compared with those who undergo on-pump procedures," says co-researcher Dr. Anthony De Souza, a consultant cardiac surgeon at the Royal Brompton Hospital in London.

The pump is a heart-lung bypass machine. Until recently, all coronary bypass operations—and there are approximately 500,000 performed in the United States every year—were done by stopping the heart and having the machine support the body's circulation.

But many patients who had the on-pump surgery complained of symptoms such as mental confusion, memory loss and other neurological problems. Some have suffered strokes. So in recent years, more and more of these operations have been done off-pump, while the heart is still beating.

Off-pump surgery lets patients receive coronary bypass grafts without using the heart-lung machine. The technique gives surgeons access to multiple heart vessels while the heart continues to beat.

Although the quality of the cardiac bypass grafts is equal between on- and off-pump procedures, the off-pump operation is more complicated and requires more training. It is more difficult to operate on a beating heart than one that is still, De Souza notes.

THE STUDY

In their study, De Souza and his colleagues randomly assigned 50 patients to on-pump coronary artery bypass grafting and 54 to off-pump surgery.

Three months later, the researchers evaluated both groups of patients using coronary angiography.

Although the two groups fared well at the three-month checkup, 98% of the grafted arteries remained open in the on-pump group, compared with 88% of the grafts in the off-pump group, De Souza says.

"Off-pump surgery may not be the nirvana everyone professes it to be," De Souza says. "It is a good technique, but it may not completely replace on-pump surgery."

"Both operations are safe, but there are benefits and disadvantages to off-pump surgery. Patients should not demand off-pump surgery. The surgeon needs to make the decision on the basis of what is best for the individual patient," he notes.

FINDINGS RAISE QUESTIONS AND DOUBTS

Dr. Gus J. Vlahakes, from the division of cardiac surgery at Massachusetts General Hospital in Boston, says he reserves off-pump surgery for high-risk patients.

However, he finds the difference between the two techniques surprising. "This study has raised the question that graft [openness] might not be as good in patients done off-pump," Vlahakes says.

Dr. Nirav Patel, a cardiac surgeon at Lenox Hill Hospital in New York City, where 98% of the operations are done off-pump, has a different opinion.

"This paper does not really make any sense, because it is done by [a group of] surgeons who are not experienced at doing off-pump surgery," Patel explains.

He notes that De Souza's group of surgeons had only two years' experience in off-pump surgery on a total of only 98 patients before the start of the study.

"Two years and small numbers of selected patients is not enough experience to complete the learning curve," he says.

25% of People Having Angioplasty Have Strokes

Journal of the American College of Cardiology.
Journal of the American College of Cardiology news release.

One in four people undergoing carotid angioplasty and stenting procedures to open blocked arteries may have dislodged debris travel from the vessel walls to the brain.

According to a recent study, even protection devices aren't completely effective against the stroke that may result from that debris.

Carotid angioplasty and stenting each use a catheter with a balloon tip to widen the areas of reduced blood flow in the carotid artery, which runs along the neck into the head. A wire mesh tube, like a tiny scaffold, is left behind to help hold the blood vessel open.

Although angioplasty and stenting are designed to widen the artery and thereby lower heart attack and stroke risk, the treatment itself does carry a small risk of both.

THE STUDY

German researchers examined magnetic resonance imaging (MRI) scans of 42 patients before and after they had the procedures. In these patients, six different types of protection systems were used. The most common was a tiny basket filter in the carotid artery designed to catch any particles that broke loose during the angioplasty and stenting procedures.

In nine cases, the MRI scans revealed particles may have lodged in the brains of patients and interfered with blood flow, even though the patients didn't have any symptoms.

SAFER STENTS?

A more frequent problem associated with the use of stents is that the arteries have a tendency to narrow again. This phenomenon is called *restenosis* and occurs in approximately 25% of patients who are treated with conventional stents.

Heart specialists have recently developed a type of stent that is designed to reduce the risk of this common complication. These stents are covered with medication that reduces inflammation and scarring.

These drug-eluting stents have shown great promise in clinical studies, preventing restenosis more often than uncoated stents. They also appear to greatly reduce the odds that patients will require additional procedures.

However, the new stents have also had setbacks. In October 2003, the US Food and Drug Administration (FDA) issued a warning stating that the first version of drug-coated stents to win regulatory approval could cause life-threatening blood clots in some patients. The FDA received reports of more than 290 clotting cases and 60 deaths associated with the device.

New Drug Boosts Failing Hearts

Mihai Gheorghiade, MD, associate chief, cardiology, Feinberg School of Medicine, Northwestern University, Chicago.
Otsuka Maryland Research Institute Inc., Rockville, press release.
Presentation, American Heart Association Scientific Sessions 2003, Orlando.

People who have congestive heart failure may soon have a new treatment to suppress the buildup of fluid that starves them of their breath.

Heart failure patients who took the drug, *tolvaptan,* lost more weight and felt better than those who did not get the pill, recent research has found. Most of the weight loss was due to a decrease in the fluid that accumulates in people with heart failure.

THE RESULTS

"The addition of tolvaptan [to heart failure therapy] reduced body weight, mainly by relieving congestion, and made [patients] feel better," says study leader Dr. Mihai Gheorghiade, associate chief of cardiology at Northwestern University's Feinberg School of Medicine in Chicago.

The effects of the drug appeared within 24 hours of starting the treatment. The regimen called for a single pill of varying dosage for seven weeks after patients were discharged from the hospital.

The trial of 319 patients wasn't large enough to detect any increase in near-term survival from the drug. However, Gheorghiade says tolvaptan appears to reduce the number of return hospitalizations and deaths within 60 days of being admitted to the hospital with heart failure. The drug is being tested in 3,600 men and women participating in an international study to see if it can save lives.

Tolvaptan is being developed by Otsuka Maryland Research Institute Inc., which funded the latest research. The Federal Drug Administration has yet to approve the drug.

In addition to reducing fluid buildup, tolvaptan also appears to stabilize salt imbalances, or *hyponatremia,* Gheorghiade says. Hyponatremia is considered an important predictor of poor outcomes in heart failure patients. To date, he adds, there are no drugs to treat this condition—a fact that could hasten the approval of tolvaptan.

■ ■ ■ ■

Congestive Heart Failure

Approximately 1 million Americans are hospitalized each year because of congestive heart failure.

Doctors treat patients in two ways: They use drugs to improve the efficiency of their heart and they use diuretics to eliminate the excess fluid buildup.

Although current therapy is often effective, approximately one quarter of patients go back to the hospital within 60 days for more treatment—and one in 10 die.

The following are signs of heart failure you should be aware of…

●**Shortness of breath,** especially if it comes on at night or when you're lying flat.

●**Sluggishness and fatigue** that does not improve with rest.

●**Swelling in the legs and ankles,** which can indicate that the right side of your heart isn't pumping blood efficiently, allowing fluid to build up in the lower extremities.

● **Angina, or chest pain** (it can also affect the arms). Angina often happens during exercise but disappears at rest as the heart is no longer straining.

● **Loss of appetite and bloating**, which can reflect the accumulation of fluid in the digestive tract.

 For more on heart failure, try Heart Failure Online at *www.heartfailure.org.*

'Silent' Heart Arrhythmia? Pump Up Your Medicine

Albert L. Waldo, MD, professor, cardiology and medicine, Case Western Reserve University, Cleveland. *Journal of the American College of Cardiology.*

Atrial fibrillation may persist in patients who seem to have the problem under control. Therefore, treatment with an anticoagulant should be continued in patients for longer than originally believed, German researchers say.

Based on the results of their study, the German researchers recommend that doctors treat atrial fibrillation patients with the anticoagulant *warfarin* (*brand name:* Coumadin), even if patients seem to be free of heart rhythm problems for more than three months.

Standard practice is to treat episodes of atrial fibrillation with rhythm-correcting drugs and with anticoagulants until a patient has not had an episode for three months.

THE STUDY

In the study, the researchers followed up 110 patients who had atrial fibrillation. Each had a pacemaker that recorded all of their heart rhythms. The research found that 38% of those study subjects who did not report any symptoms of atrial fibrillation (which can include an irregular or rapid heartbeat felt by the patient) had a recurrence that lasted longer than 48 hours.

This so-called silent fibrillation should be treated if the patient has one other risk factor for stroke—for example, high blood pressure, diabetes or advanced age, according to the researchers.

The study confirms what other studies have also suggested. "This is one of several studies suggesting that patients put on anti-arrhythmia drugs who their doctors think are fine have silent episodes of atrial fibrillation," says Dr. Albert L. Waldo, the Walter H. Pritchard professor of cardiology and medicine at Case Western University in Cleveland.

Warfarin is not an easy drug to take, he says, because it interacts with foods and other medications, such as antibiotics, so it's difficult to keep the blood level of warfarin steady enough to be constantly effective, Waldo says. Therefore, patients taking warfarin must be closely monitored by their doctors. But even with its downsides, "warfarin is very, very effective," he adds.

■ ■ ■ ■

Problems with Warfarin

Too many atrial fibrillation patients who would benefit from warfarin are not being prescribed the medication, according to Dr. Albert L. Waldo. One major reason is that warfarin is an extremely difficult drug to manage because it interacts not only with many other medicines but also with many foods. Among other restrictions, people who take warfarin can't drink alcohol or eat broccoli, lettuce or other green, leafy vegetables.

One reason for doctors' reservations about warfarin is that any patient taking it must have a blood test every two or three weeks to be sure that the blood is thin enough to avoid clotting but not so thin as to cause dangerous bleeding, Waldo notes.

The value of the risk score for stroke in patients with atrial fibrillation would increase greatly if and when a blood thinner that is easier to manage becomes available, he says.

There is hope that a new blood thinner now in advanced clinical trials will not require the intense management of warfarin, Waldo says.

The medication, Exanta, being developed by the AstraZeneca pharmaceutical company, is being used in several large-scale trials involving thousands of patients.

Initial reports of those trials have been extremely encouraging, and there is hope that the drug will be put on a fast track for approval by the US Food and Drug Administration.

Atrial Fibrillation Cases Filling Hospitals

George A. Mensah, MD, chief of cardiovascular health programs, Centers for Disease Control and Prevention, Atlanta.

Ira S. Nash, MD, associate professor, medicine, Mount Sinai Hospital, New York City, and spokesman, American Heart Association.

Circulation, online edition.

More and more Americans are being hospitalized for the heartbeat abnormality called *atrial fibrillation,* which is bad news not only for those patients, but also for the country's public health system, federal experts report.

If these trends continue, the annual number of hospital admissions that are related to atrial fibrillation will increase to more than 3.3 million by 2025, predicts Dr. George A. Mensah, chief of cardiovascular health programs at the Centers for Disease Control and Prevention (CDC).

CONDITION CAN TRIGGER BLOOD CLOTS

Atrial fibrillation is a loss of coordinated contraction between the upper chambers of the heart, known as the atria, and the lower chambers, known as the ventricles. The atria fail to beat forcefully enough, so they don't eject enough blood. Clots can form in the remaining blood, and they can eventually enter the bloodstream and block an artery in the heart or brain, causing a heart attack or stroke.

Age is a leading risk factor for atrial fibrillation. It is also common in people who have conditions such as high blood pressure, congestive heart failure or diabetes, and in those who have had heart attacks.

Mensah and his team of researchers at the CDC looked at the National Hospital Discharge Survey, which is performed annually. One significant discovery was that more than half of the people who were hospitalized were 75 years or older.

Many of those older people were later discharged to nursing homes. That finding, along with an associated high prevalence of congestive heart failure in those patients, "presages a staggering burden on the Medicare system and the quality of life for affected persons," the report says.

"What this report says is that atrial fibrillation is becoming more of a public health problem over time," says Dr. Ira S. Nash, an associate professor of medicine at Mount Sinai Hospital in New York City and a spokesman for the American Heart Association.

FIRST PRIORITY: PREVENTION

Most efforts are aimed at battling the known risk factors. "We think there is a growing need for more aggressive attention to addressing risk factors in women—especially a focus on high blood pressure—because we have found that women are hospitalized more than men," Mensah says.

It is possible for someone to be unaware that he/she has atrial fibrillation, but most of the time there are symptoms, Nash says.

Symptoms include palpitations, a sense that the heart is beating erratically. "But sometimes people just have a decline in their physical abilities," he says.

Doctors must be alert for the signs of atrial fibrillation, which can often be subtle, Mensah says.

"There are many instances when an elderly woman goes into the hospital with [a variety of] nonspecific complaints, such as chest discomfort or shortness of breath," he explains. "If an EKG [electrocardiogram] is taken, it will show atrial fibrillation. This diagnosis always should be taken seriously. We are trying to make clinicians aware of the importance of atrial fibrillation."

New Arrhythmia Treatment Saves Lives!

Journal of the American College of Cardiology news release.
Journal of the American College of Cardiology.

According to a recent study, a high-tech method is more effective than drugs at controlling atrial fibrillation, the most common type of arrhythmia. People who have atrial fibrillation have an increased risk of fainting, stroke and heart attack.

THE STUDY

Italian researchers studied 1,171 people with atrial fibrillation—589 had the new pulmonary vein ablation technique and 582 were treated with anti-arrhythmic medications.

At a median follow-up point of 2.5 years, the survival rate for the patients who had ablation was better than for the patients who were treated with drugs. The patients in the ablation group had less than half the death rate of the other group—36 deaths (6%) in the group receiving ablation compared with 83 deaths (14%) in the group receiving medication.

THE TECHNIQUE

In the new pulmonary vein ablation technique, specific parts of the patient's heart are mapped in three-dimensional form. A catheter is then threaded through the patient's blood vessels into the area where the atrium connects to the pulmonary vein.

Radio frequency pulses emitted from the tip of the catheter produce circular scars that interrupt the abnormal electrical signals that trigger atrial fibrillation.

■ ■ ■ ■

Atrial Fibrillation Symptoms

According to the US government's National Institutes of Health, the symptoms of atrial fibrillation can come on quite suddenly. *Those symptoms include…*

●**Heart palpitations** feel like your heart is pounding or racing. You may simply have an unpleasant awareness of your own heartbeat.

Or, you may feel skipped beats. Your heart rhythm may be regular or irregular. Palpitations can be felt in your chest, throat or neck.

●**Change in the pulse rate.** It may feel rapid, racing, pounding, fluttering or too slow.

You may also experience…

●**Dizziness, light-headedness.**

●**Fainting.**

●**Confusion.**

●**Fatigue.**

●**Shortness of breath.**

●**Breathing difficulty when lying down.**

●**Sensation of tightness in the chest.**

Call your doctor if you experience any of these symptoms.

Doctors Determine Who Needs Heart Rhythm Aids

Circulation.
American Heart Association news release.

Pictures of the heart and the blood flowing around it can help doctors identify people with the most to gain from electronic implants that treat heart rhythm problems.

So says a study by Dutch scientists, who used *single photon emission computed tomography* (SPECT) and ultrasound imaging to assess the hearts of 153 people who had ventricular arrhythmias—abnormal heart rhythms originating in the heart's large pumping chambers.

The researchers concluded that the patients who had the most scarring on the heart and the greatest reduction in *left ventricular ejection fraction* (LVEF) had the greatest risk of recurrent arrhythmias. LVEF is the percentage of blood ejected with each beat, and is considered one of the most reliable measures of heart function.

Using the imaging technologies to identify patients who are at the greatest risk could lead to more efficient use of lifesaving—but expensive—implantable cardioverter-defibrillators (ICDs), the study says.

"Patients who have extensive scar tissue and LVEF less than or equal to 30% are at high risk for [arrhythmia] recurrences, and ICD implantation may be preferred in these patients," says Dr. Alida E. Borger, co-author of the study.

"This [evaluation] is very important because it can help guide patient management and might serve as a gatekeeper for the use of ICDs," co-author Dr. Jeroen J. Bax adds.

VARYING LEVELS OF SEVERITY

Arrhythmias affect millions of Americans, with varying degrees of severity. Having periodic "skipped beats" and "flutters" in the chest become increasingly common with age, according to the American Heart Association.

Typically, arrhythmias don't lead to more serious health problems. But they could. An estimated 2.2 million people in this country have atrial fibrillation, one of the most common rhythm anomalies, putting them at increased risk of strokes.

Many arrhythmias, including atrial fibrillation, can be managed with medications. Pacemakers can also correct irregular beats.

Although heart disease may be the underlying cause of an arrhythmia, it often is not. Other known causes of abnormal heartbeats include stress, caffeine, tobacco and alcohol, according to the National Institutes of Health (NIH). Diet pills, cough medicines and cold remedies also can trigger an arrhythmia. Arrhythmias can start in either the heart's atria or its ventricles.

■ ■ ■ ■

Heart Rhythm Disturbances

The NIH publishes this list of rhythm disturbances that affect the heart…

- **Sinus arrhythmia.** Cyclic changes in the heart rate during breathing. This is normal and affects both children and adults.
- **Sinus tachycardia.** The sinus node sends out electrical signals faster than usual, speeding up the heart rate.
- **Sick sinus syndrome.** The sinus node does not fire its signals properly, slowing the heart rate. The rate may vary between a slow (bradycardia) and fast (tachycardia) rate.
- **Premature supraventricular contractions** or premature atrial contractions (PAC). The atria beats prematurely.
- **Supraventricular tachycardia (SVT).** A series of early beats in the atria speed up the heart rate.
- **Atrial flutter.** Rapidly fired signals cause the muscles in the atria to contract quickly, leading to a very fast, steady heartbeat.
- **Atrial fibrillation.** Electrical signals in the atria are fired quickly and erratically. Electrical signals arrive in the ventricles irregularly, leading to an irregular rhythm.
- **Premature ventricular complexes (PVC).** An electrical signal from the ventricles causes an early heartbeat. The heart then seems to pause until the next beat of the ventricle occurs in a regular fashion.
- **Ventricular tachycardia.** The heart beats rapidly because of electrical signals arising from the ventricles rather than the atria.
- **Ventricular fibrillation.** Fast, uncontrolled electrical signals in the ventricles cause the heart to quiver rather than beat and pump blood.

Important News for Women: Get the Same Critical Heart Tests as Men

Nikolaos Dagres, MD, cardiologist, Hospital of the Westfaelische Wilhelms-University, Muenster, Germany. *Journal of the American College of Cardiology.*

Here's one more aggressive treatment to which women are referred much less often than men—*radiofrequency catheter ablation therapy,* which is used for many different heart rhythm abnormalities.

A study finds women with the same severe symptoms as men are referred an average of 28 months later than men for the treatment.

"It is my opinion that this is another example of a tendency for more conservative treatment of women," says study author Dr. Nikolaos

Dagres, a cardiologist at the Hospital of the Westfaelische Wilhelms-University in Muenster, Germany. "It probably has something to do with social opinions and habits."

THE TREATMENT

In the radiofrequency ablation procedure, a catheter is threaded through a blood vessel in the heart so that high-frequency radio waves can eliminate the cells that are causing an abnormal heart rhythm. In many cases, drug treatment is tried first.

The study looked at 894 patients who had the treatment at the University during a 43-month period.

The authors found a 28-month delay, on average, in giving ablation treatment to women with the same conditions and symptoms as men, even though the women had abnormal heart rhythms more often than the men who received the therapy. The women also had been prescribed more drugs for the condition than the men.

There was no obvious medical reason to defer ablation therapy for the women, according to Dagres.

"There is no difference in the success rates, no difference in complication rates and no difference in recurrence rates, so the outcome is the same in both sexes. But women are referred [for ablation therapy] later than men," he says.

■ ■ ■ ■

Heart Disease in Women

Heart disease is the leading cause of death for American women, killing nearly one third of them, according to the National Coalition for Women with Heart Disease.

Each year, 267,000 women in this country die from heart attacks, six times as many as those claimed by breast cancer.

Women are also more likely than men to have poor outcomes after having a heart attack. Thirty-eight percent of women, but just 25% of men, are likely to be dead within a year of a first heart attack, and 35% women,

but just 18% of men, have a second heart attack within six years of the first episode.

According to the Coalition, although more women die each year of heart disease than men, they receive less care in several areas. They're less likely to be prescribed beta-blockers, ACE inhibitors and aspirin after a heart attack. They undergo far fewer procedures, such as angioplasty, stenting and cardiac bypass. They receive only 28% of defibrillator implants and 36% of open-heart surgeries. And, the group says, women make up only one quarter of the participants in all heart-related research studies.

Exercise Testing Warns Healthy Women of Hidden Heart Trouble

Roger S. Blumenthal, MD, FACC, FCCP, director, preventive cardiology, Johns Hopkins Hospital, Baltimore.

Nieca Goldberg, MD, chief, women's cardiovascular care, Lenox Hill Hospital, New York City.

Journal of the American Medical Association.

A brief exercise test can identify apparently healthy women who are at high risk of heart attack and stroke, according to a 20-year study by physicians at Johns Hopkins Medical Institutions.

THE STUDY

The test includes two simple measures: The first is endurance, or how long a woman can keep walking as the speed of a treadmill increases. The second is the time it takes her heart rate to return to normal after 30 minutes or less of exercise.

The study examined nearly 3,000 women who had no signs of heart disease. Those who ranked in the bottom quarter of the test results were 3.5 times more likely to have a cardiovascular death than those in the upper half, say Dr. Roger S. Blumenthal and his colleagues at the Hopkins Ciccarone Preventive Cardiology Center.

"While our study suggests that an exercise test can provide a good prospective into the cardiovascular risk of women whose capacity is below normal or who have a slow return rate…it is still up to the individual doctor to determine whether an exercise test should be done," Blumenthal says.

THE MESSAGE

The message for women, he says, is that "they have to realize that if they have a low level of physical capacity, they can improve their performance and improve their cardiovascular health with regular exercise."

Dr. Nieca Goldberg, chief of women's cardiovascular care at Lenox Hill Hospital located in New York City and a spokeswoman for the American Heart Association, says, "There has been a lot of controversy about the value of exercise testing in women. We are always looking for ways to determine heart disease risk in women. This test is readily available and cost-effective."

The American Heart Association and other health organizations have been trying to get women to pay more attention to the risk of cardiovascular disease, the leading cause of death in American women and men.

TEST IS APPROPRIATE FOR ALL WOMEN

Women should undergo an exercise test if they have heart disease. But the test should also be considered for symptom-free women "who have multiple risk factors, such as obesity, smoking or diabetes, those women who are totally sedentary and over 50, and those who are thinking of starting an exercise program," Goldberg says.

A poor result on this exercise test should prompt a woman to begin a regular exercise program under a doctor's supervision. And it also should serve as a warning sign that "it is time to start paying attention to all the risk factors, keeping blood pressure under control, lowering cholesterol and not smoking," Goldberg says.

A brisk half-hour walk every day can be enough to promote heart health for most people, cardiologists say.

Air Travel Blood Clot Risk Only Slightly Elevated

Thomas Schwarz, department of vascular medicine, University Hospital of Dresden, Germany.
Archives of Internal Medicine.

Sitting in a cramped plane for hours may be more than just uncomfortable and tiring. Three studies have confirmed that air travel increases the risk of potentially deadly blood clots. Advanced age, oral contraceptive use and being overweight heighten the risk even more. But overall, the risk is mild, the researchers say, adding that the findings do "not justify social alarm."

THE STUDIES

In one study from the University of Milano in Italy, researchers evaluated 210 patients who had *venous thromboembolism* (VTE)—a syndrome in which blood clots form in the veins—and compared them with 210 healthy people. During the month before the study, 15% of those with clots had flown, compared with 8% of the control subjects.

Although 15% may sound like a high percentage, the researchers concluded that air travel is a "mild risk factor" for VTE. In comparison, they found that oral contraceptive use increased the risk of blood clot problems 14-fold, and those with genetic or other risk factors for VTE were 16 times more likely to get clots.

In another study, researchers from Germany evaluated 964 passengers who had returned from flights of eight hours or more, comparing them with 1,213 people who didn't fly. Long-haul flights doubled the risk for isolated calf muscle VTE, the researchers say.

In the third study, Spanish researchers reviewed cases of lung blood clots—called pulmonary embolisms—in passengers arriving at Madrid-Baraja Airport. They found 16 cases of pulmonary embolisms over a six-year span. All of the people who had pulmonary embolisms had been on flights of more than six hours.

SELF-DEFENSE

"More research is necessary in this field," says Dr. Thomas Schwarz, in the department of vascular medicine at University Hospital of Dresden, Germany, who led the German study. "For passengers at risk [those who have a high body mass index, are older or have had previous clots], stretching exercises are important." Also important is drinking nonalcoholic beverages to stay hydrated.

"Videotapes on how to practice stretching exercises should be mandatory on all airlines on long-haul flights," he adds.

info For information on blood clot problems, visit the British Heart Foundation at *www.bhf.org.uk/questions*. Click on "Heart Block" under the "Medical" category.

Deaths from Lung Clots Are Dropping

Samuel Z. Goldhaber, MD, director, Venous Thromboembolism Research Group and Anticoagulation Service, Brigham and Women's Hospital, and associate professor, medicine, Harvard Medical School, Boston.

Kenneth T. Horlander, MD, physician, pulmonary and critical care medicine, department of pulmonary medicine, Clarke-Holder Clinic, LaGrange, GA.

Archives of Internal Medicine.

Deaths from pulmonary emboli—blood clots in the lungs—have been steadily declining in recent decades. And a new study has found that the rate fell about 30% over a 20-year period.

Nevertheless, the number of deaths caused by these clots remains consistently higher among the African-American population and among men, according to the study.

The findings point out the need for more prevention in high-risk groups, experts say.

"The encouraging news is that the death rate from pulmonary embolism is falling," says Dr. Samuel Goldhaber, director of the Venous Thromboembolism Research Group and Anticoagulation Service at Brigham and Women's Hospital in Boston.

It's not clear why an overall decrease took place. Better preventive measures, detection and treatment along with a decrease in risk factors might be at least partially responsible.

"The death rate is still substantial," says Goldberg, "and we should probably start shifting our focus more to prevention. In my opinion, we still have an unacceptably high death rate for pulmonary embolism."

Health care practitioners often fail to recognize clotting of a lung artery, or pulmonary thromboembolism (PTE). "They're one of the masqueraders," says study author Dr. Kenneth T. Horlander, a pulmonary and critical care medicine physician with Clarke–Holder Clinic in LaGrange, Georgia. "It can go untreated and then we have higher mortality."

The other issue that is confusing is that no one seems to know exactly how many people die from pulmonary embolism. Estimates vary from 50,000 to 100,000 deaths annually. Horlander undertook this study largely to try to narrow this wide range of estimates.

THE STUDY

Horlander's group reviewed almost 43 million death certificates that listed PTE as a cause of death. These death certificates were part of files that were compiled by the National Center for Health Statistics over a period of 20 years. Almost 600,000, or 1.3%, listed PTE as the cause of death and, of those, almost 200,000—or about one third—listed PTE as an underlying cause of death.

During the 20-year period, mortality rates for African-Americans were consistently 50% higher than the mortality rates for Caucasians. And the mortality rates for Caucasians were consistently 50% higher than those for people of other races, such as Asian and American Indian. Within each racial group, mortality rates were 20% to 30% higher for men than for women.

Horlander speculates that how long a person waits to seek care and their initial treatment might affect outcomes.

Surgery, many forms of cancer, old age, trauma, obesity, inflammatory bowel disease and long plane trips appear to be risk factors for PTE.

info For information on the prevention of pulmonary embolism, visit the Mayo Clinic's Web site at *www.mayoclinic.com*. Click on "Pulmonary Embolism" under "Diseases & Conditions."

'Hot Pepper' May Treat Angina

Journal of Physiology.
Penn State news release.

The same type of nerve receptors that are in your mouth that tell you peppers are scorchers may also be responsible for chest pain during a heart attack, a Penn State College of Medicine study says.

"Our study is the first to demonstrate that the 'hot pepper' receptor exists on the heart and may be responsible for triggering heart attack chest pain," says researcher Dr. Hui-Lin Pan, a professor of anesthesiology.

"Until now, the capsaicin, or hot pepper receptor, was only known for sensing heat and pain from the skin. Our data suggest that the hot pepper receptors could become a new target for the treatment of some types of chronic chest pain, such as angina pectoris, that are resistant to other treatments," Pan says.

THE STUDY

Working with rats, Pan and his team found evidence that suggests these receptors—called VR1 receptors—trigger the cardiovascular and nerve responses of a heart attack, including chest pain.

Pan plans to search for the chemicals produced by the heart tissue during a heart attack and examine how they interact with the VR1 receptors.

Valvular Heart Disease Is Often Missed During Annual Physicals

Jeffrey Borer, MD, director, Howard Gilman Institute for Valvular Heart Diseases, Weill Medical College of Cornell University, New York City.

By age 70, half of all Americans have valvular heart disease. Caused by either a leaky aortic valve or a stenotic valve (when the valve doesn't open properly), this condition can lead to heart failure or sudden death. If a doctor uses a stethoscope only on the front of the chest he/she may not detect the telltale sounds of a heart murmur.

Better: Your doctor must examine you in the *left lateral decubitus* position, in which you're lying on your left side at a 45-degree angle to the examining table.

If a murmur is detected, you should receive an echocardiogram. Treatment includes medication or surgery.

11

Natural Remedies

Grandma Knows Best: Old-Fashioned Cures Are Best for Kids!

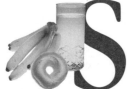Some old-fashioned home remedies may work as well, or better, than commercial remedies for treating common ailments, a doctor says. Dr. Kenneth Haller, an assistant professor of pediatrics at Saint Louis University School of Medicine in Missouri, suggests that sometimes you should "turn back the clock and listen to what your Grandma recommended."

Following are some of Haller's favorite old-fashioned treatments…

•**Dab a bit of roll-on antiperspirant on mosquito bites.** The aluminum salts that are in the antiperspirant help the body reabsorb the fluid in the bug bite, and thereby reduce the swelling and itching.

•**Freeze a bagel or washcloth** and give it to a teething child to gum.

•**Mix a quarter teaspoon of salt in a half cup of water** and use a dropper or spray the solution into a stuffy nose. It helps clean out nasal mucus that holds pollens and virus bugs.

•**Drink plenty of fluids when you have a sore throat.** A dried-out throat is more likely to get infected.

•**Mix a solution of half vinegar and half water for swimmer's ear.** Put the solution in the ear and then let it drain out.

•**For a child with diarrhea,** feed him/her plenty of starches and the BRAT (bananas, rice, applesauce and toast) diet. For constipation, avoid starchy foods and serve plenty of fruits and vegetables, other high-fiber foods and water.

•**Massage the bridge of the nose** a few times every day and alternate warm compresses on each eye to treat pink eye. This condition is often caused by a blockage in the

---

St. Louis University Health Sciences Center news release.

The National Center for Complementary and Alternative Medicine.

212

ducts that drain tears away. If it does not clear in two days, call your doctor.

●**To prevent ear wax accumulation,** put a solution of half water and half peroxide in the ears once a month. Never use cotton swabs to remove ear wax—they just push wax deeper into the ears.

The medical establishment is more accepting of these time-tested treatments. In fact, the US government's National Institutes of Health (NIH) has begun extensive research into what natural remedies really work.

■ ■ ■ ■

The Official Word on Alternative Therapies

Here are the National Institutes of Health's (NIH) answers to questions people frequently ask about complementary and alternative medicine (CAM)…

●**How can I find reliable information about a CAM therapy?** Talk to your health care practitioner. Tell him/her about the therapy you are considering and ask questions about safety, effectiveness or interactions with medications (prescription or nonprescription). Your health-care provider may know about the therapy and be able to advise you on its safety and use.

●**How can I do research?** Use the Internet to search medical libraries and databases for information. Visit your local library or a medical library for books or publications that contain scientific articles discussing CAM or the treatment in which you are interested. Thousands of articles on health issues are published every year. A reference librarian may be able to help you search for ones on the therapy that interests you.

●**Are dietary supplements safe?** The manufacturer of a dietary supplement is responsible for ensuring the safety and effectiveness of the product. The US Food and Drug Administration (FDA) cannot require testing of dietary supplements prior to marketing. However, the FDA can remove a product from the marketplace if the product is found to be dangerous to the health of Americans.

●**How can I determine whether statements made about the effectiveness of a CAM therapy are true?** Visit the FDA online at *www.fda.gov* for information about the product or practice. Information about dietary supplements can be found on the FDA's Center for Food Safety and Applied Nutrition Web site at *www.cfsan.fda.gov.* Or visit the FDA's Web page on recalls and safety alerts at *www. fda.gov/opacom/7alerts.html.*

Check with the Federal Trade Commission (FTC) at *www.ftc.gov* to see if there are any fraudulent claims or consumer alerts regarding the therapy. Visit the Diet, Health, and Fitness Consumer Information Web site at *www.ftc. gov/bcp/menu-health.htm.*

info Visit the National Center for Complementary and Alternative Medicine (NCCAM) Web site at *http://nccam.nih.gov,* or call the NCCAM Clearinghouse toll-free at 888-644-6226 to see if NCCAM has information or scientific findings about the therapy.

Vitamin C May Help Block Ulcers

Joel A. Simon, MD, MPH, FACN, associate professor, clinical medicine and epidemiology, University of California, San Francisco School of Medicine, and staff physician, San Francisco Veterans Affairs Medical Center.
James Everhart, MD, chief, epidemiology and clinical trials branch, division of digestive diseases and nutrition, National Institute of Diabetes & Digestive & Kidney Diseases, National Institutes of Health, Bethesda, MD.
Journal of the American College of Nutrition.

People who consume large amounts of vitamin C to try to protect themselves from colds might also be defending their stomach and intestines against ulcers.

The higher a person's blood levels of ascorbic acid, another name for vitamin C, the lower their risk of gastrointestinal trouble, according to a study.

"We are not the first to show this," admits Dr. Joel A. Simon, an associate professor of clinical medicine and epidemiology at the University of California San Francisco School of Medicine and a staff physician at the San Francisco Veterans Affairs Medical Center. "But it could be the largest study" so far.

Simon and his team of researchers examined the Third National Health and Nutrition Examination Survey (NHANES III), and discovered almost one third of the 6,746 adults who were evaluated had antibodies against *Helicobacter pylori*. This strain of bacteria is now believed to cause most peptic ulcers. Chronic infection with *H. pylori* is an important risk factor, Simon notes, for both peptic ulcer problems and gastric cancer.

Researchers found that higher blood levels of ascorbic acid in the people studied were associated with lower rates of H. pylori infection, Simon says.

After the researchers accounted for factors that might affect the relationship, including age and body mass index, they still found that the subjects with the highest blood levels of ascorbic acid, had a 25% lower risk of having the infection.

When the researchers looked at infection with especially virulent strains of H. pylori, there was a 69% lower risk for those with higher blood levels of ascorbic acid.

NO CAUSE-EFFECT LINK DISCOVERED YET...

Simon does not know why vitamin C may work, although animal studies have found that ascorbic acid inhibits the growth of H. pylori. If there is a true association, he says, higher intakes of vitamin C might help prevent infection and, in turn, ulcers. Simon's study was supported by a donation from Roche Vitamins Inc. and a Public Health Service grant.

"It's an interesting finding," says Dr. James Everhart, chief of the epidemiology and clinical trials branch of the division of digestive diseases and nutrition at the National Institute of Diabetes & Digestive & Kidney Diseases. "But I think the results were not terribly strong." And it still doesn't prove cause and effect, he adds.

Every year, there are as many as 500,000 new cases of peptic ulcer disease in the United States, according to the American Gastroenterological Association. In addition to infection, many ulcers are the result of irritation from nonsteroidal anti-inflammatory drugs (NSAIDs), such as aspirin and ibuprofen.

Contrary to popular belief, ulcers are not caused by eating spicy food.

info For information on H. pylori and ulcers, visit the National Digestive Diseases Information Clearinghouse at *http:// digestive.niddk.nih.gov*.

■ ■ ■ ■

Food Sources Plentiful for Vitamin C

The National Institutes of Health Medline-Plus library says there's no shortage of vitamin C available in foods...

Vitamin C is found in green peppers, citrus fruits and juices, strawberries, tomatoes, broccoli, turnip greens and other greens, sweet and white potatoes and cantaloupe.

Most other fruits and vegetables contain a small amount of vitamin C. Fish and milk also contain small amounts.

The current Recommended Daily Allowance (RDA) for vitamin C is 60 milligrams (mg) a day, a number originally set in 1980 and reviewed in 1989 by the Food and Nutrition Board, a part of the National Academy of Sciences.

The RDA is based on the amount of vitamin C that is needed to prevent scurvy, a potentially fatal disease that is marked by fatigue and bleeding.

However, research from the National Institutes of Health (NIH) shows that healthy adults may benefit from a daily intake of 100 to 200 milligrams of vitamin C.

SUPPLEMENTS MAY HELP, TOO

There also has been much debate regarding the use of vitamin C supplements in cancer and heart disease prevention. Although the evidence is mixed, it is still encouraged that individuals maintain adequate intake.

And—surprise!—most of the current evidence does not support vitamin C's role in the prevention or treatment of the common cold.

Fight Secondhand Smoke With Vitamin C

Marion Dietrich, PhD, epidemiological researcher, University of California at Berkeley.

Linda Ford, MD, allergist and immunologist, Omaha, NE, and former president, American Lung Association.

Nutrition and Cancer.

Vitamin C already has a great reputation for its health benefits, and now research shows it may ward off some of the effects of secondhand smoke. But don't rush to the vitamin aisle yet. Although the author of the study says the findings are reason enough to embrace vitamin C, other experts are more cautious.

Previous research has suggested vitamin C may prevent some of the destructive effects of molecules known as free radicals. These molecules, found in tobacco smoke, damage cells by exposing them to dangerous amounts of oxygen. The oxidation is associated with smoking-related disorders such as clogged arteries, cancer and heart disease.

THE STUDY

California researchers studied the effects of vitamin C on 67 nonsmokers, who are regularly exposed to secondhand smoke. Most were spouses of smokers, and most were exposed to the smoke of at least nine cigarettes per day, says study author Marion Dietrich, an epidemiological researcher at the University of California at Berkeley.

One group of the nonsmoking subjects took 500 milligrams (mg) of vitamin C each day. That's a common amount found in over-the-counter supplements. Another group took a placebo, and the final group took daily doses of a specially created supplement made of vitamin C, vitamin E and an antioxidant called *alpha-lipoic acid.*

After two months, researchers analyzed the level of a chemical linked to oxidation, called F2-isoprostanes. Its level dropped by 11% and 13%, respectively, for the nonsmokers who took vitamin C or the vitamin mixture compared with those who took the placebo.

Meanwhile, the level of vitamin C in the bloodstream increased by 32% among those study subjects who took the plain vitamin C and by 41% among those who took the combination supplement.

"If you cannot escape secondhand smoke, then you should at least have a very healthful diet with lots of fruits and vegetables that can give you a good amount of vitamin C," Dietrich says. An alternative would be to take a vitamin C supplement, she adds.

"It's taking a big leap of faith to go that far," says Dr. Linda Ford, an allergist and immunologist and former president of the American Lung Association.

She isn't convinced by the data because it doesn't show that vitamin C reduces any kind of disease. Only a long-term study in humans would prove that, she says. Instead, she recommends stepping up your efforts to avoid tobacco smoke.

info For more information on the many benefits of vitamin C, go to the Food and Drug Administration's Web site at *www.fda.gov.*

■ ■ ■ ■

Secondhand Smoke, Firsthand Disease

As more and more information has emerged through research, the dangers of secondhand smoke have become more evident. The risk to children is especially significant.

These findings from the US Environmental Protection Agency (EPA) outline the government's position on the dangers of secondhand smoke...

●**Infants and young children** whose parents are smokers among the most seriously affected by exposure to secondhand smoke, being at increased risk of lower respiratory tract infections such as pneumonia and bronchitis. The EPA estimates that passive smoking is responsible for between 150,000 and 300,000 lower respiratory tract infections annually in infants and children younger than 18 months, resulting in between 7,500 and 15,000 hospitalizations each year.

•**Passive smoking** can lead to a buildup of fluid in the middle ear, the most common reason for the hospitalization of children for an operation.

•**Children who have asthma** are especially at risk. EPA estimates that exposure to secondhand smoke increases the number of episodes and severity of symptoms in hundreds of thousands of asthmatic children. The EPA estimates that between 200,000 and 1,000,000 asthmatic children have their condition made worse by exposure to secondhand smoke.

Vitamin D May Protect Against Colon Cancer

Durado Brooks, MD, director of colorectal cancer, American Cancer Society, Dallas.

David A. Lieberman, MD, professor of medicine, and chief of gastroenterology, Portland VA Medical Center, Oregon.

Journal of the American Medical Association.

A new study says vitamin D can help you avoid the polyps that can lead to colon cancer.

"Because of the interplay between calcium and vitamin D, it has been difficult to tease out what was important. And this study goes a good way toward strongly suggesting that vitamin D is an important protective factor, while the calcium question still remains somewhat open," says Dr. Durado Brooks, director of colorectal cancer at the American Cancer Society.

Colorectal cancer—or cancer that begins in either the colon or the rectum—is the second-leading cancer killer in America. Because virtually all colon cancers start as polyps, the key is to find these abnormal growths before they become malignant.

Many doctors believe that screening—as well as healthy lifestyle factors—could prevent many of the 57,000 deaths caused by colon cancer each year.

THE STUDY

Researchers looked at 3,121 people aged 50 to 75 years from 13 Veterans Administration medical centers across the country. All the participants were symptom-free and almost all were men. Each person was first given a screening colonoscopy to detect the presence of polyps.

"About 10% had serious colon polyps, the kind that could develop into cancer over time," says Dr. David Lieberman, lead author of the study and the chief of gastroenterology at Portland VA Medical Center in Oregon.

"We have evidence that if we detect and remove polyps we can actually prevent most cancers. This data emphasizes the importance of getting screened when you feel perfectly fine," he says.

The study participants also gave detailed information regarding family history of colon cancer, as well as diet and exercise.

Participants who had a first-degree relative with colon cancer had a 66% increased risk of polyps; those who smoked had an 85% increased risk. People who drank at least seven alcoholic drinks every week had a slightly increased risk.

On the positive side, participants who consumed more than 4.2 grams of cereal fiber per day had a lower risk of serious colon polyps, as did people who took a daily aspirin and more than 645 international units (IUs) of vitamin D each day.

Physical activity, daily multivitamins and calcium had smaller positive effects. Overall, though, the effects were mild.

Although the study didn't prove that any particular factors changed the risk of getting cancer, the authors suggest taking steps that may lower your risks.

Those steps are: getting regular exercise, taking multiple vitamins and adding more fiber and vitamin D to your diet. Vitamin D can be found in fortified milk and in cod liver oil, salmon, mackerel and sardines. You also can get the optimal amount of vitamin D by taking a multivitamin and a calcium/vitamin D supplement, Lieberman says. And you can increase your fiber intake by eating more fruits, vegetables and whole grains.

info For more information on colon cancer, visit the National Cancer Institute at *www.cancer.gov.*

Three Minerals that Help Lower Blood Pressure

Daniel Jones, MD, dean, School of Medicine, University of Mississippi Medical Center, Jackson.

Marlene Most, PhD, RD, associate professor, Pennington Biomedical Research Center, Louisiana State University, Baton Rouge.

Abstract, American Heart Association meeting, Washington, DC.

I f you have high blood pressure, you might be scouring food labels for the sodium content. But you might want to broaden your search.

Researchers explain that while salt may raise blood pressure, its effect appears to be worsened in people who fail to take enough calcium, potassium, magnesium and some other beneficial nutrients.

THE STUDY

The research looked at diet and high blood pressure in tens of thousands of Americans participating in a series of nutrition surveys between 1980 and 2000.

In the surveys, sodium intake did not seem to have a major impact on blood pressure—though calcium consumption drove it down. People who reported eating more calcium, potassium and magnesium tended to have lower blood pressure than those who ate less of these nutrients.

When salt does have an impact on blood pressure, the researchers say, it appears to reflect a poor intake of the other nutrients.

But, Dr. Daniel Jones, dean of the School of Medicine at the University of Mississippi and a spokesman for the heart group, says more convincing evidence in other studies points to a stronger effect of salt on blood pressure. "The best data available from clinical trials simply tells us something different," Jones says. "This shouldn't sway medical practice."

DANGERS OF HIGH BLOOD PRESSURE

A quarter of all American adults, and two-thirds of those older than 65 years, have high blood pressure—considered a reading of at least 140/90 millimeters of mercury (mmHg). Elevated blood pressure is linked to strokes, heart attacks, kidney failure and a host of other serious health problems.

Obesity, stress, alcohol abuse and lack of exercise all raise the risk of high blood pressure. Heavy salt intake has also been linked to the condition, though the effect appears to be greater in certain people with a genetic susceptibility to salt.

CONFIRMS OTHER FINDINGS

Marlene Most, a dietitian at Louisiana State University's Pennington Biomedical Research Center has studied the impact of nutrition on blood pressure. The latest work, Most says, mirrors what she and colleagues have found in previous research.

One prior study compared the effects on blood pressure of different diets with varying amounts of salt. It found that while reducing sodium intake did seem to lower blood pressure, increased consumption of potassium, calcium and magnesium did, too.

"It seems to be the combination of those nutrients, working in concert," that keeps blood pressure in check, Most says. "My feeling is that there might be other things in food that we don't know about" that also control blood pressure—unstudied chemicals in vegetables, for example.

WHAT TO DO

So why not load up on diet supplements to drive down blood pressure? "It won't work," Most says. "You need this multitude of minerals or perhaps these other components from foods" to get the effect.

To get these nutrients in your diet, load up on fruits and vegetables. Milk and other dairy products are excellent sources of calcium.

The National Institutes of Health (NIH) recommends that people eat a maximum of 2,400 milligrams (mg) of salt a day, or about two teaspoon's worth. Ideally, the experts say, salt intake should be about 1,500 mg per day, or about two thirds of a teaspoon.

Although it may be relatively easy to stop salting food at the table, the trick is avoiding sodium in packaged and processed items such as soups and frozen dinners.

info For more on the dangers of high blood pressure, visit the National Heart, Lung and Blood Institute at *www.nhlbi.nih.gov/hbp.*

■ ■ ■ ■

Beneficial Minerals for Your Diet

Here are the most healthful minerals, according to the National Medical Library.

Caution: The toxicity level describes the symptoms you might experience if you take too much, showing there *can* be too much of good thing.

CALCIUM

Sources: Milk and milk products (yogurt, cheese, etc.), tofu, broccoli, calcium-fortified orange juice, some fortified cereals.

Benefits: Helps build strong bones and teeth; involved in muscle contractions and nerve function.

Toxicity level: Muscle and abdominal pain; calcium kidney stones.

CHROMIUM

Sources: Egg yolks, meat, whole grains, cheese.

Benefits: Works with insulin for proper glucose metabolism.

Toxicity level: None known.

IRON

Sources: Red meat, seafood and fish, dried apricots, dried beans, fortified cereals.

Benefits: Helps carry oxygen to body tissues including muscle; supplement usually recommended during pregnancy.

Toxicity level: Liver disease, arrhythmias.

PHOSPHORUS

Sources: Dairy products, egg yolks, meat, poultry, fish, legumes, soft drinks.

Benefits: Works with calcium to build and maintain bones and teeth; helps convert food to energy.

Toxicity level: Lowers blood calcium.

POTASSIUM

Sources: Milk and yogurt, many fruits and vegetables (especially oranges, bananas, and potatoes).

Benefits: Vital for muscle contractions and nerve transmission; important for heart and kidney function; helps regulate fluid balance and blood pressure.

Toxicity level: Slower heart beat, kidney failure.

ZINC

Sources: Seafood, meats, eggs, whole grains.

Benefits: Important in function of many enzymes; important for wound healing.

Toxicity level: Nausea, vomiting, abdominal pain.

Fish Oil May Prevent Severe Weight Loss in Cancer Patients

Gut.
BMJ Specialist Journals news release.
Go Ask Alice!, Columbia University Health Question and Answer Internet Service.
Neurology.

Fish oil may help prevent a condition that leads to the severe weight loss experienced by people with some types of advanced cancer, a British study says.

The condition, called *cachexia,* is caused by changes in metabolism and appetite loss, and is a major factor in the illness and death of patients who have advanced cancer.

THE STUDY

A study of fish oil included 200 people with pancreatic cancer. Slightly more than half the patients (105) received a high-calorie, high-protein liquid supplement, and the other 95 received an energy-dense, high-protein liquid supplement enriched with fish oil (an omega-3 essential fatty acid) and vitamins E and C. Each group drank 480 milligrams (mg) per day for eight weeks.

Omega-3 essential fatty acids can also be found in flax oil, pumpkin seeds and walnuts.

Prior to the study, the patients had lost approximately 17% of their body weight and were losing more than 3 kilograms of weight per month. After eight weeks of taking the supplements, the weight loss had stopped in both groups.

When the researchers examined the data more closely, they found a significant association between the amount of weight and muscle bulk gained and the amount of fish oil supplement consumed.

Patients taking the fish oil supplement also reported a much-improved quality of life.

The researchers say further research is necessary to confirm their findings.

Previous studies have shown that fish oil consumption lowers blood pressure and reduces the risk of heart attack and stroke. There's also strong evidence that the omega-3s can help memory.

Researchers from University Medical Center Utrecht found that people who ate large amounts of foods rich in omega-3 polyunsaturated fatty acids and consumed a lot of fatty fish had a 19% lower risk for impaired brain functioning and a 28% lower risk for impaired brain speed than those who didn't follow a similar diet. Conversely, those with diets high in cholesterol were found to have a "significantly" increased risk (27%) of impaired memory.

■ ■ ■ ■

Where to Find Omega-3s

According to Columbia University's *Go Ask Alice!* column, the best fish to eat for the omega-3 essential fatty acids are…

- **Salmon.**
- **Mackerel.**
- **Rainbow and lake trout.**
- **Sardines.**
- **Halibut.**
- **Oysters albacore,** blue fin and yellow fin tuna.
- **Striped sea bass.**
- **Turbot.**
- **Swordfish.**

info For more information about cachexia and how to cope with it, visit the American Cancer Society at *www.cancer.org*.

Cheers! Red Wine Wards Off Breast Cancer

Shiuan Chen, PhD, director of surgical research, City of Hope Cancer Center, Los Angeles.
Cancer Research.

Red wine may do more than reduce the risk of heart disease. The grape skin and seeds appear to contain a natural cancer-fighting chemical that could block the development of breast tumors, California researchers have found.

THE RESEARCH

Scientists at City of Hope Cancer Center in Los Angeles isolated a plant substance, or phytochemical, called procyanidin B dimer, that reduced the size of tumors when given to mice with breast cancer.

Although there are drugs available that can slow the growth of breast cancers that thrive on the hormone estrogen, this is the first naturally occurring phytochemical that appears to have the same effect, says study author Shiuan Chen.

"It was surprising that we were able to identify this chemical in a natural source," says Chen, director of surgical research at City of Hope. "Further, there was a pretty significant reduction of tumor size in all the mice, and a number of animals ended up with no tumors."

However, Chen explains that natural phytochemicals are more likely to be used in a preventive way than as treatment for breast cancer because existing drugs are far stronger.

"We are talking about prevention," he says. "By having this in the diet, one can keep the estrogen at a lower level, which can be preventive for breast cancer."

For postmenopausal women who have breast cancer tumors that are fueled by estrogen (approximately 75% of breast cancers in this age group), estrogen-suppressing therapy is aimed at the estrogen produced outside of the ovaries, in peripheral tissue like fat and skin cells, Chen says.

Medications such as anastrozole, letrozole and exemestane, which are taken in pill form, reduce the activity of an enzyme called *aromatase* that is key to the production of estrogen. The estrogen is no longer available to breast cancer tumors, inhibiting their growth.

The phytochemicals work in the same way as these drugs, but have the advantage of naturally occurring in the skins and seeds of grapes, Chen says.

Chen cautions that the research is based on an animal study, and that he's conducting clinical trials on postmenopausal women to confirm any benefit to humans.

He notes that, for normal, healthy women, a glass of red wine a day or eating grapes with skins and seeds may just reduce the overall circulation of estrogen in the body.

WHY NOT WHITE?

Why does red wine, not white, confer this potential benefit?

Chen says red wine is made by fermenting not just the juice from a wine grape, but the skin and seeds as well, which is where the phytochemical is located. White wine is most often made by using just the juice from the grape and discarding the skin and seeds, he says.

info For more news on treating breast cancer, visit the National Institutes of Health at *www.nih.gov*.

Protect Yourself from Infections—and Perhaps Cancer—with Tea!

Jack F. Bukowski, MD, PhD, assistant professor, medicine, Harvard Medical School, and staff rheumatologist, Brigham and Women's Hospital, both in Boston.

Hasan Mukhtar, PhD, Helfaer professor of cancer research and director and vice chairman, research, department of dermatology, University of Wisconsin, Madison.

Joseph Simrany, president, Tea Council of the USA, New York City.

Presentations, American Chemical Society national meeting, New York City.

D rink tea. And drink lots of it. Black tea. Green tea. Iced or hot. If you don't want to drink it, rub it on your skin.

Approximately a dozen studies presented to the American Chemical Society expounded on the health benefits of the beverage, ranging from trimming fat to fighting cancer.

IMMUNE SYSTEM PROTECTION

In what might be the first study that links immunity with tea, researchers in Boston discovered people who drank five to six cups of black tea each day appeared to get a boost in that part of the immune system that acts as a first line of defense against infection.

Dr. Jack F. Bukowski, an assistant professor of medicine at Harvard Medical School and staff rheumatologist at Brigham and Women's Hospital, and his colleagues asked non-tea drinking, non-coffee drinking volunteers to consume five to six cups of black tea infusion or instant coffee for either two or four weeks. They took blood samples and tested the activity of the immune system against bacteria.

THE RESULTS

"We found that the samples taken after they drank tea were able to react against the bacteria fivefold better," Bukowski says. "But we did not go on to show that drinking tea actually protects you against getting sick." That will be the subject of the next study.

Although the tea can't be viewed as a cure, it could be viewed "almost as a vitamin for the immune system," Bukowski says.

TUMOR PROTECTION?

Another study discovered that mice that had been genetically engineered to develop prostate cancer, and drank the equivalent of about six cups of tea a day, did not develop tumors. "Those animals who drank tea were substantially protected and they lived longer," says study author Hasan Mukhtar, a professor of cancer research at the University of Wisconsin in Madison. No one knows if the same mechanism will be at play in humans, but Mukhtar says he suspects that tea will have some effect in some patients.

"China has the lowest prostate cancer rate in the world and Japan's rate is also very low, and they drink much more tea," he notes.

REDUCES BODY FAT

Another study found that a green tea extract reduced body fat in mice, possibly by inhibiting the absorption of fats and starches, and that drinking green tea may mitigate DNA damage from smoking that leads to mouth cancer. Still other researchers are working on developing a cream made up of tea polyphenols, which would ward off skin cancer.

Finally, researchers in Boston found that drinking tea improved the function of blood vessels and platelets, and consequently, may reduce the risk of heart attack and stroke. This result adds to an already large body of knowledge on tea and heart health.

"The results of studies on tea have been quite positive along a whole array of human ailments with the strongest appearing to be cardiovascular," says Joseph Simrany, president of the Tea Council of the USA in New York City.

info To learn more about the benefits of tea, visit the UK Tea Council at *www.teahealth.co.uk.*

∎ ∎ ∎ ∎

A Good Cuppa

A good cup of tea may be more than just a pleasurable drink, especially if it's black, green or red tea. According to John Hopkins' *Health After 50* newsletter, highly concentrated forms of these teas may lower LDL or "bad" cholesterol. *Here's how you can maximize the flavor of your home brews…*

- **Using one tea bag or one teaspoon of loose tea per cup.**

- **Using fresh, cold water.**

- **For black tea,** heat the water to a rolling boil, but for green tea, heat the water only to the boiling point.

- **Pre-warm your cup or pot.**

- **Steep green tea for about two minutes,** black for five to 10 minutes.

Cranberries May Stop Stroke Damage

Catherine C. Neto, PhD, assistant professor, chemistry and biochemistry, University of Massachusetts–Dartmouth, North Dartmouth.

Presentation, American Chemical Society national meeting, New York City.

Scientists have found preliminary evidence that cranberries may reduce the cellular damage left by strokes.

Cranberries contain high levels of antioxidants and have previously been shown to have health benefits with regard to urinary tract infections and possibly even cancer and heart disease.

"What they're looking at is neuroprotection, which is trying to minimize damage at the time the stroke is happening," says Dr. Keith Siller, director of the New York University Comprehensive Stroke Care Center. "This study tries to do this."

THE STUDY

The authors of this study, which was partially funded by the Cranberry Institute, an industry group, cultivated rat brain cells and exposed them to conditions similar to those experienced by a human brain during and after an *ischemic* stroke (one that cuts off the blood supply to the brain). One group of cells was deprived of oxygen and glucose in order to simulate a stroke. The other group of cells was exposed to hydrogen peroxide, which simulates what happens after oxygen to the brain starts flowing again. During this latter phase, even more brain cell damage occurs.

The cells were further divided into groups that each received different concentrations of cranberry juice. Exposure to the highest concentration of extract (about the same as half a cup of whole cranberries) caused a 50% reduction in brain cell death.

The researchers aren't sure exactly why the berries have this salutary effect, but they do have theories.

"Cranberries have numerous compounds that are really strong antioxidants which neutralize free radicals that cause damage to tissues and cells," says study author Catherine C. Neto, an assistant professor of chemistry and biochemistry at the University of Massachusetts –Dartmouth.

After blood flow reestablishes itself after a stroke, there appears to be a high concentration of free radicals that add to the damage caused by the stopped blood flow. "Antioxidants might be neutralizing free radicals that are generated and reducing oxidative damage," Neto says.

OTHER BERRIES GOOD, TOO

A separate study, conducted by one of the coauthors of this study, found blueberries had a similar effect.

info The National Stroke Association has information on preventing and recovering from a stroke at *www.stroke.org*.

■ ■ ■ ■

Tasty Cranberry Recipes That Are Good for You

Dried cranberries are a no-fat, no-cholesterol, no-sodium food. One-quarter cup of dried cranberries provides ½ serving from the fruit group of the Food Guide Pyramid. *Here's what to do with sliced and dried cranberries…*

●**Add to trail mix,** quick breads, muffins, desserts, sauces, salsa and salads.

●**Sprinkle dried cranberries over cold or cooked cereals** or cook in the cereal.

●**Add to chopped chicken salads.**

The US Department of Agriculture has some tasty, nourishing recipes using cranberries…

CRANBERRY GRANOLA BARS

½ cup honey

2 tablespoons + 2 teaspoons brown sugar

1 tablespoon + 1 teaspoon oil

1½ cups oats

1¼ cups toasted rice cereal

1¼ cups dried cranberries

1. Combine honey, brown sugar and oil in a small saucepan. Heat over low heat until it is well mixed.

2. Mix oats, rice cereal and cranberries. Add the honey mixture and stir until all the ingredients are thoroughly combined.

3. Pat firmly into an 8" x 8" baking pan.

4. Bake in 350°F oven for 15 minutes; press mixture firmly, once more, into the bottom of the pan. Bake 5 more minutes.

5. Cool completely. Refrigerate, at least one hour, for easier cutting. Cut 4" x 6" for 24 bars.

CRIMSON SLAW

½ head (1 pound 8 ounces) red cabbage, shredded

½ red onion, thinly sliced

¼ onion, thinly sliced

4 tablespoons oil

2 tablespoons vinegar

2 tablespoons sugar

½ teaspoon salt

¼ teaspoon black pepper

1½ cups dried cranberries

1. Toss cabbage and onions together in a large mixing bowl.

2. Mix oil, vinegar, sugar, salt, and pepper together in a small bowl to make a dressing.

3. Pour dressing over cabbage mixture; toss with cranberries.

4. Marinate in refrigerator for 1 hour. Serves 6.

Source: Recipes from Ocean Spray.

Eat Dark Chocolate to 'Beat' Heart Trouble

Robert H. Eckel, MD, chairman, Council on Nutrition, Physical Activity and Metabolism, American Heart Association, and professor of medicine, University of Colorado College of Medicine, Denver.

Samantha Heller, MS, RD, senior clinical nutritionist, New York University Medical Center, Joan and Joel Smilow Center for Cardiac Rehabilitation and Prevention, New York City.

Journal of the American Medical Association.

It's said that chocolate can mend a broken heart—and it may actually be true, in a physiological sense.

Two studies suggest that dark chocolate and drinkable cocoa have beneficial effects on certain measures of heart function. Both were small studies, however, and experts warn it's not yet time to substitute dark chocolate for tried-and-true fruits and vegetables.

We are not yet ready to change nutrition policy, says Dr. Robert H. Eckel, chairman of the American Heart Association's Council on Nutrition, Physical Activity and Metabolism. "Not only is chocolate high in calories, but one third of it is fat that can be converted to a monounsaturated fatty acid. This doesn't give us enough information to give the green light to chocolate consumption."

THE FIRST STUDY

The first study tried to ascertain the beneficial properties of polyphenols, compounds that are found in various plants including cocoa plants.

Thirteen people, aged 55 to 64, who had recently diagnosed and untreated hypertension, were randomly assigned to receive either dark chocolate bars with 500 milligrams (mg) of polyphenols and 480 calories, or white chocolate, also with 480 calories but no polyphenols. (Because white chocolate does not contain cocoa solids, the Food and Drug Administration does not classify it as chocolate.) After 14 days, the participants in the study abstained from chocolate for seven days, then switched groups.

Subjects taking the polyphenol-rich chocolate saw a reduction in their blood pressure

within 10 days. Those in the white chocolate group had no reduction.

"The way we process chocolate tends to reduce the concentration of healthful compounds," says Samantha Heller, senior clinical nutritionist at the Joan and Joel Smilow Center for Cardiac Rehabilitation and Prevention at New York University Medical Center.

THE SECOND STUDY

The second study involved 26 participants who were asked to drink cocoa, which is high in flavonoids called *flavan-3-ols*. In this study, just one drink had a beneficial effect on endothelial function. The endothelium is the inner lining of the blood vessels.

"Chocolate is still chocolate in terms of fat composition," Eckel adds. "Even though there could be some properties of cocoa that are beneficial, we still have lots of downsides of caloric consumption that may cut across the grain of benefit."

Choose fruits and vegetables for their natural cardioprotective qualities, but don't despair. "If you want a chocolate treat once in a while, the bitterer the better and don't feel badly about it," Heller says.

info The American Heart Association has more on polyphenols and flavonoids at *www.americanheart.org.*

Incredible Breakthrough: Better Blood Thinner Comes from Cobras!

Jonathan Halperin, MD, professor, medicine, Mount Sinai Medical Center, New York City.

Howard Herrmann, MD, director, cardiac catheterization and interventional cardiology, University of Pennsylvania, Philadelphia.

Warfarin, the widely used but problematic blood thinner first used as a rat poison, may soon have to make way for a new drug that seems to work more predictably and safely.

Patients will have researchers to thank, along with an unusual suspect—the cobra.

The drug, derived from cobra venom, is called *ximelagatran,* or Exanta. Its manufacturer, AstraZeneca, is awaiting approval by the US Food and Drug Administration (FDA).

"It would bring a dramatic change to how cardiologists practice," says Dr. Jonathan Halperin, a professor of medicine at Mount Sinai Medical Center in New York City.

PROBLEMS WITH WARFARIN

Warfarin, also known by the brand name Coumadin, has been available for almost 60 years. It thins the blood, reducing the formation of blood clots that can block arteries and contribute to a stroke or heart attack.

The drug is often a second line of defense after aspirin, which prevents blood clots in a different way and is not as powerful.

But taking warfarin isn't as simple as merely popping pills. "The problem with warfarin is that everybody absorbs it a little differently. People have to have frequent blood monitoring to adjust the dose," says Dr. Howard Herrmann, director of cardiac catheterization and interventional cardiology at the University of Pennsylvania in Philadelphia.

The blood tests are typically required at least once every month. If patients and doctors do not work together to keep an eye on warfarin levels, the blood can become too thin (raising the risk of internal bleeding or hemorrhaging after an accident) or too thick (raising the risk of a clot).

Since warfarin works by interfering with the body's absorption of vitamin K from food, even a minor change in a person's diet can disrupt warfarin levels.

Complicating matters further, warfarin interacts with a long list of drugs, affecting the action of either or both of them.

NEW DRUG PROMISES EASIER USE

Recent studies report that unlike warfarin, Exanta thins the blood without major fluctuations. Patients would not need to undergo regular blood tests to check the thinness of their blood.

"It's given in a fixed dose, and has no significant food or drug interactions," says Halperin. "It's almost like one-size-fits-all."

POSSIBLE SIDE EFFECTS

Experts caution that while Exanta may be a great improvement over warfarin, it won't be perfect. The drug appears to affect liver enzymes in approximately 6% of patients, although they did fine later, Halperin says.

"It will be appropriate for people who take [Exanta] to have certain blood tests from time to time to make sure they and the medicine are getting along well with one another," Halperin says.

Then there's the matter of cost. New drugs typically cost much more than drugs that are more than a half-century old. But experts say doctors will save time and money by not having to order and review monthly blood tests. More cost savings could come if fewer people have strokes because more of them take the easier-to-use drug.

According to the manufacturer of Exanta, studies have shown blood thinners reduce the incidence of stroke by 62% in patients at risk, but only half of them get the optimal treatment.

On the whole, Halperin says, "there's a good chance that a drug like this could replace warfarin for most people."

info For more information about how blood thinners like warfarin work, visit *www. nlm.nih.gov/medlineplus/druginfo.*

Attention Folks Over 50: Boost Your Flu Vaccine With Green Algae

Canadian Medical Association Journal.
Ocean Nutrition Canada, news release.

Green algae extract may increase the body's immune response to flu vaccine, according to a recent study by Canadian scientists.

Researchers from Dalhousie University in Nova Scotia, and Ocean Nutrition Canada, a nutritional biotechnology company, found that taking a carbohydrate extract of green algae in pill form greatly boosted the immune response to the flu vaccine in people aged 50 to 55 years.

"These results have raised the bar, showing that natural products can be studied for clinical effect in a pharmaceutical-caliber study," says researcher Dr. Scott Halperin, a professor at Dalhousie.

THE STUDY

Halperin and his colleagues gave two different doses of green algae extract to two groups of 41 healthy people for 28 days. Another 42 people received a placebo. All the study volunteers were at least 50 years old.

After 21 days, all subjects received a flu vaccine. The vaccine contained three different flu strains.

The researchers found the people taking 400 milligrams (mg) per day of the algae extract had much greater antibody responses to the vaccine at seven and 21 days after vaccination. The algae extract caused no adverse effects, the study says.

ABOUT FLU

Flu is a respiratory infection that is caused by influenza viruses. These viruses can lead to symptoms like muscle aches, fevers and chills, and can sometimes be life-threatening. The Centers for Disease Control and Prevention (CDC) says that between 10% and 20% of Americans catch the flu each year, resulting in approximately 114,000 hospitalizations and 36,000 deaths.

■ ■ ■ ■

How to Avoid the Flu

The CDC offers the following tips for reducing your risk of contracting flu and other respiratory viruses...

• **Avoid close contact with sick people.** When you are sick, keep your distance from others to protect them from getting sick too.

• **Stay home** when you are sick.

• **Cover your mouth and nose** when you cough or sneeze. Doing so may prevent those around you from getting sick.

• **Wash your hands frequently.** It will help shield you from germs and protect others from your germs.

• **Avoid touching your eyes,** nose or mouth. Germs are often spread when a person touches something that is contaminated with germs and then touches his or her eyes, nose, or mouth.

Flu has no cure, but there are a few things you can do to make yourself more comfortable if you catch the virus. Get plenty of rest, drink a lot of liquids, and avoid using alcohol and tobacco. You can take fever-reducers and pain-killers, but never give aspirin to children or teenagers who exhibit flu-like symptoms—especially fever—without first consulting your doctor. There are now several flu-fighting drugs available by prescription. They include Symmetrel, Tamiflu, Flumadine and Relenza.

info For more tips on flu prevention, visit *http://familydoctor.org/073.xml*.

Getting Rid of Nagging Coughs

Jamison Starbuck, ND, a naturopathic physician in family practice and a lecturer at the University of Montana, both in Missoula.
Bottom Line/Health.

Cough tops the list of bothersome medical complaints. A cough is annoying, not only to the sufferer, but also to everyone within earshot.

Acute coughs are most often the result of a viral upper respiratory illness. Allergy, asthma, environmental irritants and sinusitis also can cause cough. In most cases, we cough because our body is trying to heal itself by getting rid of mucus or other irritants in the respiratory tract. Unfortunately, this isn't always successful —acute coughs can last for three to six weeks, long after other viral symptoms, such as runny nose and sore throat, have disappeared. If you have a cough that has lasted longer than six weeks—or longer than three to four days if accompanied by pain, fever or other symptoms—see your doctor for a physical exam. Such coughing can indicate serious illness, such as emphysema, lung cancer, tuberculosis or pneumonia. If your cough is not due to a life-threatening condition, natural remedies can provide substantial relief.

Coughs usually are worse when your mucus membranes and the air around you are dry. You can begin to ease your cough by drinking enough fluids (at least eight 8-ounce glasses of water daily) and by using a humidifier in your home or office.

To soothe your respiratory tract and make expectoration of mucus more effective, try a cough "elixir" that contains honey and the herbs elecampane (*Inula helenium*), marshmallow root (*Althaea officinalis*), mullein (*Verbascum thapsus*) and wild cherry bark (*Prunus serotina*). Most natural-food stores will have a cough formula that contains these ingredients.

If your cough still persists, it might be helpful for you to try one of the following homeopathic remedies...

•**Rumex.** Use when cough causes a tickling sensation in the back of the throat. This type of cough is usually dry, worsens while talking and prevents sleep.

•**Spongia.** Use when cough sounds croupy (like a seal's bark) and when it causes a dry throat. This type of cough usually improves after the sufferer consumes warm foods or beverages. It may be accompanied by shallow breathing or panting.

•**Phosphorus.** Use when cough is accompanied by hoarseness, sore throat pain and/or tightness and weight in the chest. This type of cough often worsens when the sufferer goes from warm to cold temperatures.

Purchase 30C potency pellets of the remedy that most closely matches your symptoms. Take two pellets, and let them dissolve under the tongue, two times per day for up to three days. If you have selected the right remedy,

your cough should improve within that time. You can then discontinue the treatment.

Boost Brain Power with This Meat Molecule

Proceedings B.
Royal Society, a research institute of the United Kingdom's National Academy of Science news release.

Creatine, a chemical that's popular among bodybuilders and athletes, can bulk up your brain power, according to a study by Australian researchers.

The study found that taking creatine, which is found naturally in meat, as a dietary supplement boosts memory and general intelligence.

Creatine, which is a fundamental form of stored energy in the muscle tissue, is sold in nutrition stores, mainly to athletes and weight lifters who are looking for a performance edge. Whether it truly provides one is unknown. However, physiologists say creatine supplements do appear to increase a person's short-term workout capacity.

The Australian researchers monitored the effects of a 5 gram-per-day supplement of creatine on 45 young adult vegetarians. A 5-gram supplement is the amount usually taken by fitness buffs.

Vegetarians were chosen for the study because they do not get creatine through meat consumption.

THE STUDY

The subjects were divided into two groups. One group received the creatine supplement while the other group received a sham supplement for six weeks. For another six weeks, both groups took no supplements. In the final six weeks, the two groups were swapped so that those who had taken creatine first now received the placebo.

The memory and intelligence of the subjects were tested at the start of the trial, at the end of the first six-week period and at the start and end of the final six-week period.

"The results were clear with both of our experimental groups and in both test scenarios: creatine supplementation gave a significant measurable boost to brain power," according to lead researcher Dr. Caroline Rae.

The study findings echo previous research showing that increased brain creatine levels correlate with improved memory and reduce mental fatigue.

However, it is not clear that taking creatine would have any long-term effect on memory or intelligence.

"Creatine supplementation may be of use to those requiring boosted mental performance in the short term—for example, university students," Rae says.

Although the brief use of creatine appears to be safe, little is known about its side effects over time.

Some evidence suggests that creatine supplements may cause at least temporary kidney damage in certain people. In addition, there have been some anecdotal reports of other side effects, including nausea, cramping and stomach upset.

info To learn more about creatine, visit *http://muscle.ucsd.edu/musintro/crea tine.shtml.*

Easiest Way to Improve Your Memory

Matthew Walker, PhD, instructor, psychiatry, Harvard Medical School, Boston.
Daniel Margoliash, PhD, professor, psychology and organismal biology, University of Chicago.
Nature.

Improving your memory is easier than you think—all you need to do is get a good night's sleep, according to two studies on sleep and human memory.

The studies focused on memory for different tasks—one tested participants on motor skills and the other on speech memory—but participants in both studies performed better after sleeping.

"A full night of sleep is critical to enhancing learning," says an author of one of the studies, Matthew Walker, an instructor of psychiatry at Harvard Medical School in Boston.

THE STUDY

Walker and his team randomized 100 healthy young adults into eight different groups that learned finger-tapping sequences. The only difference between the groups was the point in the sleep-wake cycle in which they learned the task.

Walker says they discovered three stages of memory creation. The first stage is compared to a computer file, where information could be lost until it is saved. Saving a file on a computer takes only seconds, but it can take up to six hours in a person, Walker says. During this time, the memory becomes more stable and is less likely to be forgotten.

The second stage of memory processing happens during sleep. Walker says the last two hours of an eight-hour night of sleep are the most critical for memory storage. During this stage the file is reopened and reorganized. This stage, he explains, enhances the memory and prepares it for recall.

The last stage of memory occurs when you recall a memory. Walker says it's as if you've reopened the file and can modify it. Slight changes to the memory can then be saved.

This information about memory could be useful when treating people with problems such as post-traumatic stress disorder. Walker says that as a memory is brought up in therapy, it could be altered slightly, making it less traumatic each time.

THE SECOND STUDY

The author of the second study, Daniel Margoliash, a professor of psychology and organismal biology at the University of Chicago, says two things happen during sleep—the brain recovers parts of memories that have been lost during the day, and memories are stabilized for long-term storage.

Margoliash and his colleagues, Howard Nusbaum and Kimberly Fenn, had volunteers listen to simple words on a speech synthesizer, and were asked to identify the sounds. Twelve participants were tested in the morning and re-tested 12 hours later. Another 12 volunteers were tested in the evening and then 12 hours later, after a night's sleep. The final group of 24 were tested and then re-tested immediately.

The researchers found performance was better for the participants who had a chance to sleep before their second tests. Those who received testing in the morning and then again 12 hours later, lost about half of what they had learned during the intervening hours, Margoliash says.

info Visit the New York University School of Medicine's Sleep Disorders Center at *www.med.nyu.edu/sleep.*

Natural Sleep Remedies

Jamison Starbuck, ND, a naturopathic physician in family practice and a lecturer at the University of Montana, both in Missoula.
Bottom Line/Health.

A good night's sleep is truly one of life's blessings. Unfortunately, one out of three adults has insomnia, which affects not only their emotional well-being and autoimmune health, but also their vulnerability to infectious disease.

Medical doctors often use prescription sedatives, such as *zolpidem* (Ambien), or antidepressants, such as *trazodone* (Desyrel), to treat insomnia. These drugs generally work in the short-term, but their safety may diminish if they are used for more than 30 consecutive days. Both types of drugs can cause side effects, such as constipation and drowsiness.

Unlike prescription drugs, which simply knock you out, natural medicine treats the cause of your insomnia. *Here's my natural approach to treat this condition**...

The chief triggers of insomnia are emotional stress, pain and hormone irregularity. Decide which of these fits your situation and select one or more of the remedies listed below.

*Some of these remedies may be inappropriate for pregnant women or some people who have chronic health conditions. Consult your doctor.

EMOTIONAL STRESS

If you know that your sleeplessness is caused by emotional stress, my favorite homeopathic treatment is Calms Forté (Hylands). This formula contains key ingredients, such as passionflower, oat and chamomile, and is available at health-food stores.

Two pellets, dissolved under the tongue at bedtime, quell both mild anxiety and the tendency to over-think. If you awaken frequently, you can repeat this dose up to three times throughout the night.

I also recommend the herbs valerian and hops for stress-related insomnia. Take 60 drops of each herb together, in tincture form, in four ounces of hot water at bedtime. Both herbs are mildly sedating, generally safe and can be combined with Calms Forté.

PAIN

Insomniacs who suffer from joint and back pain can improve their sleep by relaxing their muscles at bedtime. Start with a warm Epsom salts bath just before bed (use at least two cups Epsom salts per tub). For even greater relaxation, also take a magnesium supplement (300 milligrams [mg]) and a homeopathic preparation of magnesium known as Mag. Phos 6X (four pellets under the tongue), both at bedtime immediately after the Epsom bath.

HORMONE IRREGULARITY

Menopause, premenstrual syndrome, thyroid hyperactivity or a surge in stress hormones that may be precipitated by life changes or excessive exercise can all cause insomnia. Hormone-related insomnia should be evaluated carefully and treated by your medical doctor or naturopathic physician.

One hormone-related insomnia that most people can treat themselves is linked to *seasonal affective disorder* (SAD), a condition that causes mild to moderate depression from the autumn season until spring. A dose of 0.5 mg to 2 mg of the hormone *melatonin,* taken at bedtime, may well correct the insomnia that is linked to SAD. Melatonin is available at health-food stores and pharmacies. Start with the 0.5 mg dose and increase after five days, if necessary. I recommend discontinuing melatonin for SAD-related insomnia by late March.

All About the Amazing Power of Acupuncture

Gary Kaplan, DO, past president of the Medical Acupuncture Research Foundation.

Bottom Line/Personal.

Acupuncture is no longer considered a "fringe" treatment. Since 1997, when it was formally recognized as a legitimate medical technique,* acupuncture's uses in Western medicine have been growing. *Here's what it can do for you…*

HOW IT WORKS

Acupuncture involves the insertion of hair-thin needles into one or more of the body's 2,000-plus acupuncture points. In traditional Chinese medicine, it's thought that the needles rebalance the flow of energy (chi) through 14 major pathways, or meridians. Acupuncture used to be considered questionable because meridians couldn't be readily identified.

Fact: Acupuncture points actually do exist. Each one is located near a vascular bundle that contains a nerve, artery, vein and lymphatic vessel in the space between muscles. The effects of stimulating specific points have been scientifically verified.

Example: One acupuncture point on the foot has traditionally been linked to eye disorders. Brain scans performed at the University of California, Irvine, showed that stimulating that point increased activity in the brain's occipital region, the area involved with vision.

Acupuncture therapy generally involves a series of six to 12 treatments over a period of weeks or months. Cost per treatment is $45 to $150, with the average around $90. It sometimes is covered by insurance.

It used to be thought that acupuncture provided only short-term relief. But in some cases, acupuncture appears to permanently alter the way cells function—for example, by increasing the ability of nerve cells to release painkilling neurotransmitters. This shows promise for the

*By the National Institutes of Health Consensus Development Conference.

treatment of chronic conditions, such as osteoarthritis, tendinitis, headaches and irritable bowel syndrome.

The World Health Organization has identified more than 40 conditions that may be helped by acupuncture. *The best evidence is for the following conditions…*

BACK PAIN

Many physicians routinely recommend acupuncture for pain in the lower back, and insurance companies often pay for it. Acupuncture works at least as well as some over-the-counter drugs—and without causing stomach upset or other side effects.

Acupuncture seems to increase blood supply to injured areas and promote faster healing. It also may encourage the release of painkilling endorphins and stimulate nerve fibers to block pain sensations. Patients with acute back sprains or spasms who are treated with acupuncture in addition to conventional treatments (ice packs, massage, physical therapy, etc.) can cut their healing time in half, from an average of about four weeks to two.

TOOTH EXTRACTION

Patients who have their teeth extracted or other oral surgeries experience less postsurgical pain and require lower doses of analgesics when they are given acupuncture afterward. They also have less swelling and inflammation. In addition to causing an increase in painkilling endorphins, acupuncture lowers levels of prostaglandins, inflammatory chemicals that cause nerve and tissue irritation.

SURGICAL PAIN

Studies have shown that patients who are given acupuncture during surgery require lower levels of anesthesia—and therefore, have fewer anesthesia-related complications, such as nausea. Acupuncture also can be used postsurgically to help control pain.

NAUSEA AND VOMITING

More than three dozen randomized controlled studies have shown that acupuncture is effective for treating and preventing nausea and vomiting—important for cancer patients getting chemotherapy. A study of 104 women undergoing high-dose chemotherapy found that those who received acupuncture had significantly less nausea and vomiting than those who didn't get the treatments. Acupuncture also may be helpful for reducing morning sickness during pregnancy.

PAINFUL MENSTRUATION

A number of studies have also shown that women with dysmenorrhea (painful menstrual periods) can get long-lasting relief with acupuncture. In a typical case, a woman might receive several treatments prior to her period, then additional treatments afterward. A total of six to 12 treatments can potentially eliminate the problem for good.

The uterine contractions that result in menstrual cramps are caused by an increase in prostaglandins. Acupuncture can calm the nervous system and potentially cause a permanent reduction in prostaglandins.

ADDICTION

Acupuncture has been used to treat nearly every form of addiction—tobacco, alcohol, heroin, etc. It may reduce physical and emotional withdrawal when combined with conventional approaches, such as psychotherapy and medication.

Example: Studies have shown that about 60% of addicts drop out of traditional treatment programs, but the dropout rate declines to approximately 40% when acupuncture is included.

ACUPUNCTURE SAFETY

To get proper treatment...

●**Get a diagnosis from a medical doctor** before getting acupuncture treatments. Otherwise you might be misdiagnosed. *Example:* My brother-in-law had a high fever and went to an acupuncturist, who treated him for flu and a urinary tract infection. What he really had was prostatitis with early sepsis, a potentially life-threatening infection that required antibiotic treatment.

●**See a qualified acupuncturist**—either a medical acupuncturist (MD or DO), a practitioner who is a member of the American Academy of Medical Acupuncture (AAMA, 323-937-5514, *www.medicalacupuncture.org*) or one who is board-certified by the American

Board of Medical Acupuncture, an independent entity within the AAMA...or a licensed acupuncturist, a practitioner who has completed the state or national exams conducted by the National Certification Commission for Acupuncture and Oriental Medicine (NCCAOM, 703-548-9004, *www.nccaom.org*).

●**Ask how many treatments you will need.** If it's more than 12 or the practitioner won't be specific, get a second opinion.

●**Avoid acupuncture if you are taking anticoagulant medications,** such as Coumadin or heparin, or if you have a bleeding disorder (such as hemophilia).

Acupuncture Calms Moms and Kids

Shu-Ming Wang, MD, associate professor, anesthesiology, Yale University School of Medicine, New Haven, CT. Presentation, American Society of Anesthesiologists annual meeting, San Francisco

A cupuncture can quell a parent's anxiety before his or her child has surgery —and it can calm the child, as well.

The problem of parental anxiety before a child's surgery is common, says Dr. Shu-Ming Wang, an associate professor of anesthesiology at Yale University School of Medicine. "We not only have to take care of the kids, but the parents are important, too," she says. Helping parents control their anxiety before their child has an operation is important because anxious parents can upset the child.

If a sedative is prescribed for the parents, it can hamper their ability to help care for the child after surgery, she notes.

THE STUDY

Wang inserted tiny acupuncture needles, called *press needles,* into three areas of the ears of 34 mothers approximately 30 minutes before their children received anesthesia for surgery.

Another 33 mothers received sham acupuncture, with the needles inserted into areas with no acupuncture effect.

Wang measured the anxiety levels of the mothers and children before the needles were placed, and then measured the children's anxiety during induction of anesthesia and the mother's anxiety after the induction.

The children were aged two to seven years and none got pre-surgery sedatives. The mothers stayed with the children while the anesthesia was begun.

The acupuncture groups fared better. The mothers' anxiety scores were six points lower than in the sham treatment group. And the children in the acupuncture group scored 33 out of 100 on anxiety measures, compared with 47 out of 100 in the sham group (higher scores indicate more anxiety).

The intervention group mothers wanted to keep the needles, Wang says.

Wang used auricular acupuncture, "a little different than traditional Chinese acupuncture," she says. In auricular acupuncture, points on the outer ear are treated. Wang chose points known as relaxation, valium and master cerebral points.

The outer ear acts "like a switchboard to the brain," according to the Society of Auricular Acupuncturists, a British-based organization. It's believed that an acupoint on the ear, when treated, triggers electrical impulses from the brain to the specific body part being treated.

■ ■ ■ ■

Research on Acupuncture

According to information from the National Center for Complementary and Alternative Medicine, other studies have found acupuncture to have proven, positive health effects…

●**In one small, randomized controlled clinical trial,** more than half of the women who experienced a major depressive episode and who were treated with acupuncture improved significantly.

●**In another controlled clinical trial,** of seven children with attention deficit hyperactivity disorder who underwent acupuncture treatment, nearly half showed some improvement in their symptoms.

●**In a third small controlled study,** eight pregnant women were given moxibustion, a traditional Chinese remedy in which medicinal herbs are burned just above an acupressure point, to reduce the rate of breech births, in which the fetus is positioned for birth feet-first instead of the normal position of head-first. Researchers found the treatment to be safe, but they were uncertain whether it was effective. However, a later study that applied moxibustion to 130 pregnant women who were presenting breech found that the acupuncture significantly increased the number of normal head-first births.

info For information on auricular acupuncture, try the Society of Auricular Acupuncturists Web site at *www.auricular acupuncture.org.uk.*

Magnets No Relief for Aching Feet

Glenn Gastwirth, DPM, executive director, American Podiatric Medical Association, Bethesda, MD.
Todd Schlifstein, DO, clinical assistant professor, rehabilitation medicine, New York University School of Medicine, New York City.
Journal of the American Medical Association.

Shoe inserts containing magnets don't provide more relief for heel pain than regular inserts, so says a recent study, funded by a grant from Spenco Medical Corp.—a leading maker of nonmagnetic insoles and other orthotic devices.

Although magnets are considered safe when applied to the skin, there's very little scientific evidence to support their use to relieve pain. Even so, more and more people are turning to magnets, with sales in the US estimated at $500 million annually and worldwide sales near $5 billion.

THE CONDITION

Plantar heel pain, or plantar fasciitis, is a common foot problem that often manifests as knife-like pain in the heel area. It usually results from abnormalities in the way people walk, by placing too much stress on the heel bone and its surrounding tissues. The condition is often associated with an inflammation of the connective tissue along the bottom of the foot.

"Heel pain and plantar fasciitis are often due to the excessive rolling in of the foot which puts a strain on the plantar fascii, which is the band of connective tissue on the bottom of the foot," says Glenn Gastwirth, executive director of the American Podiatric Medical Association. This condition can last several months or years, and can also be aggravated by injury, being overweight or by wearing poorly constructed footwear.

THE STUDY

Researchers at the Mayo Clinic in Rochester, Minnesota, randomly assigned 101 adults with plantar heel pain to wear shoe insoles with an active magnet or insoles with a sham magnet for at least four hours each day, four days a week, for eight weeks. The participants kept diaries in which they rated their pain on a scale of one to 10, with 10 being the most severe pain. The strength of the magnets was comparable with magnets that are available to the public.

Both groups reported improvements in symptoms, but there were no significant differences between the groups at the end of eight weeks. By the end of the study, 33% of the nonmagnetic group and 35% of the magnetic group reported being all or mostly better.

Although the study authors claim regular insoles have been found to be effective in relieving the pain of plantar fasciitis, others, like Gastwirth, disagree.

"Flat insoles with or without magnets are going to be of little value," Gastwirth says. "Generally [heel pain and plantar fasciitis] are treated more effectively not by insoles but by orthotic devices that control the mechanics of the foot."

Ideally, that orthotic device would be custom-made for your foot after a podiatrist has conducted a gait analysis, but nonprescription devices are a good start, Gastwirth says.

"By far, the most effective way to treat the condition is through the proper support and control of the foot by orthotic devices," Gastwirth says. Sometimes a person will also need to take an anti-inflammatory medication.

As for the value of magnets, some experts feel the jury is still out.

"[The magnet] wasn't helpful in this study, but might it be helpful for other things?" asks Todd Schlifstein, clinical assistant professor of rehabilitation medicine at New York University School of Medicine located in New York City. "Plantar fasciitis is what we call musculoskeletal pain. Maybe magnets would be better for neuropathic pain."

info The American Podiatric Medical Association at *www.apma.org/top10.html* has information on heel pain and on the top 10 foot problems.

Treating Chronic Skin Problems...Naturally

Mark A. Stengler, ND, associate clinical professor, Bastyr University, Kenmore, WA.

Bottom Line/Personal.

Chronic skin problems, such as eczema, psoriasis and acne, are a few of the most common reasons people visit dermatologists. Conventional topical treatments (ointments and lotions) are helpful, but many people find they work only temporarily.

Most chronic skin problems need to be addressed internally as well as externally because they often are the result of internal problems that are related to digestion, detoxification and liver function.

Several natural remedies are effective, and they rarely have side effects. Allow four weeks for improvement of chronic skin problems ...one to two days for acute flare-ups. For each condition, you can use all the remedies recommended. Unless otherwise noted, they prevent as well as treat the condition. All are available in drugstores and/or health-food stores.

Important: Never start a new treatment without consulting your doctor, especially if you are taking any medications or are pregnant.

ECZEMA

•**EPA (*eicosapentaenoic acid*).** This long-chain fatty acid in the omega-3 family has potent anti-inflammatory properties. The highest concentrations are found in fish and fish oils, but EPA also is prevalent in other foods, such as flaxseed and walnuts.

It is difficult to get enough EPA from fish and/or walnuts, so I suggest that adults take fish oil in a dosage containing 1.8 grams of EPA daily or two tablespoons of flaxseed oil daily, whichever you prefer.

•**Evening primrose oil.** This contains a different essential fatty acid known as *gamma linolenic acid* (GLA), which reduces skin inflammation. Take 2,000 milligrams (mg) of primrose oil daily.

•**Probiotics.** These good bacteria prevent food sensitivities that are often connected to eczema. Friendly bacteria are found in yogurt (look for products with live cultures, such as Horizon Organic and Stonyfield Farm). Good bacteria also are in sauerkraut, kefir (a cultured milk product, like yogurt), miso and cottage cheese. It is hard to get enough from food, so I suggest taking a supplement. Take four billion organisms (usually one to two capsules) daily between meals.

•**Sulphur.** This homeopathic remedy works to soothe skin and relieve itching. It is particularly helpful if eczema is worse after bathing and in warm environments. For acute flare-ups, take two pellets of a 30C potency twice daily for one week. Then stop taking the remedy unless symptoms return.

•**Chamomile (*Matricaria chamomilla*).** Chamomile contains a group of phytonutrients that have strong anti-inflammatory properties. Apply a cream to the affected areas two to three times daily until symptoms disappear.

•**Oatmeal baths soothe itchy skin.** Tie up one-quarter cup of oats in cheesecloth or a leg from nylons, and let water from the tap run over it before you soak. Oatmeal also can be purchased as a powder and added to your bath. Pat, don't rub, yourself dry.

PSORIASIS

•**Fish oil.** Take five grams twice a day. It significantly reduces the itching, scaling and redness of psoriasis lesions.

•**Dandelion root (*Taraxacum officinale*).** This supports liver detoxification, which improves psoriasis. Take 300 mg of the capsule form three times daily with meals.

•**Aloe vera.** One study has shown that a 0.5% aloe vera cream used for four weeks significantly relieved psoriasis lesions. Apply twice daily.

ACNE

•**Zinc.** One double-blind study found that taking 30 mg of zinc for three months was an effective treatment for acne for almost one-third of patients. Adults should take 45 mg of zinc twice daily with meals for three months and then reduce the dosage to 30 mg daily for long-term supplementation. To maintain mineral balance, take zinc in conjunction with copper at a dose of 3 mg to 5 mg once a day.

•**Burdock root (*Arctium lappa*).** This herb treats many causes of acne, including hormonal imbalance, inefficient liver activity and skin bacteria. Take 300 mg of the capsule form, 30 drops of tincture or one cup of tea three times daily.

•**Fish oil.** Take supplements or flaxseed oil in the dosages recommended for eczema (see information on EPA).

•**Tea tree oil gels or creams.** Tea tree oil is an antiseptic as well as an anti-inflammatory. Apply topically once daily.

WOUNDS/BURNS

•**Aloe vera.** Apply topically twice each day until the burn or wound is healed. Look for a product that contains a high concentration of aloe (80% or higher).

•**Calendula officinalis.** This soothing herb is an antiseptic. Apply it in gel or cream form twice every day.

•**Vitamin C.** Take 1,000 mg twice daily to promote wound healing. For quicker healing, take 400 international units (IU) of vitamin E and 30 mg of zinc daily as well.

12

Nutrition, Diet & Fitness

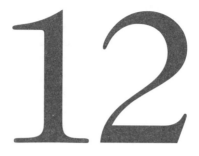

High-Protein Diet Pumps Up Heart Patients' Health

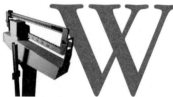

When Delaware researchers saw their patients with diabetes shed pounds on a high-fat, carbohydrate-restricted diet, they tried the same diet on a group of obese patients with heart disease.

ENCOURAGING RESULTS

The regimen—very similar to the controversial Atkins Diet—yielded encouraging results. The heart patients lost an average of 5% of their body weight over six weeks.

And these patients did not see measurable increases in their blood-fat levels—a concern for experts skeptical about this dietary approach to weight loss.

Although the researchers say more study is needed, they believe the results help substantiate the high-fat, high-protein, low-carb diet made popular by the late Dr. Robert Atkins.

"Lo and behold, we ended up with something very close to what Dr. Atkins had been saying for years," says Dr. James H. Hays, the endocrinologist and researcher who led the study at Christiana Care Health Services in Wilmington, Delaware.

Other studies have shown that the Atkins approach is effective for short-term weight loss. But a key question is whether the dieters will achieve results over a longer period of time and avoid a harmful buildup of artery-clogging fat that could boost their risk of cardiovascular disease.

THE STUDY

Hays' study focused on a small sample of patients—17 men and six women with atherosclerotic heart disease. All were obese and had been treated with cholesterol-lowering medications before entering the trial. Patients with diabetes were excluded.

James H. Hays, MD, endocrinologist, Christiana Care Health Services, Inc., Wilmington, DE.

Amy Joy Lanou, PhD, nutritionist, Physicians Committee for Responsible Medicine, Washington, DC.

Mayo Clinic Proceedings.

Subjects were instructed to get half of their daily calories from saturated fat, primarily red meat and cheese. Fresh fruit and nonstarchy vegetables were allowed in restricted amounts, but starches, such as bread and potatoes, were forbidden. Participants were not required to record their fruit and vegetable intake.

THE RESULTS

Overall, the diet resulted in decreases in weight and body fat and participants kept blood-fat levels in check, the study found.

Not everyone will be persuaded by the results of the study, Hays says. "[The study is] very small, it's very short and it's uncontrolled," he concedes.

SOME REMAIN UNCONVINCED

Amy Joy Lanou, nutrition director at the Physicians Committee for Responsible Medicine, is among the skeptics.

"I'd be very interested to see what happens with these individuals if the study was taken out over a year," she says.

Lanou's committee called on a US advisory panel to warn the public about the dangers of high-protein, low-carb diets—including the risk for cardiovascular disease—in its next update of federal dietary guidelines.

MORE FINDINGS

Hays is heartened by the diet's positive results with two other groups of patients who were tracked for longer periods. They included women with polycystic ovary syndrome, a hormonal condition, and people with reactive hypoglycemia, whose blood sugar drops after a meal.

Those with polycystic ovary syndrome lost 14.3% of their total body weight over 24 weeks. Reactive hypoglycemia patients dropped 19.9% of total body weight over a year. Neither group showed any significant change in blood-fat levels, Hays says.

Lanou advises people concerned about their weight to consider a diet proven to be safe and effective over a longer period of time. "We do know that choosing a plant-based diet will result in better health, as well as weight loss," she says.

info For more about the Atkins Diet, see the University of Arizona's Sarver Heart Center at *www.heart.arizona.edu.*

Myths of Low-Carb Dieting

Sandra Woodruff, RD, author of *Secrets of Fat-Free Cooking, The Good Carb Cookbook* and *Secrets of Good-Carb/Low-Carb Living.* Avery.
Bottom Line/Health.

These days, supermarket shelves and restaurants are filled with low-carbohydrate food choices, which many people believe virtually guarantee weight loss. Not true.

Just as many consumers assumed a few years back that they could load up on low-fat cookies, cakes and crackers and still lose weight, the low-carb craze has perpetuated many potentially dangerous myths...

Myth: All carbohydrates are "bad."

Reality: Carbohydrates—the sugars and starches in foods—have gotten an undeservedly bad reputation.

One reason is that consuming too much of the *wrong* kinds of carbohydrates causes the body to produce too much insulin, the hormone that helps regulate sugar (glucose) in the body.

High insulin levels encourage the body to store fat rather than burn it. Excess insulin production has been linked to heart disease, type 2 diabetes and breast, colon, prostate and other cancers.

However, not all carbohydrates are bad. It's true that some, including those found in processed foods, such as white bread, white rice, low-fiber breakfast cereals, many snack foods, sodas and sweets, enter the bloodstream quickly, causing a rapid increase in blood sugar and insulin levels.

But the carbohydrates found in vegetables, whole grains and many fruits enter the bloodstream more slowly, and, unlike processed foods, these "good" carbs are loaded with fiber and disease-fighting nutrients.

Myth: Eating "low-carb" versions of high-carbohydrate foods, such as bread and pasta, will help you lose weight.

Reality: Manufacturers have succeeded in taking out carbs by replacing flour with wheat gluten and other proteins, plant fibers, poorly digested starches and other bulking agents. However, these foods still contain *calories*. Ounce for ounce, these modified foods may contain fewer carbs but may—or may not—have fewer calories.

The same can be said for "sugar-free" desserts, which often contain generous amounts of added fat to make up for qualities lost when sugar is removed. Ultimately, calories still count, and it pays to compare labels.

Myth: A low-carb diet is "heart-healthy" because it helps lower cholesterol.

Reality: The truth is that cholesterol levels typically drop on any reduced-calorie diet (including a low-carb/high-saturated-fat diet). That's the body's response to being in a state of semistarvation.

This does not mean that a regular diet of bunless bacon cheeseburgers is healthy. Diets high in saturated fat have been linked to serious health problems, including colon cancer, type 2 diabetes and Alzheimer's disease. Moreover, when weight loss stops or the pounds creep back on, cholesterol levels often will rise again.

Myth: When cutting carbs, there's no such thing as too low.

Reality: Some diets—most notably Atkins—initially suggest a carbohydrate intake of as little as 20 grams (g) per day. This type of diet can cause health problems, especially for people who have kidney disease or gout or those who take medications for diabetes or high blood pressure.

Anyone interested in following a very-low-carb diet should do so only under a physician's supervision.

A reduced-carb diet is a much healthier option that provides more flexibility and is easier to stick with over the long term. Reduced-carb diets provide about 40% of their calories from carbs—about 120 to 160 g per day—during the weight-loss phase. The carbohydrates should come from nutrient-dense vegetables, fruits and whole grains. Reduced-carb diets leave ample room to eat at least eight servings of vegetables and fruits a day.

Myth: You don't have to worry about the fat content of high-protein foods.

Reality: If you eat a low-carb, high-protein diet that allows greasy meats, high-fat cheese, butter, cream and similar foods, you're still consuming artery-clogging saturated fats that will increase your risk for heart disease and many other health problems.

On the other hand, eating a low-carb diet that includes skinless poultry, fish, lean meats, unsaturated fats, low-fat dairy products, nuts, seeds and fiber-rich fruits and vegetables will lower your risk for many diseases.

Myth: If you are on a diet that limits carbohydrates, it always is a good idea to eliminate dairy products.

Reality: Unfortunately, many low-carb diets do not recommend dairy foods, such as milk and yogurt.

Not only does this create a calcium deficit, it also may thwart weight-loss efforts.

Researchers have found compelling evidence that the calcium that is contained in dairy products helps stimulate the fat-burning machinery in the body through a complex series of hormone reactions.

One recent study published in the *Journal of the American College of Nutrition* found that each 300-milligram (mg) increase in daily calcium intake—the equivalent of one cup of low-fat milk—was associated with approximately six fewer pounds of body fat in adults.

The best way to meet your calcium intake requirements is to eat low-fat versions of milk, yogurt and cheese.

It is best to aim for three one-cup servings of milk or yogurt or 1.5 ounces of low-fat cheese per day. Some good nondairy sources of calcium include kale and calcium-fortified soy foods.

Skipping Breakfast Makes You Fat

Yunsheng Ma, PhD, assistant professor, epidemiology, University of Massachusetts Medical School, Worcester.

Ruth Kava, PhD, RD, director, nutrition, American Council on Science and Health, New York City.

Gail Frank, DrPH, RD, professor, nutrition, California State University at Long Beach, and spokeswoman, American Dietetic Association.

American Journal of Epidemiology.

Many people believe that eating right before bedtime is a sure method for getting fat. But research suggests that late eaters are no more likely to be overweight than anyone else.

It's what you consume the rest of the day—especially in the morning—that counts.

Americans who regularly skip breakfast are 4.5 times more likely to be overweight, researchers found.

But, the good news for nibblers is that those who eat four or more small meals a day are actually on the thinner side.

THE STUDY

Led by Yunsheng Ma, an assistant professor of epidemiology at the University of Massachusetts Medical School, the researchers examined a national cholesterol study that took place over five years.

A total of 499 people reported five times a year on what they ate over 24-hour periods. They found that people who ate more than three times a day were about half as likely to be overweight as those who ate three or fewer times a day.

Ma suspects the difference may be related to consistent blood sugar levels among the frequent eaters.

Insulin levels climb when blood sugar rises, contributing to hunger and the buildup of fat, Ma says.

What's the link between skipping breakfast and tipping the scales? People who skip breakfast will often overcompensate for that missed meal throughout the day, taking in more calories than they would have if they'd eaten a sensible breakfast.

Gail Frank, a professor of nutrition at California State University at Long Beach and a spokeswoman for the American Dietetic Association, says if you do not break the fast soon enough to need a moderate amount of calories, you'll be starving. How does the normal person respond? They eat, and they keep eating.

info The American Dietetic Association offers plenty of resources about healthy eating at their Web site *www.eatright.org.*

Diet Bars and Drinks Really Do Help You Lose Weight!

Presentation, the North American Association for the Study of Obesity annual meeting, Fort Lauderdale, FL.

North American Association for the Study of Obesity news release.

Replacing conventional food with prepackaged diet bars and vitamin drinks can help you lose weight over the long haul, experts say.

People who followed a meal replacement plan for 10 years weighed, on average, approximately 33 pounds less than dieters who didn't use a meal replacement plan, according to a recent study.

THE STUDY

The study, presented to the North American Association for the Study of Obesity, was among the longest studies ever to evaluate particular weight control programs—Slim-Fast shakes and bars in this case—over a long period of time. The study was sponsored in part by Slim-Fast.

The study's senior author is Dr. George L. Blackburn, director of the Center for the Study of Nutrition Medicine at Beth Israel Deaconess Medical Center and associate professor of surgery at Harvard Medical School.

People who were trying to shed pounds were instructed to eat a small meal of conventional food and two meal substitutes per day—say, two shakes—to bring their caloric intake to 1,200 to 1,500 calories per day.

The 130 people who used meal replacements as part of their weight management program maintained an average weight loss of six pounds after 10 years.

The 154 people in the control group who didn't use the meal replacements gained an average of almost 27 pounds over the same time period.

■ ■ ■ ■

Obesity Epidemic

Over the last 20 years the rate of obesity in the United States has risen at an "epidemic" pace, according to the Centers for Disease Control and Prevention (CDC).

Nearly two thirds of American adults are now overweight, and almost one third are obese, according to the National Institutes of Health.

Obesity is defined as being a Body Mass Index (BMI) score of 30 or higher, indicating a frame that's carrying far too much weight for its height.

Both excess weight and obesity are important risk factors for many serious health problems, including diabetes, heart disease, cancer, stroke and high blood pressure.

Shedding excess pounds—through diet, exercise and even surgery—can significantly reduce a person's risk of weight-related illness.

Although some drastic diets may lead to impressive short-term weight loss, most crash dieters end up regaining the weight that they were so happy to lose.

The best way to lose weight and keep it off is to change the lifestyle choices that promote poor health—eating too many calories and failing to exercise.

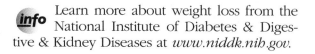 Learn more about weight loss from the National Institute of Diabetes & Digestive & Kidney Diseases at *www.niddk.nih.gov.*

Natural Protein Cuts Your Urge to Eat by 30%

Stephen Bloom, MD, professor, medicine, Hammersmith Hospital, Imperial College, London.

David Cummings, MD, associate professor, medicine, University of Washington, Seattle, Seattle VA Puget Sound Health Care System.

New England Journal of Medicine.

Injections of a natural protein significantly trimmed a person's urge to eat, a study found. The discovery could lead to effective obesity treatments.

The protein, normally secreted in the intestine, is called *peptide YY* (PYY), and it cuts food intake by sending satiety signals to the brain. Previous research had shown that normal-weight people don't eat as much when injected with PYY prior to a meal. The latest study finds the effect is equally potent for the obese, cutting short-term food intake by about 30% in both groups.

"We didn't know whether PYY would work in the obese," says Dr. Stephen Bloom, a diabetes expert at London's Imperial College and leader of the study.

"But when we administered PYY it was fully effective. That is the first step for trying to establish it as a therapy for obesity," he adds.

THE STUDY

Bloom and his colleagues studied the effects of PYY in 12 fit and 12 obese men and women. The obese subjects had roughly 40% lower levels of the peptide than their slim peers.

Bloom calls that difference "very important" since it gives the obese a greater tendency to eat. "They don't have the same level of satiety hormone that thin people have."

Why PYY was so low in the obese study subjects, however, isn't clear. It could reflect prolonged overeating or it could be the cause of the overeating.

Dr. David Cummings, an appetite expert at the University of Washington in Seattle, is concerned about touting the results of Bloom's study. "Does PYY help you avoid one meal, or is it a regulator of body weight over the long haul?" asks Cummings, who studies another appetite hormone called *ghrelin*. Ultimately, he says, drug treatment for obesity will likely be a cocktail of medicines that target several pathways to appetite regulation.

Eating Disorders Not Just For Teens Anymore

Shari Lusskin, MD, reproductive psychiatrist, New York University Medical Center, New York City.

Eating disorders such as anorexia or bulimia, which once affected mostly teenage girls, are a problem for a growing number of baby-boomer women.

Anorexia is characterized by weight loss due to excessive or compulsive dieting, often coupled with self-induced vomiting and chronic laxative use. Bulimia is defined as excessive binge eating, followed by purging or vomiting, and frequently, using laxatives.

Because the trend is so new, experts say there are no reliable studies to document how many women have eating disorders.

NEW FORM OF DISORDERS

A relatively new expression of eating disorders is what some experts are calling "anorexercise," and it's attracting a substantial number of older women. They calculate every calorie consumed, and devise a workout designed to burn those exact number of calories—and within 12 hours or less after eating.

"Some women will get up at 5 AM to run, just to burn off what they ate the night before. And they can go to some very unhealthy extremes in using exercise to control their weight," says reproductive psychiatrist Dr. Shari Lusskin, an associate professor at New York University School of Medicine.

HORMONAL CONNECTION?

Although the causes of eating disorders are not fully understood, some experts believe hormones may play a role, particularly since the number of women affected far outweighs the number of men. According to the National Institutes of Mental Health, some 7 million

American girls and women battle eating disorders, compared with 1 million boys and men.

And like the hormone fluctuations that occur during puberty—when young women are at risk for eating disorders—hormonal changes take place during perimenopause, when older women appear vulnerable as well.

Sometimes, undiagnosed depression is to blame, Lusskin says. "Because eating and depression can be so intimately entwined, it's likely that at least some older women with an eating disorder are really suffering from an undiagnosed depression, with a basic thread of unhappiness that ran through their lives for a long time and probably didn't come to the forefront until they hit middle age," she says.

The good news is that older women generally respond to treatment for eating disorders faster than younger women, and they are generally more motivated to seek help.

Treatment for all age groups includes counseling, medication, and, for older women, having a spouse involved in treatment.

Most important, say experts, is to join a support group. Studies show that sharing feelings with others facing a similar problem plays a major role in helping women of all ages overcome eating disorders.

info To learn more about eating disorders, visit the National Eating Disorders Association at *www.nationaleatingdisorders.org*.

What Are the Symptoms of Eating Disorders?

The National Institutes of Health (NIH) offers this explanation of different types of eating disorders and their symptoms…

•**Anorexia nervosa.** People who have anorexia develop unusual eating habits, such as avoiding meals, picking out a few foods and eating them in small amounts, weighing their food and counting the calories of everything they eat. They may also exercise excessively.

•**Bulimia nervosa.** People who have bulimia eat an excessive amount of food in a single episode and almost immediately make themselves vomit or use laxatives or diuretics to get rid of the food in their bodies. This behavior is referred to as the "binge/purge" cycle. Like people who have anorexia, people who have bulimia also may have an intense fear of gaining weight.

●**Binge-eating disorder.** People who have this recently recognized disorder have frequent episodes of compulsive overeating, but unlike those with bulimia, they do not purge their bodies of food. During these food binges, they often eat alone and very quickly, regardless of whether they feel hungry or full. They often feel shame or guilt over their actions. Unlike anorexia and bulimia, binge-eating disorder occurs almost as often in men as in women.

Even Moderate Exercise Helps Drop Pounds

John M. Jakicic, PhD, director, Physical Activity and Weight Management Research Center, University of Pittsburgh, PA.

Rachel Ballard-Barbash, MD, associate director, National Cancer Institute applied research program, Bethesda, MD.

I-Min Lee, ScD, MPH, associate professor, medicine, Harvard Medical School, Boston.

Journal of the American Medical Association.

R ecent research has been able to put some fairly precise numbers into the equation of exercise and weight loss.

The study found that women do not need to engage in hours of vigorous exercise to reap the weight-loss benefits, provided they also watch what they eat.

"There is currently a controversy over the amount of exercise you need," says study leader John M. Jakicic, director of the University of Pittsburgh Physical Activity and Weight Management Research Center. "Some people say this number, some people say that number. This is the first big clinical trial to address the issue."

Jakicic says, "If you can get people to exercise 30 minutes a day and reduce calorie intake by 20%, you get a reasonable reduction

in weight. If you increase that to 60 minutes a day, you dramatically increase weight loss."

NOT BY EXERCISE ALONE

For women who do not like to exercise, the good news from the Pittsburgh study is that a brisk 30-minute walk every day fills the bill, Jakicic says. "While 60 minutes gives better results, 30 minutes is pretty good."

But, he cautions, exercise alone doesn't do it. "If you do exercise without a change in eating habits, you won't see the benefit," says Jakicic. "It's really about the calories. Anything you do to reduce calories is good."

And although the effects of weight reduction on the risk of conditions such as heart disease and diabetes are obvious, another report adds another potential benefit—a lessened risk of breast cancer.

BREAST CANCER STUDY

The role of exercise in reducing the risk of breast cancer is outlined in a study by Dr. Anne McTiernan and colleagues at the Fred Hutchinson Cancer Research Center in Seattle. It is a big study, looking at exercise patterns of more than 74,000 women.

Again, a good benchmark was a daily brisk walk, adding up to between 75 and 150 minutes a week. Women who walked that much lowered their breast cancer risk by 18%, compared with women who did no exercise. More vigorous exertion, up to 10 hours of walking a week, reduced the risk slightly more. Starting exercise early in life gave the most benefit, but women of all ages benefited —and the greatest benefits were found in the thinnest women.

This is not startling news, says Dr. Rachel Ballard-Barbash, associate director of the National Cancer Institute applied research program. A review published last year found more than two dozen studies showing "convincing evidence that physical activity protects against breast cancer."

The new study provides evidence that exercise at any age is good, Ballard-Barbash says. "Many women between the ages of 50 and 79 saw benefits."

The mechanisms of protection appear clear, says Dr. I-Min Lee, an associate professor of medicine at Harvard Medical School. "Weight reduction favorably alters estrogen levels in the body," Lee says. "It also affects insulin and growth factor levels."

Exercise Your Way to Better Sex

Eric Rimm, ScD, associate professor, nutrition and epidemiology, Harvard School of Public Health, Boston.

Andrew McCullough, MD, director, male sexual health, fertility and microsurgery, New York University Medical Center, and assistant clinical professor, urology, New York University School of Medicine, New York City.

Annals of Internal Medicine.

Working out is not only good for a man's heart, it can benefit his love life as well.

Erectile dysfunction, or ED, is common in men older than 50 and is even more common with increasing age, but keeping fit seems to counter the problem. ED is defined as the inability, without treatment, to have and maintain an erection adequate for sexual intercourse.

One third of the men surveyed in a study reported having problems with an erection in the prior three months. Although the incidence of ED increased about 5% each year for all men, the problem was less common among men leading healthy lifestyles. For these men, there was about a 10-year delay before ED became a problem.

"There's a clear increased risk of erectile dysfunction as people age," confirms study author Eric Rimm, an associate professor of nutrition and epidemiology at the Harvard School of Public Health in Boston.

The same measures that prevent or delay health problems like cardiovascular disease and diabetes can help delay the onset of ED— keep your body lean and don't smoke.

THE STUDY

Rimm and his team looked at 31,742 men between the ages of 53 and 90 who participated in a study group of dentists, optometrists, osteopaths, podiatrists, pharmacists and veterinarians. The study was partially funded by Pfizer Inc., which makes the anti-impotence drug Viagra.

Thirty-three percent of the participants reported having ED in the past three months. Less than 2% of the men who reported ED said those incidents had occurred before the age of 40, while 4% had problems between the ages of 40 and 49. After age 50, however, erectile problems increased substantially, with 26% of men reporting difficulty between 50 and 59 years of age, 40% noting ED between 60 and 69 years, and 61% of men older than 70 reporting a problem.

Seventy-four percent of men younger than 59 reported "good" or "very good" sexual function, but only 10% of men older than 80 could say the same.

Men who ran three hours or more each week or played five hours of singles tennis reported a 30% lower risk of ED than those who did little or no exercise. Watching more than 20 hours of television each week, excessive consumption of alcohol, smoking and being overweight were associated with higher levels of ED. Having diabetes, a previous stroke or taking antidepressants or beta-blockers were also factors.

The bottom line is that risk factors for ED are about the same as those for heart disease. Rimm hopes that this news may help change behavior. "A lot of people have known about exercise and obesity and cardiovascular disease and the message is not getting through. The population is getting more overweight," says Dr. Andrew McCullough, director of male sexual health, fertility and microsurgery at New York University Medical Center. "Maybe people think of cardiovascular disease as too far off, but ED is much more immediate and affects the quality of life.

"Since ED is intimately associated with the health of the vascular system, a man needs to have his cardiovascular risk factors thoroughly examined so that maybe we can do some prevention. This clearly shows that prevention can affect erectile function," he says.

info For more information about erectile dysfunction, visit the American Foundation for Urologic Disease at *www.afud.org.*

Fat Facts: New Food Labels May Save Lives

Alice H. Lichtenstein, DSc, professor of nutrition, Tufts University, Boston.

Henry Anhalt, DO, director, division of pediatric endocrinology, Infants and Children's Hospital of Brooklyn, Maimonides Medical Center.

Food and Drug Administration.

The United States government will soon require food manufacturers to list the amount of unhealthy trans fatty acids contained in their products. Mounting scientific evidence shows that consumption of trans fat, along with saturated fat and cholesterol, raises LDL ("bad") cholesterol levels, thereby increasing the risk of heart disease.

The ruling has been "eagerly anticipated" for years, says Alice Lichtenstein, a professor of nutrition at Tufts University in Boston.

CHANGE IN EFFECT BY 2006

Under the new regulations, by January 1, 2006, all food labels must carry information on trans fats, located directly under the information about another dangerous substance, saturated fat. This is the first major change in labeling requirements in a decade.

The Food and Drug Administration estimates that the changes will save between $900 million and $1.8 billion each year in medical costs, lost productivity and pain and suffering.

UNHEALTHY FAT

Trans fats develop during the process of hydrogenation, in which hydrogen is added to vegetable oil to make it more solid. They are often found along with saturated fat in foods such as vegetable shortening, some margarines, crackers, candy bars, cookies and fried and other processed foods.

Americans consume about 1.5% to 2% of total calories in trans fats, while intake of saturated fat is running at about 12% to 14% of calories. The combined total intake of trans and saturated fats should probably be under 10%, Lichtenstein says.

Manufacturers of dietary supplements will be required to list trans fat content, as well as saturated fat and cholesterol on the Supplement Facts panel when their products (such as nutrition bars and energy bars) contain more than trace amounts (more than 0.5 grams).

The ruling may reduce liability for manufacturers. "If I have told everybody what's in there and they still want to eat it, then let the buyer beware," says Dr. Henry Anhalt, director of pediatric endocrinology at Infants and Children's Hospital of Brooklyn at Maimonides Medical Center. "But if I hide what's in there because it tastes good, that's a horse of another color."

info The US Food and Drug Administration offers more information on trans fats at their Web site, *www.fda.gov/oc/initiatives/transfat.*

■ ■ ■ ■

What Foods Contain Trans Fats... And How Much?

Trans fat is made when manufacturers add hydrogen to vegetable oil—a process called *hydrogenation.* This process usually turns liquid oils into solids, and increases the shelf life and flavor stability of foods.

Trans fat is found in vegetable shortenings, some margarines, crackers, cookies, snack foods and other items made with or fried in partially hydrogenated oils. A small amount of trans fat occurs naturally in dairy products and in some meat.

Trans fat raises LDL ("bad") cholesterol, although saturated fat is the main dietary culprit of high cholesterol.

The following table compiled from information from the Food and Drug Administration (FDA) and the US Department of Agriculture (USDA) shows the trans fat content of some everyday food products.

Product	Common Serving Size	Trans Fat (g)
French Fried Potatoes (Fast Food)	Medium	8
Butter	1 tbsp	0

Product	Common Serving Size	Trans Fat (g)
Margarine, stick	1 tbsp	3
Mayonnaise (Soybean Oil)	1 tbsp	0
Shortening	1 tbsp	4
Potato Chips	Small bag (42.5 g)	3
Doughnut	1	5
Cookies (cream filled)	3	2
Candy Bar	1	3
Cake, pound	1 slice	4.5

Don't assume similar products are the same. Be sure to check the Nutrition Facts panel on every product because similar foods can vary in calories, ingredients and nutrients.

■ ■ ■ ■

How to Interpret a Food Label

People read food labels for different reasons. But whatever the reason, many consumers would like to know how to use this information more effectively and easily.

The following guidance is intended to make it easier for you to use nutrition labels to make quick, informed food choices that contribute to a healthy diet.

THE SERVING SIZE

Serving sizes are provided in familiar units, such as cups or pieces, followed by the metric amount.

Serving sizes are based on the amount of food people typically eat, which makes them realistic and easy to compare to similar foods.

Pay attention to the serving size, including how many servings there are in the food package, and compare it to how much you actually eat.

CALORIES AND CALORIES FROM FAT

Calories provide a measure of how much energy you get from a serving of this food. The label also tells you how many of the calories in one serving come from fat.

Nutrition Facts

Serving Size 1 cup (228g)
Servings Per Container 2

Amount Per Serving

Calories 250   Calories from Fat 110

	% Daily Value*
Total Fat 12g	**18%**
Saturated Fat 3g	**15%**
Trans Fat 1.5g	
Cholesterol 30mg	**10%**
Sodium 470mg	**20%**
Total Carbohydrate 31g	**10%**
Dietary Fiber 0g	**0%**
Sugars 5g	
Protein 5g	
Vitamin A	**4%**
Vitamin C	**2%**
Calcium	**20%**
Iron	**4%**

*Percent Daily Values are based on a 2,000-calorie diet. Your Daily Values may be higher or lower depending on your calorie needs:

		Calories	2,000	2,500
Total Fat	Less than		65g	80g
Sat Fat	Less than		20g	25g
Cholesterol	Less than		300mg	300mg
Sodium	Less than		2,400mg	2,400mg
Total Carbohydrate			300g	375g
Dietary Fiber			25g	30g

THE NUTRIENTS

The nutrients listed first are the ones Americans generally eat in adequate amounts, or even too much. Eating too much fat, saturated fat, trans fat, and cholesterol, or sodium may increase your risk of certain chronic diseases, like heart disease, some cancers, or high blood pressure. Eating too many calories is linked to obesity.

Note: Health experts recommend that you keep your intake of saturated fat, trans fats and cholesterol as low as possible as part of a nutritionally balanced diet.

GET ENOUGH OF THESE

Americans often don't get enough dietary fiber, vitamin A, vitamin C, calcium, and iron in their diets. Eating enough of these nutrients can improve your health and help reduce the risk of some diseases and conditions.

Remember: You can not only use the food label to help limit those nutrients you want to cut back on, but also to increase those nutrients you want to consume in greater amounts.

THE PERCENT DAILY VALUE (%DV)

This part of the Nutrition Facts panel tells you whether the nutrients (fat, sodium, fiber, etc) in a serving of food contribute a lot or a little to your total daily diet.

%DVs are based on recommendations for a 2,000 calorie diet. For labeling purposes, FDA set 2,000 calories as the reference amount for calculating %DVs. The %DV shows you the percent (or how much) of the recommended daily amount of a nutrient is in a serving of food. By using the %DV, you can tell if this amount is high or low. You, like most people, may not know how many calories you consume in a day. But you can still use the %DV as a frame of reference, whether or not you eat more or less than 2,000 calories each day.

■ ■ ■ ■

Here Are the Foods To Watch Out for

In addition to trans fats, other foods, if eaten to excess, could precipitate heart and other health problems.

• **Saturated fats.** Foods high in saturated fats tend to raise blood cholesterol. They include high-fat dairy products (like cheese, whole milk, cream, butter and ice cream), fatty fresh and processed meats, poultry skin and fat, lard, palm oil and coconut oil. Keep your intake of these foods low.

• **Dietary cholesterol.** Foods that are high in cholesterol also tend to raise blood cholesterol. These foods include liver and other organ meats, egg yolks and dairy fats.

The USDA also explains the benefits of food containing unsaturated fats…

• **Unsaturated fats.** Unsaturated fats (oils) do not raise blood cholesterol. They occur in vegetable oils, most nuts, olives, avocados and fatty fish like salmon. Olive, canola, sunflower and peanut oils are high in monounsaturated fats. Vegetable oils such as soybean oil, corn oil and cottonseed oil and many kinds of nuts are good sources of polyunsaturated fats. Some fish, such as salmon, tuna and mackerel, contain omega-3 fatty acids that are being studied to determine if they offer protection against heart disease. Use moderate amounts of food high in unsaturated fats, taking care to avoid excess calories.

Experts: Don't Rush Into Gene-Based Diets

Abdallah Daar, MD, PhD, professor, public health sciences, and director, Program in Applied Ethics and Biotechnology, Joint Centre for Bioethics, University of Toronto, Canada.

Peter A. Singer, MD, MPH, professor, medicine and director, Joint Centre for Bioethics, University of Toronto, Canada.

Helen Wallace, PhD, deputy director, GeneWatch UK, Tideswell, England.

Science is uncovering more and more about the role of genetics in the development of diseases such as diabetes, obesity, birth defects and food allergies.

Researchers are discovering how chemicals in foods can affect genes—or even how genes can predict whether particular foods are likely to cause health problems.

Studies show that some of the variations in a person's blood pressure and bone density, for example, also are genetically determined. In some people, food may even cause genes to malfunction.

The issue of genetics and diet, or nutritional genomics (nutrigenomics), is a growing field of research on how nutrients and genes interact and how genetic variations may cause people to respond differently to nutrients.

Scientists are predicting that it could bring about radical changes in how food is grown, processed and consumed.

Some corporations, for instance, might be as interested as doctors in knowing that you have a higher genetic risk of getting a certain health condition.

"We could see food companies, which are very powerful, who might say, 'Hey, buy this because it might help you genetically,'" says Dr. Abdallah Daar, a professor of public health sciences at the University of Toronto.

EXPERTS UNCONVINCED

Some experts warn against such a headlong rush into nutrigenomics before there's been a more detailed examination of its ethical implications.

A report titled Nutrition and Genes: Science, Society and the Supermarket, a joint undertaking by the University of Toronto Joint Centre for Bioethics and the philosophy department at the University of Guelph, Ontario, stops short of prescribing guidelines for the development of the field.

"If even part of its promise is realized, nutrigenomic testing and the labeling of foods for specific subpopulations on the basis of their genetic makeup could become highly important public health tools," Peter A. Singer, director of the Joint Centre for Bioethics, says in the report.

"But this research raises many of the ethical concerns now associated with genetic testing," he says.

Genetic test kits can be ordered online. According to several vendors, consumers need only to take a cheek swab, answer a lifestyle questionnaire and send it to the company, which for a fee, will send you a list of genetic indicators and corresponding nutritional guidelines.

However, as genetic profiling is still in its infancy, not all experts agree with confidence on the capability of current knowledge to recommend dietary changes.

Lower Cholesterol Right From Your Kitchen

David J.A. Jenkins, MD, professor, department of nutritional sciences, University of Toronto.
Nieca Goldberg, MD, director, women's cardiac care, Lenox Hill Hospital, New York City.
Journal of the American Medical Association.

G rab a spoon and get healthier! Adding fiber-rich plants such as oats, barley and nuts to a standard low-fat diet can reduce cholesterol levels by nearly 30%. That's just about as much as a statin drug, researchers report.

In a four-week trial with 46 participants, it was shown that diet alone can produce impressive cholesterol-lowering results, says study leader Dr. David J.A. Jenkins, a professor in the University of Toronto's nutritional sciences department.

THE STUDY

Jenkins and his colleagues assigned 16 people with dangerously high blood cholesterol levels to a standard cholesterol-lowering diet —low in saturated fat and rich in whole-wheat cereals. Another 14 people ate the same diet and also took cholesterol-lowering *lovastatin*. A third group of 16 followed the experimental diet, which included ample amounts of oats, barley, psyllium, soy foods and almonds.

Those foods were chosen because they are rich in plant sterols, viscous fiber and soy protein. The US Food and Drug Administration now allows that sterols, viscous fiber, some nuts (including almonds) and soy protein can reduce the risk of heart disease. But "this dietary combination had never been directly compared with the use of a statin," note the researchers.

After four weeks, participants following the standard diet had an average reduction of 8% in blood levels of LDL cholesterol, the "bad" kind that clogs arteries. The reduction in LDL was a much higher 30.9% for those taking the statin and 28.6% for those eating the experimental diet.

"The main message of the experiment is that unlike before, when most reductions of cholesterol by diet alone were modest, we can put together a number of components with a much broader appeal that for many people can be an alternative to the older statins," such as lovastatin, Jenkins says.

Jenkins says it's now necessary to study the diet against the newer statins, which tend to be more effective than the older ones.

THE AHA AGREES

The diet "is consistent with the new guidelines of the American Heart Association," says Dr. Nieca Goldberg, director of women's cardiac care at Lenox Hill Hospital in New York City and a spokeswoman for the association. "The guidelines recognize the importance of adding fiber and soy protein and nuts to your diet," she says. "This diet is not exactly the same as the American Heart Association's diet, but they are similar."

Some caution is needed when interpreting the study results because the study was a small one, Goldberg says, and "the diet is pretty restrictive." But it does provide guidance for doctors and people worried about their cholesterol levels, she adds.

The issue of compliance—can people follow this diet for a long time?—is important to both Jenkins and Goldberg. Jenkins is optimistic because the added foods are familiar to most people. "Many people eat bran on a regular basis," he says. "We're not talking about foods that have never been introduced before."

info Find the current guidelines on healthy eating from the American Heart Association at *www.americanheart.org.*

Sweet Relief—Hot Cocoa, A Healing Drink

Journal of Agricultural and Food Chemistry.

That steaming mug of cocoa may do more than just warm your body and spirit on a cold winter day. It may provide you with some health benefits, too.

Hot cocoa contains more antioxidants per cup than a similar serving of red wine or tea and may be a healthier choice, says a Cornell University study.

Antioxidants are chemicals believed to help fight cancer, heart disease and aging.

The researchers found that, on a per-serving basis, the antioxidant concentration in cocoa was almost two times stronger than in red wine, two to three times stronger than in green tea, and four to five times stronger than in black tea.

BETTER HOT THAN COLD

The study also says hot cocoa triggers the release of more antioxidants than cold cocoa.

Many other popular beverages, such as cranberry juice and orange juice, also contain high levels of antioxidants, but they weren't evaluated in this study.

Experts say the best way to obtain plenty of antioxidants is to eat a variety of fruits and vegetables.

HOW ANTIOXIDANTS WORK

Antioxidants retard the damage to cells caused by so-called free radicals, renegade molecules that have been linked to cancer and other ailments.

Antioxidants—including beta-carotene, lycopene and the vitamins C, E and A—make free radicals stable and prevent them from harming healthy cells.

Antioxidants are found in many foods, such as fruits and vegetables, as well as in nuts, grains and even meats, poultry and fish. They are also available in supplement form. According to the American Heart Association, 30% of people in this country now take some form of antioxidant supplement.

Although scientists have plenty of laboratory evidence showing that antioxidants block the kind of cell damage associated with cancer, studies in humans have yielded mixed results.

Some results have suggested that people who consume more of these molecules may protect themselves from certain cancers and other diseases, but other studies haven't found such an effect.

■ ■ ■ ■

More Antioxidant Research

There are currently three large ongoing studies looking at the link between antioxidants and cancer, according to the US National Cancer Institute. *These are...*

● **The Women's Health Study (WHS)** is assessing whether vitamin E can help prevent cancer among female health workers 45 years and older.

● **The Selenium and Vitamin E Cancer Prevention Trial (SELECT)** is trying to learn if taking selenium or vitamin E supplements can prevent prostate cancer in men 50 years or older. The SELECT trial is expected to finish recruiting patients in the spring of 2006.

● **The Physicians' Health Study II (PHS II)** is evaluating the effects of vitamins E and C, and multivitamin supplements on prostate cancer and overall cancer incidence. This study is expected to conclude in August 2007.

info You can learn more about antioxidants from the Centers for Disease Control and Prevention at *www.cdc.gov/nccdphp/dnpa/ 5aday/faq*. Go to "Fruits and Vegetables and Our Health."

Forget Apples— Try a Tomato a Day

Howard Sesso, ScD, MPH, Brigham and Women's Hospital, Boston.
American Society for Nutritional Sciences.

Just one serving a day of tomato-based foods, such as pizza or tomato sauce, might be a tasty way to lower your risk for heart disease by as much as 30%, according to a recent study.

"The results are pretty enticing," says study author Howard Sesso, an assistant professor at the Harvard School of Public Health and Brigham and Women's Hospital in Boston.

THE STUDY

Sesso and his colleagues reviewed the diets of about 40,000 women from the ongoing Women's Health Study, which for 11 years has followed women who were initially free from cancer and cardiovascular disease.

The researchers found that women who consumed seven or more servings of tomato-based foods a week—including tomato juice, tomatoes, tomato sauce or pizza—had a nearly 30% reduction in risk for cardiovascular disease compared with women who ate less than one and one-half servings a week.

The study was sparked by research that has shown a connection between a dietary increase in the antioxidant lycopene and a reduction in prostate cancer risk, Sesso says. Since tomatoes are a rich source of lycopene, he and his colleagues were interested to learn if eating tomatoes might also lower heart disease risk.

TOMATOES HEART-HEALTHY

Interestingly, however, when the researchers tabulated the result, the lycopene intake itself was not significantly associated with reduced heart disease risk.

However, when they looked at self-reported food intake, they found a clear cardiovascular benefit for those who consumed the tomato-based products regularly.

Sesso also points out that those people who showed the benefit from eating the tomato foods might just have an overall healthier diet than those who had fewer servings of tomatoes.

"It could be that the diet itself is protective if it includes more fruits and vegetables," he says. "Those people would have a better cardiovascular profile."

Whatever the cause, Sesso says, "our study suggests preliminary evidence that consuming a number of servings of tomato-based foods per week may lower the risk of cardiovascular disease."

info The American Academy of Family Physicians's Web site at *www.aafp.org* has helpful recommendations for healthy eating and other ways to reduce heart disease risk.

Tomatoes—Not Lycopene —Lower Prostate Cancer Risk

Steven K. Clinton, MD, medical oncologist, director, molecular carcinogenesis and chemoprevention, Ohio State University Comprehensive Cancer Center, Columbus.

Peter H. Gann, MD, associate professor, preventive medicine, Robert H. Lurie Comprehensive Cancer Center, Northwestern University, Chicago.

Journal of the National Cancer Institute.

Lycopene, a compound found in tomatoes, has been linked to many health benefits. But a new animal study suggests that whole tomato products, rather than just lycopene, would be a better choice for men who want to reduce their risk of prostate cancer. Eating fewer total calories also helps reduce that risk.

In the study, rats fed diets that contained whole tomato powder, including lycopene and other compounds, had a 26% lower risk of prostate cancer death than those that were fed diets containing pure lycopene or standard diets without either lycopene or tomato products, researchers said.

"Since lycopene is the carotenoid that gives a tomato its red color and has antioxidant properties, many assume the reasons tomatoes may protect, if they do, from cancer is because of the lycopene," says study author Dr. Steven K. Clinton, an oncologist at Ohio State University Comprehensive Cancer Center.

THE RESEARCH

The rats in the project were divided not just into the lycopene and tomato powder groups, but into groups that got unlimited access to food and those in which calories were reduced by 20%.

The rats that ate 20% fewer calories had a 32% lower risk of prostate cancer death than those with unlimited access to food, the researchers say.

"This reinforces the importance of preventing obesity," Clinton says. A study published in the *New England Journal of Medicine* reported that being overweight or obese seems to be responsible for 14% of cancer deaths in men and 20% in women; prostate cancer is one of the cancers associated with being overweight.

PASS THE SALSA!

Although many Americans would prefer to take a lycopene pill, Clinton says, his study points to the benefit of having tomato products in your diet in the form of the tomato itself, or as juice, soup, sauces or salsa.

So how much tomato is protective? "In the rat diet, it was 10 percent of the entire diet," Clinton says. However, he believes it would be reasonable to advise men who want to reduce their risk to eat about one tomato serving a day, or five to seven servings a week.

"Tomato juice, soup, sauce, they all fit in," he says.

Dr. Peter H. Gann, associate professor of preventive medicine at the Robert H. Lurie Comprehensive Cancer Center at Northwestern University in Chicago, notes Americans may be on their way to fulfilling the "eat more tomatoes" recommendation—they average 91 pounds of tomatoes per capita per year.

info For more on prostate cancer, see the National Library of Medicine's MedlinePlus site at *www.nlm.nih.gov/medlineplus/ prostatecancer.html.*

Is It Time to Become A Vegetarian?

Neal D. Barnard, MD, president and founder of the Physicians Committee for Responsible Medicine, Washington, DC.

Bottom Line/Health.

The average American consumes 220 pounds of meat each year, but the recent mad cow scare has made many people think twice about this practice.

Even before the latest questions were raised regarding the safety of the US meat supply, 10 million Americans identified themselves as vegetarians.

Here are answers to some commonly asked questions about vegetarianism from Dr. Neal D. Barnard, president and founder of the Physicians Committee for Responsible Medicine, an independent, nonprofit health research and advocacy group…

●**Why do you favor a meat-free diet?** It's been scientifically proven—in epidemiological studies of people who selected their own diets, and in clinical trials where people were assigned vegetarian diets—that a vegetarian regimen is the most healthful diet.

Studies of Seventh-day Adventists—people who don't smoke, use alcohol or eat meat and who exercise regularly—have shown that a vegetarian diet (excluding their other healthful lifestyle practices) allows them to live about 10 years longer than nonvegetarians.

Other studies show that vegetarians have a lower incidence of cardiovascular disease, diabetes and hypertension. Vegetarians also are 40% less likely to develop cancer, especially of the colon and prostate.

●**In your opinion, what are the greatest health risks associated with meat-eating?** Many factors should discourage you from eating meat. Cooking meat at higher temperatures, such as those used during grilling or broiling, generates *heterocyclic amines,* carcinogens that can be formed when animal tissue is heated. Because of these carcinogens as well as the harmful effects of fat and cholesterol, a meat-eater has three times the risk for colon cancer as a person who rarely eats meat.

Meat also is devoid of key nutrients, like fiber and vitamin C. Because it consists of little more than fat and protein, meat is one of the most calorie-dense foods. Fat contains nine calories per gram of weight, whereas protein, such as beans, and carbohydrates, such as breads and pasta, have only four calories per gram.

●**What do you consider to be the most healthful type of vegetarian diet?** A *vegan* diet—one that includes no animal or dairy products whatsoever—is the most healthful. From a health standpoint, there is no reason to add these foods to your diet. They typically

are high in cholesterol and fat, and can be easily replaced with healthier alternatives, such as soy products or rice milk.

There's plenty of protein in most types of beans…and grains, such as rice and oats. If your concern is calcium, green vegetables and beans are a better source than milk because they also provide antioxidants and fiber.

As for meat being "low-fat," that's simply not true. The leanest beef is 28% fat. The leanest chicken—breast, with the skin removed—is 23% fat. The fat content of fish varies widely, from 10% to more than 50%. Compare that with beans, at 4%.

In a study of 59 people who ate either a vegan diet or less than six ounces of meat per day, the vegans got more iron from eating green vegetables and beans.

●**What foods are allowed on a vegan diet?** If you adopt this form of vegetarianism, you'll be eating from four food groups—whole grains, vegetables, fruits and legumes, such as beans and peas. Eat these in whatever proportions you like, and you'll lose weight as well.

Eat spaghetti marinara, bean burritos, vegetarian chili, many kinds of Asian dishes—the list of possibilities is almost endless. If you're time-pressured, have a Veggie Delite (on Italian bread) at Subway or a veggie burger (without mayonnaise) at Burger King.

To ensure that you're consuming all your essential nutrients, take a multivitamin specifically formulated for vegetarians (marked on the label). Also take a vitamin B-12 supplement (6 micrograms daily) or eat B-12–fortified foods, including some cereals and some meat substitutes.

●**What's the best way to start a vegetarian diet?** First, speak to your doctor. If you get his/her okay, then jump in all at once, rather than simply cutting back on meat. This is safe to do, but be aware that you may experience intestinal gas if you eat a lot of beans.

Within three weeks, your taste buds will have adjusted, you'll have lost a few pounds and you'll be glad you made the change. Chances are you'll stick with a meat-free diet for the rest of your life.

●**What basic food items should be included in a vegetarian's pantry?** Pasta, rice and couscous are good staples to have on hand. For legumes, I recommend dried lentils, split peas and pinto beans, as well as canned chick peas and black beans.

My favorite produce items include potatoes, carrots, celery, yellow onions and raisins.

Baked tofu, vegetarian hot dogs and veggie burgers are delicious meat substitutes. Tortillas and pita bread also are convenient. If you want snack foods, rice cakes, popcorn and pretzels are excellent choices.

IBS? Your Problem Could Be Fat and Fructose

Nancy Kraft, RD, clinical dietitian, University of Iowa, Iowa City.

Theodore M. Bayless, MD, professor, medicine, The Johns Hopkins University, Baltimore.

Presentation, American College of Gastroenterology annual meeting, Baltimore.

Cutting back on sugar and fat makes sense for people trying to control their weight, but there may be another health benefit. Two studies suggest that fat and fructose, the sugar in fruits and honey, also can contribute gastrointestinal discomfort.

IBS is a common disorder of the intestines that leads to pain, gassiness, bloating and changes in bowel habits, according to the American Gastroenterological Association. The disorder can lead to constipation in some and diarrhea in others. Some sufferers experience both. Another common symptom may be a crampy urge to move the bowels.

In the first report, Nancy Kraft, a clinical dietitian from the University of Iowa, and her colleagues say some patients with irritable bowel syndrome (IBS) are fructose-intolerant, and restricting that type of sugar can improve their symptoms.

Kraft says fructose intolerance often is an overlooked component of IBS.

Her colleague, Dr. Young Choi, says that, "a fructose-restricted diet significantly improved symptoms in patients with IBS and fructose intolerance. Fructose intolerance is yet another piece of the IBS puzzle."

THE STUDY

In the study, the 14 patients with IBS who followed a fructose-free diet for one year, experienced a significant reduction in abdominal pain, bloating and diarrhea.

However, IBS symptoms remained the same for the 12 patients who did not stick with the diet, the researchers report.

Kraft believes these results are encouraging, because "people who limit their intake of fructose see their symptoms improve or disappear," but that further study is needed.

SECOND STUDY

Researchers from the Mayo Clinic in Rochester, Minnesota, led by Dr. Yuri Saito, collected data on the diets of 221 adults, aged 20 to 50 years. Of these patients, 102 had gastrointestinal disorders and 119 were healthy.

The research team found patients with IBS or dyspepsia (indigestion) reported eating more monounsaturated fats compared with healthy patients. These patients also ate fewer carbohydrates than their healthy counterparts.

The Mayo investigators concluded that "future studies are needed to determine whether fat intake causes gastrointestinal symptoms."

Dr. Theodore M. Bayless, a professor of medicine at The Johns Hopkins University, finds both reports of value. He is not surprised fat and fructose are linked with IBS and dyspepsia.

He notes that both fat and fructose are hard to digest and can aggravate both conditions. Bayless, however, does not believe that restricting fructose cures IBS; it may only relieve the symptoms.

Bayless says "anyone who is gassy with or without IBS will benefit by decreasing the intake of fructose."

He advises his patients to avoid fatty foods and foods that contain high levels of fructose such as grapes, dates, nuts, honey and apple or pear juice.

He also advises patients to increase fiber intake to help their bowels perform regularly.

Surprising Finding—
Calcium Lowers
Risk of Kidney Stones

Gary Curhan, MD, associate professor, medicine, and nephrologist, Brigham and Women's Hospital, Boston.

Khalid Zafar, MD, nephrologist, William Beaumont Hospital, Royal Oak, MI.

Presentation, American Society of Nephrology annual meeting, San Diego.

Young women who eat foods rich in calcium may reduce their risk of getting painful kidney stones, according to a recent study.

Dietary calcium, whole grains and vegetables all appear to lower the chances of kidney stones, while a high sugar intake may increase the risk, the study found.

Kidney stones form from substances in the urine. The most common type forms from calcium oxalate in the urine. Other substances that contribute to stone formation include uric acid, struvite and cystine.

Stones come in varying sizes—from a grain of sand to the size of a golf ball. Some stones pass through the urinary tract system on their own, but some get stuck and block the flow of urine. When this happens, medical intervention is necessary.

Contrary to what was believed in the past, diets high in calcium and protein don't increase your risk of kidney stones, the researchers say. The study also found no additional risk from taking calcium supplements.

"Dietary factors are important," says study author Dr. Gary Curhan, an associate professor of medicine and a nephrologist at Brigham and Women's Hospital in Boston. "Dietary modification may reduce an individual's risk of kidney stones. Our findings challenge the belief that calcium should be restricted."

THE STUDY

Curhan and his colleagues gathered data from the large Nurses Health Study II, which includes more than 100,000 women. For this study, the researchers focused on 96,000 women who were between the ages of 27 and 44 years when the study began.

At the end of an eight-year study period, 1,223 women had developed kidney stones.

The researchers found that women who had the highest dietary calcium intake from foods such as milk, cheese and yogurt reduced their risk of kidney stones by 27%. Consumption of phytate, a naturally occurring substance found in whole grains and vegetables, lowered the risk of kidney stones by 37%. And a higher fluid intake also appeared to reduce the risk of kidney stones.

MORE SUGAR IS WORSE

Sugar did raise the risk of developing kidney stones in young women by slightly more than 30%. Protein and calcium supplements didn't appear to significantly increase or decrease the risk.

Dr. Khalid Zafar, a nephrologist at William Beaumont Hospital in Royal Oak, Michigan, says, "The take-home message is that people with kidney stones should not decrease dietary calcium and they can take supplements and eat meat."

He says the finding that supplements don't increase the risk of kidney stones in young women is especially important, because women need calcium to prevent osteoporosis, and many don't get sufficient amounts from their diet.

info To learn more about kidney stones, visit the National Kidney and Urologic Diseases Information Clearinghouse at *www. kidney.niddk.nih.gov.*

Fiber Supplements
Do the Job

Mayo Clinic Health Letter.
Mayo Clinic, Rochester, MN, news release.

If you're having trouble getting enough fiber from the foods in your diet, consider supplements, according to the *Mayo Clinic Health Letter.* Foods such as oatmeal, cauliflower, broccoli, beans and peas are all good sources of fiber.

HIGH FIBER, LOW RISK

In addition to helping digestion and regularity, a high-fiber diet may reduce your risk of certain health problems, such as diabetes, colorectal cancer, gastrointestinal disorders, high cholesterol and obesity.

But some people find it difficult to get the recommended 20 to 30 grams of fiber per day from their diet because they don't like high-fiber foods or because those foods cause cramping or flatulence.

If that's the case, consider fiber supplements, which are bulk-forming substances available as powders, tablets, wafers, biscuits or toasted granules.

Fiber supplements, which are labeled as "bulking agents" on over-the-counter products, are safe for the long-term treatment of constipation.

■ ■ ■ ■

Advice for Taking Fiber Supplements

The *Mayo Clinic Health Letter* offers the following advice for people who decide to try fiber supplements…

●**Go slowly.** Start with a small dose and progress gradually.

●**Be consistent.** Fiber supplements are most effective when taken daily for at least one month.

●**Drink plenty of fluids.** If you don't drink enough, fiber supplements can sometimes make you constipated.

●**If you are overweight,** take fiber supplements before meals because they create a feeling of fullness. If you are underweight or normal weight, take them after meals.

●**Remember that supplements can't do it all.** They contain only part of the required amount of daily fiber. You still need to include high-fiber foods in your diet.

Unbelievable! You Can Eat Your Doggie Bag…

Tara McHugh, PhD, research leader, processed foods research unit, US Department of Agriculture's Western Regional Research Center, Albany, CA.

Althea Zanecosky, dietician, Lafayette Hill, PA, and spokeswoman, American Dietetic Association.

Soon you might not have to throw away your sandwich wrapper; you'll just eat it instead. Scientists at the US Department of Agriculture (USDA) have created edible food wraps made of vegetables and fruits.

Lead researcher Tara McHugh says that the wraps would be a healthy alternative to plastic or aluminum foil and environmentally friendly, because they'd reduce waste produced by synthetic wrapping.

The edible wrap consists of a flexible, paper-thin film made entirely of fruits or vegetables. Wrap flavors may include broccoli, carrots, tomatoes, peaches, pears, apples, papayas and strawberries.

McHugh says the wraps are biodegradable, unlike plastic and aluminum foil, and thus would help prevent waste and environmental damage to land and water.

USDA researchers make the wraps by pureeing and diluting fruits or vegetables to free-flowing mixtures, which are then spread onto Teflon sheets to dry overnight. Lipids—in this case, vegetable oils—could be used to make the wraps more water-resistant, she says.

WRAP UP YOUR VITAMIN INTAKE

McHugh says many Americans do not get the minimum five recommended daily servings of fruits and vegetables. The wraps—a few of them would equal one serving—could boost consumption, she says.

You might cover leftover pasta with a tomato wrap, which would melt into the pasta when heated. Wrap your pork chops in an apple film that would become a glaze. Try a strawberry wrap on cut bananas, or eat a carrot wrap with the salad it preserves.

Althea Zanecosky, a dietitian based in Lafayette Hill, Pennsylvania, agrees the wraps could help people, especially children, reach the recommended daily fruit and vegetable intake. Kids are drawn to fun and colorful products, such as purple yogurt, blue applesauce and colorful sports drinks, adds Zanecosky, a spokeswoman for the American Dietetic Association.

"Children are part of this group of people that could use more fruit or vegetables in their diet, and this might be one way to get one more extra fruit or vegetable into a child's diet," she says. "So if you could wrap a sandwich in strawberry wrapping that was edible, lots of kids would think that was very cool."

But Zanecosky wonders whether nutrients—including vitamins, minerals and fiber—could be lost while processing the fruits and vegetables into the wraps.

McHugh says she's confident the fiber from fruits and vegetables would be retained, but adds that the wraps have not been analyzed for nutrient retention. Any nutrients lost during processing, she says, could be replaced through fortification.

Microwaving Vegetables Destroys Nutrients

Cristina Garcia-Viguera, PhD, research scientist, department of food science and technology, Center of Edaphology and Applied Biology, Seguera-High Council of Scientific Research, Murcia, Spain.
Bottom Line/Health.

I n a recent study, broccoli that was cooked in a microwave lost more than 97% of its disease-fighting compounds, *flavonoids,* and up to 40% of vitamin C.

Although veggies that were boiled retained more nutrients than those cooked in a microwave, they still lost 66% of flavonoids and up to 40% of vitamin C.

To minimize nutrient loss: Microwave or boil vegetables on the lowest possible temperature and for shorter periods of time.

Best: Steaming vegetables reduces their nutrients by only 10%.

13

Pain Treatments

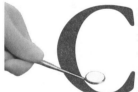

Tiny Dental Device May Stop Migraines

Can a little mouth device prevent your head from throbbing? Maybe. The US Food and Drug Administration (FDA) has approved the *nociceptive trigeminal inhibition-tension suppression system* (NTI-tss) for the prevention of migraine and tension-type headache pain.

Dr. Marvin Mansky, a Manhattan dentist, admits he "didn't think [the NTI device] was a great idea" at first. But now, after he's used it to treat 350 patients—and wears one himself occasionally—he's a believer.

"It reduces the frequency and intensity of migraines dramatically," Mansky says. "For some, it stops the migraines completely."

Chronic headaches afflict an estimated 45 million Americans, resulting in more than 8 million visits to the doctor every year, according to the National Institute of Neurological

Disorders and Stroke. For relief, people who have headaches turn to a variety of treatments, including over-the-counter and prescription medicines, dietary controls, exercise, yoga, biofeedback, stress-reduction techniques, whirlpool baths, cold packs and more.

THE DEVICE

Made of clear plastic, the inch-wide NTI device fits over two front teeth—usually, but not always, the top teeth.

It stops the teeth in the back from coming together and thus, prevents clenching—which the developer of the device, also a dentist, claims is the cause of many headaches.

According to the proponents of the NTI device, prolonged, intense clenching stresses the temporal muscles that work to open and close the jaw, often triggering migraine and tension headaches.

Some people who have tried it swear by the NTI device. The first person Mansky fitted with

Marvin Mansky, DDS, New York, NY.

Stephen Silberstein, MD, professor, neurology, Jefferson Medical College, and director, Jefferson Headache Center, Thomas Jefferson University, Philadelphia.

one was a woman who had severe head pain. Immediately, he says, her pain, on a scale of one to 10, went from a 10 to a two, and within two weeks, all pain was gone.

For that relief, many people seem willing to pay roughly $750 for the tiny tooth protector. Mansky and other dentists around the country can mold and custom-fit the device in about an hour. Most people wear it only while sleeping, although some wear a slightly less obtrusive device during the day as well.

ANOTHER OPINION

However, Dr. Stephen Silberstein, a neurology professor at Thomas Jefferson University in Philadelphia and president of the American Headache Society, disputes the connection between clenching and headaches.

"There's scientific evidence to show that only rarely does clenching ever produce headaches," Silberstein says. "If you have a sore jaw, if you grind your teeth, [the device] will probably help you. But don't expect any more than that."

"There's no question there's a value to devices," he says. Although he is unfamiliar with this particular device, Silberstein says it's "logical" that if it stops people from grinding their teeth, it would relieve any pain that stems from teeth grinding.

"If you have tennis elbow and you put a brace on it, the problem's going to get better —but it's not going to help your foot," he says, adding that the same idea applies to teeth clenching and migraines. "You have to be very careful with devices and their magic."

Responding to criticism of the device, its inventor—California dentist Dr. James P. Boyd —cites a study from Ireland that showed the jaw-clenching muscles in migraine sufferers were nearly 70% larger, as well as stronger, than the same muscles in people who did not have migraines. Boyd believes that points to a clear link between clenching and migraine headaches.

info To learn more about headaches, check with the American Council for Headache Education at *www.achenet.org/under standing*.

Diagnosing Migraines Is as Easy as 1...2...3

Neurology.
Albert Einstein College of Medicine news release.

A simple, three-question test can identify people with migraine headaches about as accurately as widely used screening tests for other illnesses, research suggests.

According to the test, which was developed by a team of American migraine experts and validated in a national study, an answer of "yes" to two of the following three questions effectively identifies migraine sufferers. *The questions are...*

• **Has a headache limited your activities** for a day or more in the last three months?

• **Are you nauseated or sick to your stomach** when you have a headache?

• **Does light bother you** when you have a headache?

THE STUDY

The researchers used this test, called ID Migraine, at 27 primary care sites and 12 headache specialty practice sites in the United States. Their study included 443 people on a routine visit to their primary care physician for any health reason. All participants completed a nine-question survey.

All of the participants in the study either had headaches that interfered with their work, studies or quality of life, or said they wanted to discuss their headaches with a doctor. They were referred to one of 12 headache specialty centers, where experts then diagnosed them without knowing how they had answered the questionnaire.

The researchers then compared the diagnoses from the headache specialty centers with the answers the participants had given on the questionnaire. Of the patients who answered "yes" to two of the three questions, 93% received a migraine diagnosis.

"Because patients with migraine headaches often present in the primary care setting, the hope is that ID Migraine will help primary care doctors in identifying migraine quickly and easily," says lead author Dr. Richard B. Lipton, professor and vice chair of neurology at the Albert Einstein College of Medicine.

"Given the current availability of effective treatment, the use of the screening tool might represent an important step toward reducing the burden of this illness," Lipton says.

■ ■ ■ ■

Migraines Are Much More Than Just Headaches

An estimated 28 million Americans have migraines, but fewer than half have been given a clinical diagnosis by a doctor. Women are three times more likely than men to experience the attacks, which can last anywhere from 30 minutes to several days.

Approximately 15% of migraine headaches are preceded by flashes of light, blind spots or tingling limbs—signs that are collectively called "aura."

They may also be accompanied by nausea and vomiting. They may strike one side of the head or both simultaneously.

What causes migraines isn't clear, though they are thought to have a genetic component. People who have these headaches say they can be triggered by stress, certain foods (such as chocolate and wine) and a variety of other stimuli.

Research shows that migraines may leave telltale scars in the brain, evidence of cell death associated with a lack of blood. People with frequent migraines were many times more likely to have scarring than those with rarer headaches, the study found.

The scarring, detected by magnetic resonance imaging (MRI) scans, hasn't been tied to any functional problems, such as memory loss or trouble thinking. However, some researchers believe that the tests we use to detect such complications may not be sensitive enough yet.

info The National Institutes of Health Web site at *http://health.nih.gov* has more information on headaches and migraine.

Skin Sensitivity Makes Choosing Migraine Treatment Easier

Rami Burstein, PhD, associate professor, neurology, Harvard Medical School, and vice chairman, research, department of anesthesia and critical care, Beth Israel Deaconess Medical Center, both in Boston.

Roger Cady, MD, director, Headache Care Center, Springfield, MO, and member, board of directors, National Headache Foundation.

Annals of Neurology online.

As if the throbbing pain, nausea and sensitivity to light that many migraine patients experience isn't bad enough, many also suffer from something called *cutaneous allodynia,* or skin sensitivity.

This sensitivity can make routine activities, such as combing your hair, shaving and putting on glasses, excruciatingly painful.

Research claims the presence of this condition may help predict how patients respond to triptans, a major class of migraine drugs. And this information could make the treatment of migraines much more predictable.

MYSTERY SOLVED?

Migraine headaches are still a mystery—no one knows why some people get migraines and others don't. Even if a person is susceptible to migraines and has a trigger that sets him or her off, it's not clear why that trigger only spurs a migraine some of the time.

Triptans, which debuted in the early 1990s, also are perplexing, relieving a person's pain one time and then not working another time.

"[This study] explains to us why triptans work and why they don't," says study author Rami Burstein, an associate professor of neurology at Harvard Medical School.

The study was funded in part by the National Institutes of Health and GlaxoSmithKline, the pharmaceutical company that was responsible for developing triptans.

THE STUDY

To try to understand migraines better, Burstein and his colleagues looked at the effect of triptans on 34 migraines that included allodynia and 27 migraines that didn't.

The results showed that triptans relieved pain in most of the patients without skin sensitivities, regardless of when the treatment was initiated.

In those people with the skin sensitivity, the drugs worked best when they were administered early.

The findings have prompted Burstein to suggest a new classification for treating migraines.

He says, "I can predict now with about 90% accuracy which migraine attacks would be terminated by triptan before I even treat them."

ANOTHER STUDY

An accompanying study on rats, also led by Burstein, sheds light on the neurological mechanisms behind this phenomenon.

At first, migraine symptoms involve nerves that are outside the brain.

"As time goes on and the migraine intensifies and grows, that pain generation changes from outside the brain to inside the brain and it ultimately can create allodynia," explains Dr. Roger Cady, director of the Headache Care Center in Springfield, Missouri, and a member of the board of directors of the National Headache Foundation.

"Once the migraine changes from the outside nerves to the inside nerves, the effectiveness of triptans drops off dramatically because those drugs work primarily on those nerves outside of the brain," Cady says.

EARLY TREATMENT IS THE MOST EFFECTIVE

For doctors and migraine sufferers, the clear message is to act early.

"Don't wait for pain to become disabling," Cady says. "The reality is there is no penalty for early treatment. If you are someone whose headaches involve allodynia, it is critical that you treat early, otherwise you are not going to get relief."

info For more on the treatment of migraines, visit the National Headache Foundation at *www.headaches.org/consumer/topicsheets/migraine.html.*

Epilepsy Drug Relieves Chronic Headaches

Roy G. Beran, MD, department of neurology, Liverpool Hospital, New South Wales, Australia.

Stephen Silberstein, MD, professor, neurology, Jefferson Medical College, and director, Jefferson Headache Center, Thomas Jefferson University, Philadelphia.

Neurology.

A medication may offer some hope of relief for people who experience chronic daily headaches. The epilepsy drug *gabapentin,* when taken daily, relieves pain in one third of patients who have chronic daily headache, according to Australian researchers.

"Chronic daily headaches include migraines, chronic tension headaches or headaches from other causes," says lead researcher Dr. Roy G. Beran, of the department of neurology at Liverpool Hospital in New South Wales.

THE STUDY

The trial was a randomized study that was conducted by the Australian Gabapentin Chronic Daily Headache Group.

Patients received either 2,400 milligrams (mg) of gabapentin, the maximum approved dose in Australia for treating people with epilepsy, or a placebo.

After the first six weeks of treatment, there was a one-week period when no treatment was given, and then the groups switched treatments for a second six-week period. Of the 133 men and women in the study, data was available for 95, according to the report.

Beran's team found that one third of the people participating in the trial stopped having chronic daily headaches while they were receiving gabapentin.

"Those who had a response did brilliantly," Beran says. However, "there was a significant number who did not have a response."

RECOMMENDATIONS

Beran believes that with a physician's approval, gabapentin should be used to treat chronic daily headache in patients where all other treatments have failed.

For people who have chronic daily headache, Beran stresses, "there is hope out there —don't give up. Our study clearly shows that there is benefit to using gabapentin in the treatment of chronic daily headache."

HIGHER DOSES MAY BE MORE EFFECTIVE

He also speculates that higher doses of gabapentin may be even more effective and may improve the response among patients who do not respond to the dosage used in his study.

"Gabapentin is one of the safest products ever made," Beran says.

He believes that gabapentin can be given in doses of up to 5 grams per day without any harmful effects.

Beran points out that in Australia, as in the United States, gabapentin is approved only for the treatment of epilepsy.

However, it is being used "off label" as a painkiller and to treat depression, mania and anxiety, he says.

NOT EVERYONE AGREES WITH STUDY RESULTS

Dr. Stephen Silberstein, a professor of neurology at Jefferson Medical College and director of the Jefferson Headache Center at Thomas Jefferson University located in Philadelphia, calls the results of the Australian research interesting, but not very persuasive.

"In my experience, gabapentin is not a very successful medication for headache disorders," Silberstein says.

Silberstein finds fault with the study methodology because it didn't distinguish between the different types of headaches and how those various types of headaches each reacted to gabapentin.

In addition, the overall beneficial effect of the drug was not very great, he says.

info To learn more about the treatments for headaches, visit the American Headache Society at *www.ahsnet.org*.

Important News: High Blood Pressure Linked to Morning Headaches

Maurice M. Ohayon, MD, PhD, associate professor, psychiatry and behavioral sciences, Stanford University School of Medicine, Palo Alto, CA.
Seymour Diamond, MD, director, Diamond Headache Center, Chicago.
Archives of Internal Medicine.

Morning headaches afflict one of every 13 people, a recent survey shows, and these painful awakenings are closely linked to depression and anxiety.

The high incidence of morning headache "is very surprising," says Dr. Maurice M. Ohayon, an associate professor of psychiatry and behavioral sciences at Stanford University School of Medicine. "It means that a lot of people are suffering."

"With a population of 300 million in America, it means that 27 million people are suffering," he says. "These are people who do not sleep well, who wake up with pain. There are probably a lot of consequences, in their work and their personal relationships."

THE SURVEY

The survey included 18,980 residents of five European countries. In all, 7.6% of the respondents said they have chronic morning headaches—1.3% every day, 4.4% "often" and 1.9% "sometimes." Women were slightly more likely than men to have chronic morning headaches (8.4% versus 6.7%).

Heavy drinkers, people who had high blood pressure or conditions affecting muscle and skeletal function were among those most likely to start the day with a throbbing head, the survey found. But the highest incidence was among people who had depression and anxiety disorders.

RECOMMENDATIONS

Because the survey found a link between high blood pressure and morning headaches, Dr. Seymour Diamond, executive chairman of the National Headache Foundation and director of the Diamond Headache Center located in Chicago, recommends checking your blood pressure if you wake up with a headache every morning.

Despite the extensive literature about morning headaches being caused by obstructed breathing, Diamond says, "This survey does not validate that opinion."

Mainly, Diamond adds, "This survey solidifies the fact that depressive disorders can cause frequent early morning headaches."

The best medications for chronic headache sufferers are the older tricyclic antidepressants, such as *amitryptyline* (Elavil) and *amoxapine* (Asendin), Diamond says. They are available in less expensive generic versions and have been "more effective in my clinical practice" in preventing headaches than newer antidepressants such as *fluoxetine* (Prozac), he says.

New Pain Reliever Easier on Your Stomach

Stefano Fiorucci, MD, professor of gastroenterology, University of Perugia, Italy.

Brett Bernstein, MD, director of ambulatory services, division of digestive disease, Beth Israel Medical Center, and assistant professor of medicine, Albert Einstein College of Medicine, New York City.

Proceedings of the National Academy of Sciences.

A new formulation of aspirin, called NCX-4016, may be effective without damaging the stomach.

Millions of people are taking aspirin daily, largely because it has been shown to reduce the risk of heart attack and stroke. But aspirin also can damage the lining of the gastrointestinal tract.

Many people also take anti-inflammatory drugs called COX-2 inhibitors for arthritis. COX-2 inhibitors can exacerbate the stomach damage caused by regular aspirin.

"Millions of people are exposed simultaneously to COX-2 inhibitors plus aspirin, which significantly increases the risk" of stomach damage, says Dr. Stefano Fiorucci, professor of gastroenterology at the University of Perugia in Italy.

THE STUDY

To see if NCX-4016 could prevent stomach damage from COX-2 inhibitors, Fiorucci and his colleagues recruited 32 healthy volunteers. Half received the NCX-4016, plus the COX-2 inhibitor *celecoxib,* which is sold under the brand name Celebrex. The other half got regular aspirin (100 milligrams) along with celecoxib.

At the end of the trial, participants in the regular aspirin group suffered about twice as much stomach damage as people in the NCX-4016 group. The results suggest that NCX-4016 may be a safer alternative to regular aspirin for patients who also are taking COX-2 inhibitors.

WHY IT WORKS

NCX-4016 differs from the old formulation of aspirin in that it releases nitric oxide, which increases blood flow to different parts of the body. One reason traditional aspirin can cause damage to the stomach is that it may decrease blood flow to the lining of the stomach, explains Dr. Brett Bernstein, director of ambulatory services in the division of digestive disease at Beth Israel Medical Center in New York City. As a result, "substances that normally protect the stomach lining can't get to it," he says. "Nitric oxide opens up the blood flow, and therefore could protect the lining."

info The American Heart Association has more on aspirin's protective effects at *www.americanheart.org.*

■ ■ ■ ■

Make Certain You Take the Right Pain Reliever

It's been quite a while since aspirin was the only choice to relieve a headache or back pain. Today, a number of over-the-counter pain relievers are available, as are prescription medications for specific conditions.

The National Institute of Neurological Disorders and Stroke (NINDS) offers the following description of the most commonly used pain relievers…

• **Nonsteroidal anti-inflammatory drugs (NSAIDs)** (including aspirin and ibuprofen) are widely prescribed and sometimes called non-narcotic or non-opioid analgesics. They work by reducing inflammatory responses in tissues. Many of these drugs irritate the stomach and for that reason are usually taken with food.

●**Acetaminophen** is the basic ingredient found in Tylenol® and its many generic equivalents. It is sold over-the-counter, in a prescription-strength preparation, and in combination with codeine (also by prescription). Acetaminophen is used for most of the ailments that aspirin treats, but it is much safer for children.

●**Anticonvulsants** are used for the treatment of seizure disorders, but are also sometimes prescribed for the treatment of pain. Carbamazepine, in particular, is used to treat a number of painful conditions, including trigeminal neuralgia. Another antiepileptic drug, gabapentin, is being studied for its pain-relieving properties, especially as a treatment for neuropathic pain.

●**Antidepressants** are sometimes used for the treatment of pain and, along with neuroleptics and lithium, belong to a category of drugs called psychotropic drugs. In addition, anti-anxiety drugs called benzodiazepines also act as muscle relaxants and are sometimes used as pain relievers. Physicians usually try to treat the condition with analgesics before prescribing these drugs.

●**Antimigraine drugs** include the triptans —sumatriptan, naratriptan and zolmitriptan— which are used specifically for migraine headaches. These drugs can have serious side effects in some people, so, like all prescription medicines, should be used only under a doctor's care.

●**COX-2 inhibitors** may be particularly effective for individuals with arthritis. COX-2 inhibitors are less likely to have the gastrointestinal side effects sometimes produced by NSAIDs. Patients may be able to take COX-2 inhibitors in larger doses than aspirin and other drugs that have irritating side effects, such as stomach irritation. However, the long-term effects of COX-2 inhibitors are still being evaluated.

●**Opioids,** derived from the poppy plant, include codeine and morphine. Opioids induce sedation as well as pain relief, and some patients may become physically dependent upon them. For these reasons, patients given opioids should be monitored carefully; in some cases stimulants may be prescribed to counteract the sedative side effects. In addition to drowsiness, other common side effects include constipation, nausea, and vomiting.

Snail Venom Delivers 'Fast' Pain Relief

Michael G. Byas-Smith, MD, assistant professor, anesthesiology, Emory University Medical School, Atlanta.

Michel Y. Dubois, MD, professor, anesthesiology, New York University School of Medicine, and director, NYU Pain Center, New York City.

Michael S. Leong, MD, assistant professor, anesthesia, Stanford University Medical Center, Palo Alto, CA.

Journal of the American Medical Association.

Results of a study found that more than half of cancer and AIDS patients who don't respond to other painkillers got relief when they were given *ziconotide,* a drug derived from the venom of a snail. The snail uses this venom to immobilize predators and prey.

Ziconotide is pain medication that is 1,000 times more potent than morphine without the problems of addiction or withdrawal.

THE STUDY

A team led by Dr. Michael G. Byas-Smith, an assistant professor of anesthesiology at Emory University Medical School in Atlanta, treated 111 patients with cancer or AIDS who had found no relief with other pain medications. The patients were randomly assigned to receive ziconotide or a placebo. Most of the patients were already taking morphine at the start of the study and continued to do so throughout the experiment. Ziconotide and the placebo were given continuously through a pump that delivers a measured dose.

The researchers found 53% of the patients receiving ziconotide had moderate to complete pain relief, compared with 17.5% of the patients receiving the placebo. In addition, five of the patients in the ziconotide group had complete relief from pain.

The drawbacks to ziconotide are the side effects, which occur when high doses are given, Byas-Smith says. The most common side effect was an altered mental state, but others include low blood pressure and dizziness.

Patients who have severe pain from AIDS or cancer, and who do not get good relief with morphine, can use ziconotide alone or in combination with morphine and achieve better pain management, he adds.

"We have another weapon to control pain. But it remains an ongoing process to figure out who is going to respond best to this treatment," Byas-Smith says.

However, the cone snail is fast becoming a threatened species because of pollution, overfishing, development and the exploitation of its beautiful shells. Scientists fear the species could disappear before biomedical research can take full advantage of the analgesic properties of the venom.

NOT A 'MAGIC BULLET'

Dr. Michel Y. Dubois, a professor of anesthesiology at New York University School of Medicine and director of the NYU Pain Center, says ziconotide "is not the magic bullet."

Dubois notes that in his study of patients who had pain from other nonmalignant problems, the results were similar, and no one knows why. But, he adds, "When it works, the relief does last.

"Unfortunately, it's not as spectacular as we expected it to be. However, ziconotide does have a place in some patients who have uncontrolled pain from cancer and AIDS," Dubois says. "But it is not going to revolutionize pain management."

Dr. Michael S. Leong, an assistant professor of anesthesia at Stanford University Medical Center, adds that his experience indicates that ziconotide can provide significant benefit for all types of intractable pain, including back pain, neck pain and other neuropathic pain.

However, ziconotide is expensive and difficult to administer and monitor, so its use will probably be limited.

info To learn more about pain management, visit The National Foundation for the Treatment of Pain at *www.paincare.org*.

Fibromyalgia: Researchers Prove Pain Is Real

Thorsten Giesecke, MD, research fellow, University of Michigan, Ann Arbor.

Bruce Naliboff, PhD, professor, medical psychology, UCLA David Geffen School of Medicine, co-director, UCLA Center for Neurovisceral Sciences and Women's Health, Los Angeles, and staff, VA Greater Los Angeles Healthcare System.

Arthritis and Rheumatism.

Fibromyalgia, a chronic pain illness, affects up to 6 million Americans, primarily women of childbearing age, according to the American College of Rheumatology.

Some experts believe that fibromyalgia patients who are also prone to emotional problems, such as depression and anxiety, are more likely to experience greater physical pain in areas called "tender points."

Common tender points are the front of the knees, the elbows, the hip joints, the neck and spine. Some physicians also think that patients with emotional issues have more sleep disturbances, morning stiffness, irritable bowel syndrome and anxiety than patients with a more positive outlook.

But a recent study may change their ideas.

THE STUDY

Dr. Thorsten Giesecke, a research fellow at the University of Michigan, and his colleagues evaluated 85 female and 12 male fibromyalgia patients. The patients answered a series of questions about their coping strategies and personality traits—particularly about their emotional well-being. They also were tested for sensitivity to pressure and pain.

The patients fell into three subgroups that refute conventional wisdom.

The first subgroup consisted of 50 patients who had moderate levels of anxiety and depression. They also felt they had moderate control over their pain, and they experienced low to moderate levels of pain.

The second group included 31 patients with high levels of anxiety and depression. They felt they had the least control over their pain, and they had high levels of tenderness.

The third group, with 16 patients, reported the lowest levels of anxiety and depression and the highest control over their pain. Yet the testing showed that they experienced the highest levels of physical pain.

Some patients have extreme pain but no psychological problems, Giesecke explains, while others have moderate pain and fairly positive moods.

TAILORING TREATMENT

The findings may help tailor treatments to specific individuals. For example, antidepressants might not work well on group three, whose members were not depressed. They might benefit from exercise therapy instead, Giesecke says.

"To better understand fibromyalgia and to have better treatment, it's important to find out if [patients with the disease are] a homogeneous group," says Bruce Naliboff, a professor of medical psychology at the UCLA David Geffen School of Medicine and on staff at the VA Greater Los Angeles Healthcare System.

Clearly, Giesecke found it is not, Naliboff adds. Some patients who have extreme tenderness don't have many emotional issues, which was not expected.

"It's easy to say it's all in their head," says Naliboff, who works with patients who have other conditions that involve psychological components, such as inflammatory bowel disease. The study will help prove that's not so, he adds.

info To learn about the symptoms of fibromyalgia and how to manage this condition, visit *http://familydoctor.org*.

When the Pain Just Won't Go Away

Peter Moskovitz, MD, clinical professor of orthopedic surgery and neurological surgery, George Washington University, Washington, DC.

Bottom Line/Health.

It starts with an injury—a broken bone, the trauma of surgery or even a bruise. You expect the pain to go away as the wound heals, but in a matter of days or weeks, it gets worse. Perhaps it spreads to other parts of your body. In severe cases, it becomes disabling.

Sound like a nightmare? For up to 6 million Americans, this is the reality of *reflex sympathetic dystrophy syndrome* (RSDS). This disorder, which is also known as *complex regional pain syndrome,* affects more women than men and usually strikes between the ages of 40 and 60.

A MYSTERIOUS CONDITION

Doctors and scientists are unsure about the exact physiological miscues that lead to RSDS. At this point, the disorder, which was first identified about 100 years ago, is best understood as the body's natural healing systems gone awry.

Any injury stimulates the sympathetic nervous system (SNS), the network of nerve cells that rev up the fight-or-flight response to deal with demanding situations. Your breathing and pulse accelerate. Blood flow to the injured area is cut back to minimize bleeding. The immune system is activated to fight infection and initiate healing. You also feel acute pain, causing you to reflexively withdraw and warning you to deal with the situation.

Normally, the immune system spontaneously returns to normal, and the SNS quiets down when the danger is past. The pain then usually recedes over hours, days or weeks as the wound heals.

In RSDS, the systems get stuck in overdrive. The pain gets worse—often much worse—instead of better. It may spread along the injured hand, arm or leg because of activation of the central nervous system.

Other changes may take place—the affected area becomes unusually pale and/or cold to the touch or, less frequently, red and hot. An affected limb often may become swollen.

The condition may last weeks, months or, in rare cases, a lifetime. It may resist treatment or go away as mysteriously as it came (half of the cases get better spontaneously).

A DIFFICULT DIAGNOSIS

If you have RSDS, it is essential to have it treated promptly and properly.

The longer it is neglected, the greater the risk it will cause lasting damage—scar tissue may develop and nerve connections become physically altered. Pain may become more resistant to treatment.

Because there is no definitive test, the diagnosis often is delayed for an average of eight months after symptoms appear.

The details of RSDS vary greatly from person to person, making the diagnosis difficult. Severe pain that is out of proportion to tissue damage is present in all RSDS sufferers. It usually is described as burning, crushing or stabbing.

Getting a diagnosis of RSDS will depend on the presence of several of the following characteristics…

• **Hyperesthesia,** or extreme sensitivity to touch and light pressure.

• **Sensation of coolness or warmth** or a difference in color and temperature in the affected body part. This is typically caused by the widening or narrowing of blood vessels.

• **Increased swelling or an increase or decrease in sweating** in the affected part of the body.

• **Tremor, weakness or decreased range of motion** and/or changes in the hair, nails or skin.

Doctors vary enormously in their ability to diagnose and treat RSDS. If you think you may have it, seek a physician—most often a neurologist, anesthesiologist or physiatrist (a specialist in physical rehabilitation)—who is familiar with the disorder and specializes in chronic pain.

EFFECTIVE TREATMENT

There is no cure for RSDS. Instead, effective treatment must include the following three key areas…

PAIN CONTROL

Controlling the pain of RSDS often involves oral medication, such as *acetaminophen* (Tylenol) or nonsteroidal anti-inflammatory drugs (NSAIDs), such as *ibuprofen* (Advil) or *naproxen* (Aleve), or prescription NSAIDs, such as *diclofenac and misoprostol* (Arthrotec) or *diclofenac* (Voltaren).

Newer COX-2 inhibitors, including *celecoxib* (Celebrex), also may prove to be helpful.

More potent opioids (derived from opium narcotics), such as codeine, acetaminophen and *oxycodone* (Percocet) or *hydrocodone* (Vicodin), may be effective as well.

Creams and lotions containing local anesthetics, anti-inflammatories, *dimethyl sulfoxide* or capsaicin (the active ingredient in cayenne pepper) rubbed on the skin can dull sensation in the painful area.

Some drugs, such as the opioid painkiller *duragesic* (Fentanyl), are now available in transdermal patches. Because these patches are applied to the skin, they are convenient and provide a steady, even supply of the painkilling medication.

Tricyclic antidepressants, such as *amitriptyline* (Elavil), may be effective for chronic pain conditions, including RSDS.

Regional sympathetic blockade and other nerve block techniques often are used to help doctors diagnose RSDS, as well as treat it. A local anesthetic, such as *xylocaine,* is injected around the nerve cells that carry SNS signals to the affected area.

Regional sympathetic blockade is particularly effective early on in the condition. A blockade that relieves the pain is considered confirmation of the syndrome in people who also experience other symptoms of RSDS. (A blockade that is ineffective, however, does not mean you are not suffering from RSDS.)

Local anesthetics or drugs to block nerve chemicals also may be injected directly into the affected area or infused into the space around the spinal cord.

PSYCHOSOCIAL SUPPORT

Psychosocial support almost always is necessary. RSDS is a highly stressful condition, and most people who have it need help coping. High levels of anxiety and clinical depression are common symptoms in many people who have RSDS.

It's a vicious cycle—stress, anxiety and depression make the pain less tolerable, and even may worsen the disease.

For these reasons, psychotherapy, counseling and often medication are an important part of RSDS care.

The counselor may provide instruction in behavioral techniques, such as biofeedback, focused imagery or meditation, to manage stress and reduce pain.

If you suffer from RSDS, your family will suffer, too. Therapy also should provide support for spouses, children and other close family members.

PHYSICAL THERAPY AND REHABILITATION

A combination of physical therapy and rehabilitation will help you function as normally as possible, despite the pain of RSDS.

Physical therapy is likely to include treatments and exercises to restore or maintain flexibility, build strength and increase endurance.

Important: Interventions must be gentle to avoid aggravating the condition. Make sure your physical therapist is experienced in treating RSDS.

An occupational therapist can help you redesign your environment and modify the ways you dress, bathe and perform other activities of daily living.

He/she also may suggest assistive devices, such as a "grabber" for hard-to-reach objects, to minimize the pain of RSDS.

info For more information on RSDS or help in finding support groups in your area for patients, spouses and family members, contact the Reflex Sympathetic Dystrophy Syndrome Association, 203-877-3790, *www.rsds.org.*

Ouch! The Price of Pain

Press briefing, *Journal of the American Medical Association,* New York City, with Elizabeth H.B. Lin, MD, family medicine physician and researcher, Group Health Cooperative, Seattle.

Walter Stewart, PhD, director, Outcomes Research Institute, Center for Health Research and Rural Advocacy, Geisinger Health Systems, Danville, PA.

Richard Howard, MD, consultant, pediatric anesthesia and pain management, Great Ormond Street Hospital for Children, London.

Journal of the American Medical Association.

When a patient visits a doctor, his/her vital signs are taken. These include temperature, blood pressure, pulse and respiratory rate. A recent study suggests that a fifth vital sign should be added—pain.

Pain not only diminishes a person's quality of life, it is expensive. Researchers have found lost productivity from pain costs US employers approximately $61.2 billion per year, but only $14.3 billion of that total was due to absenteeism. The rest is from reduced performance on the job.

"Pain is the most prevalent health condition," says study author Walter Stewart, director of the Outcomes Research Institute located in Danville, Pennsylvania.

THE STUDY

Stewart and his team looked at data from the American Productivity Audit, a telephone survey of working adults. More than 30,000 people were asked questions about their experience with the most common types of pain —headache, back pain, arthritis and other musculoskeletal pain—during work in the previous two-week period.

The greatest loss of productivity occurred among those who had a lot of control over their jobs, as well as among those with less education.

The education dimension may be the simplest to explain, Stewart says. "Their physical environments and job stressors tend to be more severe," he says. "They have poor access to health care, lower health literacy and higher levels of depression, which may exacerbate the pain experience."

In all, 5% of the people account for 29% of the total hours lost because of pain. "A minority of individuals account for the majority of lost time," Stewart explains. In any two-week period, one in eight workers reported an average loss of five hours per week.

Long-term and short-term disability, which is carefully tracked by employers, also represented a small share of the overall cost. The biggest costs came from work absence and reduced performance on the job.

Adds Stewart, "We would like pain to be the fifth vital sign. But we haven't figured out how we can seamlessly access it in a way that is effective."

PAIN NOT LIMITED TO ADULTS

Children also suffer, but treating their pain presents different challenges, said Dr. Richard Howard of Great Ormond Street Hospital for Children in London.

"Children and children in pain rarely seem to get the attention they need," he says. And although much progress has been made in the last 20 years, much more needs to be done.

Experts are recognizing that the nervous systems of children are very different from those of adults, and few drugs are tested on younger patients, Howard says.

info For more on pain management, visit the American Pain Foundation at *www. painfoundation.org*.

'Shocking' Treatment Tames Tendonitis

Ludger Gerdesmeyer, MD, Department of Orthopedic Surgery and Sports Traumatology, Technical University of Munich, Germany.
David S. Bailie, MD, chairman, orthopedic surgery, Scottsdale Healthcare, Scottsdale, Arizona.
Journal of the American Medical Association.

Can sound waves tame tendonitis in the shoulder? German researchers say *extracorporeal shock wave therapy* (ESWT) can successfully treat chronic calcifying tendonitis of the rotator cuff in patients who would otherwise need surgery.

"For the first time in the treatment of chronic calcifying tendonitis of the rotator cuff we have found a nonsurgical technique that is effective," says lead researcher Dr. Ludger Gerdesmeyer, an orthopedic surgeon at the Technical University of Munich.

How ESWT works is not fully understood. Some theories are that the shock—or sound—waves disrupt calcium deposits, increase the spread of enzymes across blood vessel walls, stimulate blood vessel growth or promote new bone formation. One or more of these mechanisms may aid in healing, say the researchers.

THE STUDY

Gerdesmeyer and his colleagues studied 144 patients with chronic tendonitis of the rotator cuff. The rotator cuff is comprised of the muscles and tendons that surround the top of the upper arm bone and hold it in the shoulder joint. These patients had all undergone other treatments, including massage therapy and steroid injections, that did not fix the problem.

Gerdesmeyer and his colleagues divided the patients into three groups. Some patients received low-energy ESWT, some got high-energy ESWT and the remainder were given a sham procedure that had no therapeutic effect.

The patients were given two treatment sessions that were administered two weeks apart. After treatment, the patients also received additional physical therapy.

During six months of follow-up, those who received ESWT showed significant improvement, compared with patients who did not receive the treatment. And patients who received the high-energy ESWT showed greater improvement than those who got the low-energy ESWT.

RELIEF WITHOUT SURGERY

Normally, these patients would have to undergo surgery, Gerdesmeyer says. However, based on these findings, he believes "people with chronic pain of the rotator cuff should be treated with ESWT, not surgery."

Gerdesmeyer and his group are looking to refine their treatment by finding the best energy levels and the most effective number of treatments.

Dr. David S. Bailie, an orthopedic surgeon and a sports medicine expert, says, "ESWT is effective for this problem, and we have had some success in our practice with low-energy ESWT treatment."

Bailie notes that ESWT is noninvasive and takes only several treatments. "Early results from an ongoing study demonstrate about an 85% success rate thus far," he adds.

"ESWT can be viewed as an alternative to surgery with few, if any, side effects. And it's probably better and safer than repeated steroid injections," Bailie says.

"Before undergoing any treatment, patients with tendonitis of the rotator cuff should ask about all of the options and consider the risk–benefit of all treatments," he advises.

info To learn more about rotator cuff problems, visit the American Orthopaedic Society for Sports Medicine at *www.aossm.org.*

Finally! An Incredible Gadget that Relieves Heel Spur Pain

Washington University School of Medicine news release.

OssaTron might sound like a kitchen gadget, but it's a medical device that uses shock waves to treat heel pain caused by *plantar fasciitis.*

The condition, also called *heel spur syndrome,* typically involves pain and inflammation at the point where the plantar fascia attaches to the heel bone, says the Washington University School of Medicine.

HOW IT WORKS

The OssaTron is a type of device called a *lithotriptor* that generates shock waves. Lithotriptors were originally developed as a nonsurgical way to treat kidney stones. The shock waves generated by the lithotriptor create vibrations that break kidney stones into tiny pieces.

Doctors now also use the OssaTron to create a small injury area close to where the plantar fascia connects to the heel bone. The new injury increases the supply of blood and nutrients to the area. That promotes healing and relieves the pain caused by plantar fasciitis.

FIRST LINE OF TREATMENT

The majority of doctors recommend rest as the first treatment for plantar fasciitis. People who have the condition should try to keep weight off the foot until the inflammation goes away. Ice applied to the sore area for 20 minutes three or four times a day may also relieve symptoms. Often a doctor will prescribe a nonsteroidal anti-inflammatory medication (NSAID), such as ibuprofen. A program of home exercises to stretch the Achilles tendon and plantar fascia are the mainstay of treating the condition, and those stretches lessen the chance of a recurrence.

Approximately 90% of the people who have plantar fasciitis improve significantly after two months of treatment, according to the American Academy of Orthopaedic Surgeons. Some people use shoes that have shock-absorbing soles or shoes fitted with a standard orthotic device, such as a rubber heel pad. Or they may have their foot taped into a specific position.

ALTERNATIVE TO SURGERY

If those approaches fail to relieve the heel pain, some people opt for surgery. The OssaTron offers an alternative to surgery.

■ ■ ■ ■

Getting to the Bottom of Plantar Fasciitis

The plantar fascia is a broad, ligament-like structure on the bottom of the foot, running from the toes to the heel. According to the American Academy of Orthopaedic Surgeons, plantar fasciitis is most commonly an overuse injury. It causes severe pain in the heel when a patient tries to walk or run.

You are more likely to get the condition if you're a woman, if you're overweight or if you have a job that requires a lot of walking or standing on hard surfaces. You're also at risk if you walk or run for exercise, especially if you have tight calf muscles that limit how far you can flex your ankles. People with very flat feet or very high arches are also more prone to plantar fasciitis.

The condition begins gradually with mild pain at the heel bone, often referred to as a stone bruise. You're more likely to feel it after (not during) exercise. The pain classically occurs again upon getting out of bed.

If you don't treat plantar fasciitis, it may become a chronic condition. You may also develop other foot, knee, hip and back problems if you unconsciously change the way you walk in an effort to avoid the pain plantar fasciitis causes.

info Learn more about foot pain from the American College of Foot and Ankle Surgeons at *www.acfas.org*.

Leeches Take the Bite Out of Arthritis

Gunther Spahn, MD, professor, internal and integrative medicine, Essen-Mitte Clinic, Essen, Germany.

Marc C. Hochberg, MD, professor, medicine and epidemiology, University of Maryland School of Medicine, Baltimore.

Marie Bonazinga, president, Leeches USA Ltd., Westbury, NY.

Annals of Internal Medicine.

Leech treatment relieves the excruciating knee pain of arthritis more effectively than conventional drug therapy, according to a study by German scientists.

It might seem like a story from many centuries ago, but the news appears to be the result of a carefully controlled, thoroughly modern medical trial.

THE STUDY

The study included 51 patients with severe arthritis-related knee pain. The 24 patients who had leeches applied to their joints reported an average reduction in pain from 53.5 to 19.3 on a standard scale used to measure pain. The reduction for those treated with *diclofenac,* a steroid drug, was much less, from 51.5 to 42.4,

according to the report from physicians at the Essen-Mitte Clinic in Essen, Germany.

The pain relief received from leech therapy wore out after a week, but "differences for function, stiffness and total symptoms remained significant for leech therapy until the end of the study," which lasted 30 days, the report says.

There are many possible reasons for the beneficial results, says Dr. Gunther Spahn, a professor of internal and integrative medicine, who was a member of the study team.

"Leeches are a pharmaceutical company, injecting…many substances into the soft tissue," Spahn explains. "These substances may have an anti-swelling, anti-inflammatory and analgesic effect. Also, the sucking itself may have a contra-irritatory effect on knee pain."

TOO EARLY TO PRESCRIBE

Dr. Marc C. Hochberg, professor of medicine and epidemiology at the University of Maryland School of Medicine, says, "I have no information about [leech therapy for arthritis] being done in the United States. I would hope it would not be done until there are more data demonstrating safety and efficacy, especially in comparison with standard therapy."

A major problem with the study, he says, is that both groups of patients knew which treatment they were getting, which "raises concern about measurement bias," especially since the pain scores were based on patients' judgment.

A "more exciting" aspect of the study is that it might lead to better painkilling drugs based on an analysis of the molecules in leech saliva, Hochberg says. "At the moment, however, I am not ready to refer my patients with knee osteoarthritis for leech therapy on the basis of these data," he writes.

Leeches had been used for centuries to get "the bad blood out," but the practice fell into disfavor by the 19th century. Today, leeches are used medically in this country, but on a very limited basis, says Marie Bonazinga, president of Leeches USA Ltd., which sells them commercially.

"We do not sell to individuals," Bonazinga says. "We sell to plastic and reconstructive surgeons for use after surgery."

info You can learn about the medicinal leeches from the University of Michigan at *http://animaldiversity.ummz.umich.edu.*

■ ■ ■ ■

Not Just Your Joints at Risk

The term arthritis refers to a group of diseases that can cause pain, stiffness and swelling in the joints.

These diseases may affect not only the joints but other parts of the body, including important supporting structures such as muscles, bones, tendons and ligaments, as well as some internal organs.

Osteoarthritis is a joint disease that mostly affects the cartilage, the tissue that covers the ends of bones in a joint. Healthy cartilage allows bones to glide over one another, and also absorbs energy from the shock of physical movement.

In patients with osteoarthritis, the surface layer of the cartilage breaks down and wears away. This allows the bones under the cartilage to rub together, causing pain, swelling and loss of motion of the joint.

Osteoarthritis most often affects the fingers, knees and hips. Sometimes it can follow an injury to a joint. For example, a young person might receive a bad knee injury from playing soccer. Then, years after the knee has apparently healed, he might get arthritis in his knee joint.

Arthritis sufferers can find short-term relief through the use of medications, heat or cold applied to the joint, a splint or brace or massage therapy.

Long-term techniques for relief include medications, weight loss, exercise and surgery. Swimming, walking, low-impact aerobic exercise and range-of-motion exercises have been found to reduce joint pain and stiffness in some arthritis patients.

info To learn more about arthritis, visit the National Institute of Arthritis and Musculoskeletal and Skin Diseases Web site at *www.niams.nih.gov.*

The Real Cause of Osteoarthritis

Steven B. Abramson, MD, chairman, Department of Rheumatology/Medicine, New York University–Hospital for Joint Diseases, New York City.
Arthritis & Rheumatism.
Harris H. McIlwain, MD, with the Tampa Medical Group, where he specializes in pain-related diseases. Board-certified in rheumatology and geriatric medicine, he is coauthor of *Pain-Free Arthritis: A 7 Step Program for Feeling Better Again.* Henry Holt.
Bottom Line/Health.

British scientists found that nearly one third of patients ready to undergo joint replacement surgery for osteoarthritis had severe inflammation in the synovial fluid that surrounds and protects the joints. This inflammation, already known to be a factor in rheumatoid arthritis, could contribute to osteoarthritis as well, the researchers suggest.

Osteoarthritis is the most common form of arthritis, especially among older people, affecting approximately 20 million Americans. By 2030, 20% of Americans—about 70 million people—will have passed their 65th birthday and will be at risk for osteoarthritis, according to the National Institute of Arthritis and Musculoskeletal and Skin Diseases.

Also called degenerative joint disease, osteoarthritis causes the cartilage that covers the ends of the bones to erode, allowing the bones to rub together at the joints. This causes pain, swelling and the loss of motion in the joint.

"Five to 10 years ago it was thought that osteoarthritis was due to the degeneration of cartilage due to wear and tear, but this is one of a number of studies finding that inflammatory mediators" are more to blame, says Dr. Steven B. Abramson, chairman of the department of rheumatology and medicine at the New York University–Hospital for Joint Diseases.

THE STUDY

For the study, the researchers from the University of Nottingham obtained synovial tissue samples from 104 men and women (*average age:* 69 years) who were about to undergo joint replacement of hips or knees due to advanced osteoarthritis.

Thirty-two of the participants showed evidence of the most severe inflammation, 36 showed evidence of moderate inflammation, 29 had minor inflammation and seven had no inflammation.

Although these samples were taken from people with very advanced cases of osteoarthritis, Abramson says, "Other studies have looked at this in the middle stage of osteoarthritis—which is about 10 years before surgical intervention—and approximately one third to one half of those patients have synovial inflammation."

Abramson says future research will aim to find out whether drugs now used to treat rheumatoid arthritis might have a role in treating osteoarthritis.

At present the most powerful drugs that modify the progression of the disease have a fair amount of toxicities, he says, so any drug management would have to include a careful risk–benefit analysis.

info To learn more about arthritis, visit the Mayo Clinic Web site at *www.mayo clinic.com.* Click on "Diseases & Conditions."

■ ■ ■ ■

Conventional vs. Alternative Treatments

Doctors will often prescribe nonsteroidal anti-inflammatory drugs (NSAIDs), such as ibuprofen, to treat the pain and inflammation of arthritis.

Some patients opt for an alternative therapy using glucosamine or chondroitin sulfate. Some research indicates that these natural supplements might also slow cartilage damage in people with osteoarthritis. Definitive results about the effects of these supplements are expected from an in-depth clinical study currently being conducted by the National Institutes of Health.

■ ■ ■ ■

Pain Relief Strategies

Following are some suggestions to minimize arthritis pain and protect your joints…

● **When grocery shopping,** request plastic bags that can be looped over your arms, between the wrist and elbow. This shifts the weight of the bags to your shoulders and upper body, instead of the more delicate wrist and hand joints.

● **Put foam "grips" around pens and pencils** (you'll find them in office-supply stores). You can use these same covers around crochet hooks and knitting needles, too.

● **Use pump toothpastes** instead of the squeeze tubes.

● **Choose clothing with Velcro closures** instead of zippers and buttons.

● **Women should wear bras** that open in the front.

Blood Test May Predict Rheumatoid Arthritis

Clifton O. Bingham III, MD, director, Seligman Center for Advanced Therapeutics, NYU-Hospital for Joint Diseases, and assistant professor, New York University School of Medicine, New York.

Berj Nercessian, MD, rheumatologist, William Beaumont Hospital, Royal Oak, MI.
Arthritis and Rheumatology.

The presence of certain proteins in the blood may predict the development of rheumatoid arthritis years before symptoms start.

That's the conclusion of a study that found one third of people with rheumatoid arthritis had the proteins, called *anti-CCP antibodies,* in their blood long before they felt the first symptoms of the disease.

Currently, doctors can diagnose rheumatoid arthritis based on symptoms and the presence of rheumatoid factor in the blood. This means most people aren't diagnosed with the disease until they've had the disorder for some time. Additionally, not everyone who has rheumatoid arthritis tests positive for rheumatoid factor.

"The anti-CCP test may help us detect patients who have early rheumatoid arthritis, and it may also predict patients who have a more progressive disease," says Dr. Clifton O. Bingham III, director of the Seligman Center for Advanced Therapeutics, which is part of the NYU-Hospital for Joint Diseases in New York City.

THE STUDY

In the latest study, researchers at University Hospital in Umea, Sweden, looked at blood samples from 83 people who had donated blood an average of 2.5 years before being diagnosed with rheumatoid arthritis.

Thirty-four percent of the study subjects who developed rheumatoid arthritis tested positive for anti-CCP antibodies. Blood samples that were taken closer to the onset of symptoms more frequently tested positive for anti-CCP antibodies.

When the researchers looked for the presence of anti-CCP antibodies in conjunction with rheumatoid factor, their ability to predict who would eventually develop rheumatoid arthritis was nearly 100%.

Finding rheumatoid arthritis early is very important, Bingham says. "Joint damage and destruction occur early in the disease process," he says. "A growing body of data is showing that early treatment will lead to a better long-term prognosis."

SOME EXPERTS QUESTION THE TEST'S UTILITY

But not everyone believes an additional test is necessary.

Dr. Berj Nercessian, a rheumatologist from William Beaumont Hospital in Royal Oak, Michigan, says he does not believe this test will help him diagnose rheumatoid arthritis more efficiently.

"The diagnosis of rheumatoid arthritis is based on a whole constellation of symptoms that are present," says Nercessian. "The blood test is just an additional test to confirm the diagnosis."

However, he does say it might be helpful in situations where a diagnosis is not clear. For example, he says many times it's difficult to tell if someone has lupus or rheumatoid arthritis, since many of the symptoms and blood tests are similar. If anti-CCP antibodies are exclusive

to rheumatoid arthritis, it could help doctors distinguish between the two diseases.

Whether these antibodies are exclusive to rheumatoid arthritis is a question that still needs to be answered.

Bingham says that there are some limitations to this test because some people who have rheumatoid arthritis won't test positive for these antibodies and a few people who do test positive may never develop rheumatoid arthritis.

Still, Bingham believes that "the anti-CCP antibodies test is going to be very useful as a diagnostic test."

■ ■ ■ ■

Rheumatoid Arthritis Statistics and Symptoms

More than 2 million Americans have rheumatoid arthritis, according to the Arthritis Foundation. Nearly three times as many women as men have the disease. The disease begins most often in middle age, but can be seen in children and young adults.

Common symptoms of rheumatoid arthritis are joint stiffness—particularly in the small joints like those in the fingers and wrists—joint pain and swelling. Bingham says if you have joint stiffness when you first wake up that lasts for more than 30 minutes, and this symptom has been occurring for more than six weeks, you should be evaluated by a doctor.

Could Vitamin D Block Rheumatoid Arthritis?

Kenneth G. Saag, MD, associate professor, University of Alabama at Birmingham.
John Klippel, MD, rheumatologist and president and chief executive officer, Arthritis Foundation, Atlanta.
Arthritis & Rheumatism.

Could taking vitamin D protect against rheumatoid arthritis? "Yes," according to researchers from the University of Alabama at Birmingham.

THE STUDY

The researchers looked at a sample of nearly 30,000 women, aged 55 to 69 years, from the Iowa Women's Health study, a large-scale research project that started in 1986. None had rheumatoid arthritis at the study's start. The researchers followed the women for 11 years, asking them about eating habits, supplement use, smoking history and body mass index.

The researchers discovered 152 cases of RA in the women during the 11 years of follow-up. And the study results suggest that getting enough vitamin D can reduce the risk.

"If the women took in less than 200 international units [IUs] of vitamin D per day, they had roughly a 33% increased risk for developing rheumatoid arthritis compared with those who received more than 200 IUs daily," says senior investigator Dr. Kenneth G. Saag, an associate professor of medicine at the University of Alabama at Birmingham.

The daily recommended dose of vitamin D is 400 IUs from either foods or supplements.

POSSIBLE EXPLANATION

Why vitamin D might be effective in guarding against rheumatoid arthritis isn't known, Saag adds. "Vitamin D has its major effect in regulating calcium in the body," he says. "But we don't think that this would necessarily explain this [protective effect]."

Saag hopes further research will unlock the possible association between vitamin D and rheumatoid arthritis.

SOURCES OF VITAMIN D

"This is just another reason why you need to eat a healthy diet," he says.

It is best to get vitamin D from food, he advises, but if you are not getting enough in your diet, you probably need supplements. A cup of milk has about 100 IUs of vitamin D and a cup of cornflakes about 40 IUs, according to the American Dietetic Association.

PROVEN WAYS TO
REDUCE RISK

Until more research is in, there are other ways to reduce the risk of RA, says Dr. John Klippel, president and chief executive officer of the Arthritis Foundation. Smoking appears to be a risk factor as well as excess caffeine.

Early detection of RA can help reduce pain, he adds. Joint pain and swelling of the hands, wrist and feet are common symptoms and should prompt medical attention, he says.

"The longer between diagnosis and treatment, the greater the risk of joint damage and disability," Klippel says. "See a rheumatologist early and get treated early."

Good News for Arthritis Sufferers: New Scan Means Better Treatment

Robert Quinet, MD, chairman, rheumatology, Ochsner Clinic Foundation, New Orleans.

Martin Pevzner, MD, chairman, rheumatology, Beaumont Hospital, Royal Oak, MI.

Arthritis and Rheumatism.

Researchers have discovered that sophisticated body scans may predict which patients will experience aggressive rheumatoid arthritis (RA), and that may give doctors a chance to use the strongest medicines in those who need them most.

THE STUDY

The study, conducted over six years, used magnetic resonance imaging (MRI) to chart the course of RA. MRI uses magnetic field and radio waves to produce more detailed images of the body than X rays can provide.

Study author Dr. Fiona McQueen and her colleagues recruited 42 people who were in the early stages of RA. All of the volunteers had an MRI and an X ray of the wrist in their dominant hand. The tests were repeated at one year and at six years.

The results indicate that patients with bone swelling at the start of the project were 6.5 times more likely to have serious joint damage at the end of the study.

MRIs also were more effective at picking up bone erosion than were X rays. The first

MRIs showed bone erosion in 45% of the study participants, compared with only 15% found in X rays.

"MRI is proving to be a very useful tool with which to investigate the disease processes in RA," says McQueen, from Auckland Hospital in New Zealand.

COST MAY BE A FACTOR TO BE CONSIDERED

Experts in rheumatology aren't quite as sure as McQueen, however.

Both Dr. Robert Quinet, chairman of rheumatology at Ochsner Clinic Foundation in New Orleans, and Dr. Martin Pevzner, chairman of rheumatology at Beaumont Hospital in Royal Oak, Michigan, feel MRIs are too expensive to be used as screening tools.

"The problem is that MRIs are so expensive, insurance companies often won't cover them," Pevzner says.

And Quinet echoes Pevzner's feelings. There are less expensive tests that can be used to predict what course an individual's RA might take, he says, including blood tests, X rays and functional assessment questionnaires.

But, Pevzner concedes, those tests are not "an exact science" and there currently is no "definitive predictor."

STUDY MAY HAVE POTENTIAL FOR FUTURE

"There are some innovative aspects to this study," says Quinet.

But he adds, "In terms of its application, I don't think it will have a major impact now. It has potential for the future."

Pevzner agrees. "In the future, it may provide another clue to which patients need aggressive treatment," he says.

That's important, he adds, because early intervention helps control the disease and limits its damage.

info To learn more about RA, visit the Arthritis Foundation's Web site at *www.arthritis.org*. Click on "Disease Center." For more on MRI, go to the National Library of Medicine Web site at *www.nlm.nih.gov*.

How to Get the Best Rheumatoid Arthritis Treatment for You

Amy Alderman, MD, MPH, University of Michigan and University of Michigan Medical Center, Ann Arbor.

Peter Gorevic, MD, head, rheumatology, Mount Sinai Medical Center, New York City.

Steven Z. Glickel, MD, Starr Hand Surgery Center, St. Luke's-Roosevelt Hospital Center, New York City.

Journal of Rheumatology.

People who have rheumatoid arthritis (RA) have several treatment options, including medication to reduce inflammation and surgery to restore dexterity.

Hand surgery is sometimes an option for those patients who don't respond to medication or whose hands have become too twisted to perform daily activities.

So which is the best choice?

SPECIALISTS ARE MILES APART

That's still a tough call, say doctors at the University of Michigan who found that the two groups of specialists who typically treat this ailment—rheumatologists and hand surgeons—are miles apart on what's most effective for individual patients.

The result: Patients can be confused when it comes to choosing a treatment.

"We have two groups of physicians who have had intensive training, who are not in communication with each other and who are in complete disagreement with each other on the management of rheumatoid arthritis," says Dr. Amy Alderman, lead author of the study as well as a resident surgeon with the University of Michigan Health System located in Ann Arbor.

Patients who have rheumatoid arthritis usually consult their primary care physician. And that, Alderman says, "puts the primary doctor in a difficult position because he or she doesn't have the training to make an informed decision. The two specialists—the rheumatologist and the hand surgeon—need to get together and get a consensus."

THE STUDY

In addition to Alderman, the authors of the study include a rheumatologist, a senior hand surgeon and a general internist.

Alderman's research group surveyed 1,000 rheumatologists and hand surgeons, who were given questionnaires on various arthritis treatment options and then offered their views about each specialty.

The recommendations of the rheumatologists and hand surgeons varied widely, depending on where patients lived, the type of physician to whom they were referred and what the doctor thought of other specialties.

SPECIALTY PREDICTS RECOMMENDATION

Hand surgeons recommended surgery within three to six months if aggressive medical management with drugs failed.

The majority of rheumatologists said surgery should be postponed for up to a year or longer—or never done at all—to give the medications a chance to be effective.

"These are completely opposing opinions," Alderman says. "There is no consistency as to whether the procedures actually work and when to do them."

The authors also found that the rates of surgery vary tremendously from state to state, with some states reporting rates that are four times higher than others.

EXPERT REACTION

Dr. Peter Gorevic, head of the rheumatology department at Mount Sinai Medical Center in New York City, says the new study "acknowledges a problem that needs to be addressed."

However, Dr. Steven Z. Glickel, a hand surgeon in New York City, says he was shocked by this study's conclusions because in his own experience rheumatologists and surgeons work very well together in trying to provide RA patients with the best possible treatment.

Glickel says the best solution for patients is to be reasonably educated about the options open to them.

Experimental Drug Works Better for Rheumatoid Arthritis Relief

Anne Davidson, MD, professor, medicine, Albert Einstein College of Medicine, Bronx, NY.

Larry Moreland, MD, professor, medicine, University of Alabama at Birmingham.

Statement, David Karp, MD, PhD, medical advisor, Arthritis Foundation.

New England Journal of Medicine.

Rheumatoid arthritis is a disease in which the immune system attacks cartilage in the joints and tissue of the body's organs, causing pain, fatigue and swelling. What triggers RA is unknown.

RA often responds well to drug therapy. Steroids, such as *prednisone,* and the immune-suppressing drug *methotrexate* are the most common treatments.

Patients frequently use painkillers and non-steroidal anti-inflammatory drugs (NSAIDs) in combination with the stronger medications.

Although these regimens can be effective, they don't work in many patients and may lead to side effects, including infections and cancers. In addition, patients often stop responding to the standard drugs after a promising start.

BUT THERE'S NEW HOPE

An experimental medication, a protein called CTLA4Ig that prevents the immune system from "seeing" and going after its targets in joint tissue, is better than conventional care for rheumatoid arthritis, research finds.

People who took CTLA4Ig had markedly lower blood levels of a certain molecule that is called *C-reactive protein* than those who didn't receive the drug, suggesting a significant suppression of inflammation.

In addition, people who took the drug along with the conventional therapy for rheumatoid arthritis were nearly twice as likely to show a reduction in joint pain, swelling and other symptoms, as those using the conventional therapy alone.

Patients taking CTLA4Ig also reported improvements in physical function and general health, as well as social and emotional well-being. The drug did not seem to cause any serious side effects.

Dr. Anne Davidson, an arthritis expert at Albert Einstein College of Medicine in the Bronx, calls the effect of the new drug "pretty good." She says the effect comes close to that of other RA drugs that have come to market, including Enbrel.

CONFIRMING STUDIES NEEDED

Dr. Larry Moreland, a co-author of the study as well as a joint specialist at the University of Alabama at Birmingham, says CTLA4Ig will have to go head-to-head against other RA therapies before its real value is clear.

"In our placebo-controlled trial this was much better than placebo, and it appears to be an effective agent," he says.

CTLA4Ig is now being developed by Bristol-Myers Squibb, which funded Dr. Moreland's study. It has not yet been approved for sale in the United States or abroad. Additional research is under way.

The new medication, and other novel treatments now being tested, "may enable patients who fail with one class of drugs to utilize another," says Dr. David Karp, a medical adviser to the Arthritis Foundation.

Exercise Helps Folks With Rheumatoid Arthritis Live Better

Thea P.M. Vliet Vlieland, MD, PT, PhD, Leiden University Medical Center, Leiden, The Netherlands.

Arthritis & Rheumatism.

Regular workouts can help patients with rheumatoid arthritis (RA) build muscle strength and aerobic capacity, improve their ability to perform daily tasks and foster a sense of emotional well-being.

THE STUDY

Dutch researchers followed up 300 men and women for two years.

The study subjects who were assigned to the exercise group attended one-hour sessions twice a week. Each exercise session consisted of 20 minutes of bicycling; 20 minutes of exercises to build muscle strength, endurance and joint mobility; and 20 minutes of sports such as badminton, volleyball, soccer and basketball. Participants also took part in 15 minutes of required pre-exercise warm-up and post-exercise cool-down.

Those patients assigned to the nonexercise group did not attend any of these sessions, but received the traditional treatment, including physical therapy, if prescribed by their physicians.

Participants in both groups—with a median age of 54 years—had similar RA characteristics. They were evaluated at the start of the study and every six months to determine functional ability, damage to shoulders, elbows, knees, hips and ankles, and general health and emotional well-being.

THE RESULTS

The researchers say they found no significant differences between the two groups in RA symptoms such as joint swelling or pain or in use of anti-rheumatic drugs and painkillers.

Compared with patients who didn't exercise, those who did showed greater improvement in daily functioning during both years, the researchers found.

Those who exercised also had a significant improvement in physical capacity during the first year, which leveled off in the second year.

The exercise group also fared better emotionally, as measured by responses to questions about depressive feelings and anxiety, the researchers say.

"The majority of the patients enjoyed participating in the high-intensity exercise program very much," says researcher Dr. Thea P.M. Vliet Vlieland of Leiden University Medical Center in The Netherlands.

Indeed, she adds, many of the patients reported having more physical activity outside of the exercise program.

EXERCISE IS BENEFICIAL

The findings suggest high-intensity exercise programs can benefit many RA patients, Vlieland says.

"The positive effects on muscle strength and aerobic capacity could be translated into an improvement in the activities of daily living, and this is what really makes a difference in your life," Vlieland says.

Many people with RA are wary of strenuous activity. And physicians often advise patients against intense exercise, in part because of fears of damaging large joints and worsening inflammation.

The study, however, found no significant detrimental effect of vigorous exercise on weight-bearing joints, except in cases where patients already had a considerable amount of large joint damage.

These patients can still exercise, but should have regimens that are individually designed for them so that they can spare the damaged joints, says lead author, Dr. Zuzana de Jong, a rheumatologist at Leiden University Medical Center.

Vlieland stresses that before beginning any exercise program, all RA patients should seek their doctor's advice.

info For more on exercise and arthritis, visit the University of Washington Department of Orthopaedics and Sports Medicine at *www.orthop.washington.edu/arthritis/types.*

Try T'ai Chi Chih To Treat Shingles

Psychosomatic Medicine.
Center for the Advancement of Health news release.

T'ai chi chih—a simple combination of meditation and movement—may protect older people from shingles.

That's the conclusion of a study that found practitioners of the ancient Chinese set of movements got an immune system boost after performing the regimen for a few months.

Researchers at the University of California, Los Angeles, measured the immune cells that fight shingles in a group of 36 Southern California residents older than 60 years. Shingles is a painful rash caused by reactivation of the chickenpox virus. Resistance to the disease weakens as people age.

The immune cell levels increased approximately 50% in the 18 people who practiced t'ai chi chih for 15 weeks, according to the study. Their ability to move around also improved, especially among those who were having trouble walking and climbing stairs before the program started.

Determining how long the increased immunity lasts and whether t'ai chi chih might boost immunity to other diseases requires more study, the researchers say.

info You can learn all about how to perform t'ai chi chih movements at *www. taichichih.org.*

■ ■ ■ ■

Recovering from Shingles May Be Difficult

Between 600,000 and 1 million Americans are diagnosed with shingles each year, according to estimates from the National Institutes of Health (NIH). The lifetime odds of contracting the disease are one in five.

Although shingles may be mild, some people may develop severe and even debilitating forms of the illness. They may be in such serious pain that they can no longer wear clothes (the clothes irritate the rash) or perform activities of daily life.

Once the initial infection subsides, some people develop residual pain and discomfort called *postherpetic neuralgia.* This condition occurs in about 20% of all people who have shingles, but in almost 40% of shingles patients older than 60 years.

When shingles occur on the face, it can cause potentially permanent blindness and deafness. The ailment is particularly hazardous for people with weakened immune systems, such as those who have HIV or are taking drugs for cancer.

Shingles does respond to treatment—if it's caught early. Antiviral drugs such as *acyclovir, famcyclovir* and *valacyclovir* can help reduce pain as well as help resolve the rash associated with flare-ups.

Some patients also get relief from painkillers and topical creams. So far, however, no treatment has been found to prevent long-lasting pain from the disease.

info You can learn more about shingles from the US Food and Drug Administration at *www.fda.gov*.

Two Breakthrough Drugs That Fight Psoriasis

Paul Cabiran, MD, dermatologist, Ochsner Clinic, New Orleans.

Kenneth Gordon, MD, associate professor, medicine, division of dermatology, Loyola University Stritch School of Medicine, Chicago, member, medical board, and chairman, research committee, National Psoriasis Foundation.

Archives of Dermatology.

New treatments could make life a little better for people with the often painful and unsightly skin condition known as psoriasis.

An estimated 5.5 million Americans have psoriasis. And up to 15% of people with psoriasis have psoriatic arthritis, an inflammation of the joints that produces arthritis symptoms, according to the National Institute of Arthritis and Musculoskeletal and Skin Diseases.

SIGNS AND SYMPTOMS

Psoriasis is marked by a thickening of the skin with bright red patches and silvery scales. But this is just the visible manifestation of an immune process gone awry.

Defective immune system cells trigger events that cause the skin's outer layer to grow faster than normal. "In some cases, it's seven or eight times the normal rate of skin growth," says Dr. Paul Cabiran, a dermatologist with the Ochsner Clinic in New Orleans. "The process is accelerated tremendously, so the dead layers build up too quickly."

So quickly, that there's not enough time for the old layers to slough off to make room for the new ones. This causes scaly, thick patches or "plaques." The redness is due to the increased blood supply that fuels rapidly growing cells.

The majority of psoriasis cases seem to have a genetic component, though scientists are still working to find the culprit gene or genes.

"We're not only making a tremendous amount of progress understanding the immunology of psoriasis but also its genetics," Cabiran says.

The relatively recent discovery that psoriasis is an immune-based disease has paved the way for breakthroughs in treatment for more severe forms of the disease.

TREATMENTS FOR SEVERE PSORIASIS

As many as one third of the people who have psoriasis have more severe forms of the disease, measured by the amount of body surface affected.

Traditionally, psoriasis has been treated with powerful drugs that affect the whole body, such as *methotrexate,* a chemotherapy drug that is used in the treatment of cancer of the lymph system. *Cyclosporine,* which suppresses the immune system and is used to prevent organ rejection in transplant patients, is also used to treat severe psoriasis.

Over the long term, these therapies can increase the risk of cancer and may have adverse affects on the liver, kidneys and blood pressure, says Dr. Kenneth Gordon, an associate professor of medicine at the Loyola University Stritch School of Medicine in Chicago and chairman of the National Psoriasis Foundation's research committee.

But in January 2003, the US Food and Drug Administration (FDA) approved the first biologic treatment for psoriasis—*alefacept (brand name:* Amevive), which is considered a breakthrough drug. Another biologic drug, *etanercept (brand name:* Enbrel), has also been approved by the FDA for psoriatic arthritis.

"These biologic medications are designed to attack a very specific part of the immune system and leave the rest of the body intact," Gordon says.

TREATMENTS FOR MILD PSORIASIS

For milder forms of the disease, different treatments are available.

"Topical therapies [creams] are more reasonable for people with less body area involved because it takes less time to cover themselves with creams every day," Gordon says.

Cabiran says steroid creams and topical vitamin D are a common first step for people who just have a little patch on the elbow, knee or scalp.

People who have larger areas that are affected might benefit from light therapy.

info To learn more about psoriasis and various treatments, visit the National Psoriasis Foundation at *www.psoriasis.org*.

■ ■ ■ ■

Coping with Psoriasis

Psoriasis is a common skin disease that causes patches of thickened, red and scaly skin, usually on the arms or torso. The disease can be painful and, in some cases, cause disfigurement.

Psoriasis and a related condition, psoriatic arthritis, afflict an estimated 4.5 million Americans each year, according to the National Psoriasis Foundation. The diseases are noncontagious immune system disorders of varying severity that are thought to have a genetic origin in approximately one third of patients.

Psoriasis has no cure. However, many treatments can alleviate symptoms of the disease. These include topical therapies, such as steroid creams, scale lifters containing salicylic acid and coal tar lotions that have been used to treat skin irritation for centuries.

For patients whose skin troubles don't resolve with topical remedies, doctors may prescribe treatment with light. Called *phototherapy,* this may include sunlight, ultraviolet light, even lasers that can resolve stubborn plaques.

Finally, those with the most serious skin symptoms may improve with drugs that modify the immune system. Among these are *cyclosporine,* the joint medication *methotrexate* and injected "biologic" drugs (made from viruses and human and animal tissue), such as *alefacept* and *efalizumab.*

The National Psoriasis Foundation offers these tips for coping with the emotional strain of the disease…

●**Learn the facts about psoriasis.**

●**Practice responses to questions people may ask** about your skin.

●**Become comfortable hearing yourself talk about psoriasis.**

●**Join activities and groups,** either with other people who have psoriasis or not.

●**Reassure yourself that you have a scientific medical condition,** not something "weird" or a "curse."

●**Expect that you may still have negative experiences,** but each time you do, it will get easier.

●**Fill your life with the positive**—focus on your family, profession and hobbies.

●**Remind yourself that there is more to your life than psoriasis** and you are much more than just your skin disease.

Take advantage of the many services provided by the Psoriasis Foundation. By meeting other people who have psoriasis, you may find more support than you ever expected.

New Cream Fights Psoriasis

British Journal of Dermatology.
Boston University news release.

New England scientists say they've developed a skin cream that successfully treats the symptoms of psoriasis.

Boston University Medical Center researchers say the topical lotion contains a protein-based drug that soothes the red, scaling skin associated with psoriasis while shortening the average bout of a flare-up.

The salve is a combination of two substances —parathyroid hormone analog PTH (1-34) and Novasomer A cream. Novasomer A works to enhance the absorption of PTH (1-34) into the skin.

THE STUDY

The researchers tested the drug on 15 adults with chronic plaque psoriasis. Lesions treated with the PTH (1-34)–enriched lotion showed a marked improvement in scaling, redness and duration.

"The study concluded that patients who were resistant to at least one standard therapy for psoriasis had a remarkable improvement in their psoriasis when they applied PTH (1-34) in Novasomer A cream to their lesion," says Dr. Michael Holick, a professor of medicine, physiology and dermatology.

"These results suggest that topical PTH (1-34) encapsulated in Novasomer A cream may be a safe and effective novel therapy for psoriasis," he says.

Psoriasis has no cure, but there are many treatments that are available to alleviate the symptoms of the disease. These include topical therapies, such as steroid creams, scale lifters containing salicylic acid and coal tar lotions that have been used to combat skin irritation for centuries.

Dermatitis Ointment More Effective than Standard Steroid Creams

Sakari Reitamo MD, PhD, acting head, department of dermatology, Hospital for Skin and Allergic Diseases, University of Helsinki, Finland.
Bottom Line/Health.

According to a recent study, after three months of use, 73% of the patients using *tacrolimus* (Protopic) ointment had at least a 60% improvement in dermatitis symptoms compared with only 52% in those using a corticosteroid.

Less than half as many people using tacrolimus discontinued the treatment because of ineffectiveness as those in the steroid group. Patients with moderate dermatitis experienced the best results. Side effects caused by tacrolimus include skin burning, which decreased after the first week of treatment.

14

Research News

Coming Soon: Drug that Lowers Cholesterol and Makes You Thin

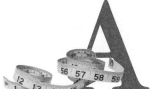

A pill that would assist people in losing weight and lowering cholesterol may be available in the future. It's only a drawing-board sketch today, but pharmaceutical company researchers say they have discovered a molecule that has been successful in reducing weight and cholesterol in laboratory animals.

The molecule resembles thyroid hormone, but it's much different from the various thyroid products that are currently on the market, says Gary J. Grover, a senior principal scientist at the Bristol-Myers Squibb Pharmaceutical Research Institute.

Most of the thyroid drugs that are currently being used are for people whose thyroid glands do not produce enough thyroid hormone. The hormone helps reduce weight by increasing the body's metabolic rate. It also works to keep blood cholesterol low. But thyroid hormone drugs can have dangerous side effects, such as an increased heart rate.

GETTING THE BENEFITS WITHOUT THE SIDE EFFECTS

The aim of Grover's research is to produce a drug that provides the benefits of thyroid hormone without the side effects. Their effort is based on the relatively new knowledge that there are two kinds of receptors that receive the hormone and pass its signal to the body.

The two kinds of receptors are called *alpha* and *beta* receptors. The newly reported molecule acts on the beta receptors, but leaves the alpha receptors alone.

"The thrust of our paper is that if you stimulate the beta subtype receptors, you get a

Gary J. Grover, PhD, senior principal scientist, Bristol-Meyers Squibb Pharmaceutical Research Institute, Pennington, NJ.

Brian Henry, spokesman, Bristol-Myers Squibb, Pennington, NJ.

Proceedings of the National Academy of Sciences.

modest increase in the rate at which energy is burned, without an increased heart rate," Grover says. "In addition to the increase in metabolic rate, we also found that beta receptor activation causes the lowering of cholesterol and lipoproteins."

Lowering blood levels of these substances can significantly reduce a person's chances of having heart or vessel problems. So the work done thus far with mice, rats and monkeys is "a first scientific step" toward a heart-friendly weight loss drug, Grover says.

He and his colleagues are now working to verify their findings. For example, they are checking to be sure that the weight reduction is due to loss of fat, rather than muscle. "Right now the consensus is that this is reasonable," Grover says.

Bristol-Myers Squibb is being cautiously optimistic about these experiments. "There are a number of things we are looking at in the obesity field, and this is one of them," says Brian Henry, a company spokesman.

info Information on thyroid hormone is available from the National Library of Medicine's MedlinePlus Web site at *www.nlm.nih. gov/medlineplus.* Click on "Drug Information."

■ ■ ■ ■

Is There a 'Magic Bullet' For Weight Loss?

Some dieters put their hopes in pills that promise to "burn," "block," "flush" or otherwise eliminate fat from the system. But science has yet to come up with a low-risk magic bullet for weight loss. Some pills may help control the appetite, but they can have serious side effects. Amphetamines, for example, are highly addictive and can have an adverse impact on the heart and central nervous system. Other pills are utterly worthless.

The Federal Trade Commission (FTC) and a number of state attorneys general have successfully brought cases against marketers of pills claiming to absorb or burn fat. The Food and Drug Administration (FDA) has banned 111 ingredients once found in over-the-counter diet products. None of these substances, which include alcohol, caffeine, dextrose and guar gum, have proved effective in weight-loss or appetite suppression.

Beware of the following products that are touted as weight-loss wonders…

● **Diet patches.** Worn on the skin, these have not been proven safe or effective. The FDA has seized millions of these products from manufacturers and promoters.

● **"Fat blockers"** purport to absorb fat and mechanically interfere with the fat that a person eats.

● **"Starch blockers"** promise to block or impede starch digestion. Not only is the claim unproven, but users have complained of nausea, vomiting, diarrhea and stomach pains.

● **"Magnet" diet pills** allegedly "flush fat out of the body." The FTC has brought legal action against several marketers of these pills.

● **Glucomannan** is advertised as the "Weight loss secret that's been in the Orient for more than 500 years." There is little evidence supporting the effectiveness of this plant root in helping people lose weight.

● **Some bulk producers or fillers,** such as fiber-based products, may absorb liquid and swell in the stomach, thereby reducing hunger. But some fillers, such as guar gum, can prove harmful, causing obstructions in the intestines, stomach or esophagus.

● **Spirulina,** a species of blue-green algae, has not been proven effective for losing weight.

PHONY DEVICES AND GADGETS

Phony weight-loss devices range from those that are simply ineffective to those that are truly dangerous to your health. *Some of the fraudulent gadgets that have been marketed to hopeful dieters over the years include…*

● **Electrical muscle stimulators,** which have a legitimate use in physical therapy treatment, do not help weight loss or body toning. In fact, when used incorrectly, they can cause electrical shocks and burns. The FDA has even taken a number of them off the market.

● **Appetite-suppressing eyeglasses** are common eyeglasses with colored lenses that claim to project an image to the retina that decreases the desire to eat. There is no evidence that these work.

• **Magic weight-loss earrings** and devices custom-fitted to the purchaser's ear purport to stimulate acupuncture points that control hunger. These claims, of course, have not been proven.

Fat Cells Tied to High Blood Pressure

Monika Ehrhart-Bornstein, PhD, researcher, German Diabetes Center, Heinrich Heine University, Dusseldorf.
Theodore Goodfriend, MD, professor, medicine, University of Wisconsin, Madison.
Proceedings of the National Academy of Sciences.

Scientists working with human fat cells called *adipocytes* have found a direct link between those cells and hormones that are known to increase blood pressure.

"Fat cells secrete products that directly stimulate the release of *aldosterone,* which is responsible for high blood pressure," says lead researcher Monika Ehrhart-Bornstein, from the German Diabetes Center at Heinrich Heine University in Dusseldorf.

"It is known that high blood pressure is present with obesity, but the [reason for the] connection between the two has remained unknown," she adds.

A malfunction in the adrenal glands—a pair of glands that is located near the kidneys—is linked to obesity. This malfunction leads to an excessive release of aldosterone, a blood pressure-elevating steroid that causes the kidneys to hold on to salt.

Although this relationship was known, how fat contributed to high blood pressure was not. Ehrhart-Bornstein and her colleagues studied whether hormones secreted by fat cells affected the production of aldosterone from the adrenal gland.

In experiments with human cells, her team found that chemicals released by fat cells spurred the adrenal gland to sharply increase its secretion of aldosterone.

These findings indicate that "fat cells are directly responsible for this increase in blood pressure," Ehrhart-Bornstein says. However, which specific factors in fat cells cause the release of aldosterone is still not known, she adds.

Ehrhart-Bornstein's team is now trying to identify which of these previously unidentified fat cell secretions might be responsible for stimulating the release of aldosterone.

Until these factors have been identified, there are no direct clinical implications to the findings, she cautions. However, in the future it could lead to new approaches for treating high blood pressure.

ANOTHER THEORY

Dr. Theodore Goodfriend, a professor of medicine at the University of Wisconsin, has a different theory on the relationship between fat tissue and high blood pressure.

He says the link between abdominal fat and high blood pressure is mysterious. "But I think it is the result of a factor or chemical released from abdominal fat that is further transformed by the liver."

The chemical stimulates the adrenal gland to make aldosterone, Goodfriend says. "We have found an association of visceral obesity with elevated aldosterone in some patients," he adds.

info To learn more about obesity and blood pressure, visit the National Heart, Lung and Blood Institute at *www.nhlbi.nih.gov.*

New Research May Prove Genetics the Key to Better Blood Pressure Treatment

Sharon Kardia, PhD, director, University of Michigan Public Health Genetics Program, Ann Arbor.
Stephen T. Turner, MD, professor, medicine, Mayo Clinic, Rochester, MN.
Eric Boerwinkle, PhD, director, Human Genetics Center, University of Texas Health Sciences Center, Houston.
Presentation, American Heart Association's 57th Annual High Blood Pressure Research Conference, Washington, DC.

Genetic tests may one day help determine the best medication for someone with high blood pressure.

US researchers hope a study—one that will take the better part of decade to complete—will lead to better treatments for one of the nation's leading causes of heart attack and stroke, says Sharon Kardia, study leader and director of the University of Michigan's Public Health Genetics Program.

THE STUDY

The study will examine the effect of two blood pressure medications on people who carry two different genes that are associated with hypertension. One of the genes—ADD2—appears to make blood pressure drugs called beta-blockers work more effectively in people who carry it. People who have the other gene—SLC9A2—appear to have better results with a thiazide diuretic blood pressure drug.

A total of 1,200 people who carry one of the two genes is being enrolled in the study, says Dr. Stephen T. Turner, a professor of medicine at the Mayo Clinic in Rochester, Minnesota. Half will take a beta-blocker, the other half will take a thiazide diuretic. They will be followed up for seven to eight years to see whether genetic makeup affects how well the drugs work.

The study is in response to observations that carriers of a certain gene did better with certain kinds of high blood pressure medications. Carriers of a specific form of the ADD2 gene who were given a beta-blocker had an average systolic blood pressure that was 20 points lower than those who were given a diuretic.

The study could help explain some of the complexities of high blood pressure incidence and treatment, Turner says. Previous studies have shown that African-American people respond better to treatment with thiazide diuretics than Caucasian people, perhaps because African-Americans are more likely to carry the SLC9A2 gene. To test that theory, the study will include people of both races.

GENETICS NOT THE WHOLE STORY

But even if the study reaches all its goals, it will be one small step in the field of hypertension research, says Eric Boerwinkle, director of the Human Genetics Center at the University of Texas Health Sciences Center.

"Hypertension is a complex process of many genes interacting with many environmental factors to affect the risk of heart attack or stroke," Boerwinkle says. The best estimate is that there may be dozens of genes involved, and that overall, genetics accounts for about 35% of risk, he says.

info The American Heart Association has more on high blood pressure and the factors that contribute to it at *www.american heart.org*. Click on "Diseases & Conditions."

Adult Stem Cell Therapy Repairs Damaged Heart

Andreas M. Zeiher, MD, chairman, department of medicine, University of Frankfurt, Germany.

William O'Neill, director, cardiology, William Beaumont Hospital, Detroit.

Circulation.

A recent study by German cardiologists has found that infusing a patient's own stem cells into a heart artery several days after a heart attack improves the heart's pumping power and speeds healing.

THE STUDY

The study found that the stem cell infusions increased the amount of blood ejected by the left ventricle, the heart's main pumping center, by nearly 20% and decreased tissue damage by 20%.

The study, by researchers at the University of Frankfurt, included only 28 patients, and the report covers just the first four months of treatment. But the results have been encouraging and have prompted a larger trial, says study author Dr. Andreas M. Zeiher, chairman of the University's department of medicine.

"We now have a 12-month follow-up, and the improvement is preserved over this time," Zeiher says. "Not a single patient in the trial developed heart failure."

Heart failure, or a progressive loss of the heart's ability to pump blood, often happens after a heart attack. The American Heart Association estimates that more than 51,500 Americans will die of heart failure this year.

ETHICAL ISSUES AVOIDED

The stem cell treatment used by the Frankfurt scientists avoids the ethical issues of fetal stem therapy because it uses the patients' own adult stem cells—Zeiher prefers the term "progenitor cells."

These cells are more limited than fetal stem cells, but they are still valuable for their ability to transform into a variety of cells, including heart muscle cells.

Some of the adult stem cells used in the study were harvested from bone marrow, and others were heart-derived cells. Both were equally effective, Zeiher says.

The long-term trial in Frankfurt includes 60 patients. Half of the patients are receiving an infusion of stem cells, the other half are getting inactive cells.

This randomized, double-blind experiment —meaning neither patients nor doctors know who is getting which treatment—is essential for verifying that the therapy works, Zeiher says.

NO DOMESTIC RESEARCH YET

Several cardiology teams in the United States are eager to start similar trials, but are waiting for approval by the US Food and Drug Administration (FDA), says Dr. William O'Neill, director of cardiology at William Beaumont Hospital in Detroit.

"Basically, all of these groundbreaking trials will be done in Europe," says O'Neill, who has submitted an application for FDA approval.

Zeiher and his colleagues clearly are leading the stem cell therapy effort, O'Neill says. The human trial was done after a number of studies in laboratory dishes and animals.

An important part of the long-term human trial will be to show that infused stem cells can migrate from an artery into the heart muscle and form new, healthy tissue, according to O'Neill. "The more likely they are to migrate, the more likely they are to hone in on damaged areas and improve heart function," he says.

Cheap, Fast Test Determines Blood Clot Risk

Ben deBoisblanc, MD, professor, medicine and physiology, Louisiana State University, New Orleans. *New England Journal of Medicine.*

A new blood test gives doctors a quick and inexpensive way to identify emergency department patients who are at high risk of life-threatening blood clots, researchers report.

The test, which costs no more than a few hundred dollars, was nearly 100% accurate in separating low-risk patients from those patients with similar symptoms who needed an ultrasound diagnostic test that can be expensive —$10,000 or more.

A DANGEROUS CONDITION

Swift diagnosis of the condition, called *deep vein thrombosis* (DVT), is critical because clots that form in the legs can travel to the lungs as a pulmonary embolism (PE), killing or crippling the patient.

The decision to use anti-clotting therapy— which has its own risk—has traditionally been made on the basis of a doctor's clinical assessment, backed up by an ultrasound scan.

THE STUDY

The study looked at more than 1,000 patients who doctors suspected had DVT.

The patients judged to be at high risk were divided into two groups.

One group went straight to ultrasound imaging, and the other had ultrasound only if the new blood test indicated danger. The new blood test measures levels of *d-dimers,* or blood clot fragments.

D-dimer testing determined that ultrasound exams were not needed for 39% of the patients given the test, so the number of ultrasound exams was cut significantly, according to the report.

And only two of the patients with negative d-dimer tests had clots, meaning that the test was 99.6% accurate.

"These tests are not now widely used, but they are poised to really gain momentum," says Dr. Ben deBoisblanc, a professor of medicine and physiology at Louisiana State University, who has done his own studies in the field. "In the next year or two, you will see this become the most common procedure for excluding patients from ultrasound."

A number of d-dimer tests have been available for years, but those that could give precise results have been too complicated to use quickly, and the simple tests have been imprecise. This study used two new tests that give precise results and that are easily performed in a clinical setting.

A negative d-dimer test result "goes a long way to telling whether a patient has a clot," deBoisblanc says. "In the right scenario, using this test means that you can stop right there. If the test result is positive, you can do the ultrasound to be sure."

START WITH YOUR DOCTOR

The selection process still starts with a doctor's clinical judgment, the report says. The doctor assigns points on the basis of conditions known to be associated deep-vein thrombosis risk—swelling of the leg, prolonged immobility, previous DVT or an active cancer.

So the combination of clinical judgment and the d-dimer test "simplifies the diagnosis of deep vein thrombosis in outpatients without compromising safety," the researchers conclude.

info The complexities of diagnosing and treating deep vein thrombosis are explained by the American Academy of Orthopaedic Surgeons at *http://orthoinfo.aaos.org*.

■ ■ ■ ■

Causes of DVT

Deep vein thrombosis (DVT) often results from orthopaedic surgery. Other factors that may contribute to this condition include age, prior history of vein disease, smoking, estrogen use, obesity and genetics.

New Study Shows a Better Way to Prevent Deep Vein Thrombosis

Yves Rosenberg, MD, MPH, project officer, National Heart, Lung and Blood Institute, Bethesda, MD.
Clive Kearon, MD, PhD, associate professor, medicine, McMaster University, Hamilton, Ontario, Canada.
New England Journal of Medicine.

A recent study tries to find the best way to prevent the potentially fatal blood clots of the condition called deep vein thrombosis (DVT).

These blood clots, which occur in a deep vein (usually in the lower leg and thigh), can cause severe discomfort and may even kill the patient by traveling to the lungs and blocking a pulmonary artery. As many as 60,000 Americans are killed each year by these pulmonary embolisms, says Dr. Yves Rosenberg, a project officer at the National Heart, Lung and Blood Institute (NHLBI) and an expert on the subject.

Recurrent clots can be prevented by taking *warfarin* (*brand name:* Coumadin), an effective blood thinner. But doses of warfarin that are too high can cause bleeding that can be damaging or fatal. Study after study has tried to determine what dose will work best to prevent clots while causing a minimum of dangerous bleeding.

Rosenberg and colleagues at the NHLBI conducted a study that showed that long-term treatment with lower-than-standard doses of warfarin effectively prevented clots over the long run with a minimum of bleeding. The results were so impressive that the study was cut short to inform doctors about it.

However, the latest research now finds that although low-dose warfarin is good, standard—that is, higher—doses are better.

THE STUDY

The study included 738 people who had DVT. The 369 patients assigned to low-dose therapy experienced 16 clots. There were only six clots in the 369 patients given standard therapy. The incidence of serious bleeding episodes was almost the same in both groups

—eight in the standard-dose group, nine in the low-dose group.

"We were surprised that the usual-dose warfarin treatment did not cause more bleeding," says study author Dr. Clive Kearon, an associate professor of medicine at McMaster University in Hamilton, Ontario.

LONG-TERM CONCERNS

However, Rosenberg is not sure this is the final word on warfarin therapy. "You cannot say that long-term treatment with the regular dose does not increase the risk of bleeding episodes," he says, arguing that the results achieved in such a carefully controlled trial might not be possible in ordinary clinical practice.

He acknowledges that the new study results are statistically significant, but points out that the study lasted only two years. "Long-term treatment has to be tailored for each individual patient," Rosenberg says. "I don't think you can say that long-term treatment with the regular dose will be effective for every patient."

Rosenberg and Kearon are in complete agreement about one thing: Patients with DVT should get long-term warfarin treatment. Some physicians stop the treatment several months after a first clot occurs, but "warfarin treatment is, without a doubt, essential to reduce the incidence of return of blood clots," Rosenberg says.

"Patients often do not stay on warfarin for the longer term," Kearon says. "This study shows that after six months, the benefit continued and the risk was low."

MRIs Can Detect Blocked Blood Vessels

Robert M. Judd, PhD, associate professor of radiology, co-director, Duke Cardiovascular Magnetic Resonance Center, Duke University, Durham, NC.

Tony Fuisz, MD, director, cardiac MRI, Washington Hospital Center, Washington, DC.

Nature Medicine.

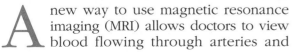

A new way to use magnetic resonance imaging (MRI) allows doctors to view blood flowing through arteries and might one day replace more invasive techniques to check for arterial blockages, new research suggests.

Currently, doctors use a procedure called an angiogram to look for a blocked artery. This requires a "contrast agent" injected into the bloodstream to highlight the artery.

Then, the angiogram images are assembled by a computer into a short movie that shows the doctor where the blockage is located.

While an angiogram is generally safe and effective, it is an invasive procedure that has a small but definite risk of harm. In addition, it requires radiation. Contrast agents occasionally have unpleasant or unwanted side effects, which may include kidney damage, according to the study authors.

ADVANTAGE OVER ANGIOGRAM

In contrast, MRI uses harmless magnetic fields and radio frequency signals to image body tissues, the researchers say.

Using this new MRI technique, "you can get images that look like those from an angiogram, but you can do it with a noninvasive MRI," says lead study author Robert M. Judd, an associate professor of radiology and co-director of the Duke Cardiovascular Magnetic Resonance Center at Duke University in Durham, North Carolina.

"The technique is still new and there are technical issues that still need to be sorted out," Judd says. "But the principle appears to be correct."

Using this technique, doctors should be able to locate a blockage in a blood vessel, as well as any partial blockage.

Judd explains that hospitals would not need new MRIs to use this new technique. All that would be needed is an upgrade in software, he says.

Now, however, the new technique works only in large vessels, such as the aorta in the heart and the renal arteries that carry blood to the kidneys.

ANOTHER OPINION

Dr. Tony Fuisz, director of cardiac MRI at Washington Hospital Center in Washington, DC, called the new research interesting. However, he says, "a new way to image segments of the aorta, renal arteries and other large vessels is like an answer to a question no one is asking. The real Holy Grail is coronary [heart arteries] imaging."

According to Fuisz, there are a number of potential obstacles to using the new technique for coronary arteries. "Some of these obstacles involve fundamental physical limitations and as such may not be able to be overcome," he adds.

info For information on magnetic resonance angiography, visit the Radiological Society of North America at *www.radiologyinfo.org*.

Scientists Strive for Breast Cancer Vaccine

Robert Vonderheide, MD, DPhil, assistant professor, Leonard and Madlyn Abramson Family Cancer Research Institute, University of Pennsylvania, Philadelphia.

Herman Kattlove, MD, spokesman, American Cancer Society.

Teresa Gilewski, medical oncologist, breast cancer service, Memorial Sloan-Kettering Cancer Center, New York City.

The prospect of a breast cancer vaccine generates tremendous hope among cancer patients and their doctors. But the reality, according to researchers, is at least a decade away.

"Probably dozens of breast cancer vaccines are under study," notes Dr. Robert Vonderheide, assistant professor at the Leonard and Madlyn Abramson Family Cancer Research Institute at the University of Pennsylvania. "It's a goal over the next decade to have a vaccine against breast cancer. But it's important to recognize how long this will take."

Most therapeutic vaccines (those that treat existing cancers) that are currently under development—including ones for breast and other cancers, such as melanoma, lung, ovarian and prostate—focus on boosting the immune system to prevent the further growth of existing cancers, block the recurrence of cancers that were treated or kill cancer cells that were not destroyed by previous treatment.

The only cancer-related vaccine approved by the US Food and Drug Administration is a prophylactic vaccine to prevent the hepatitis B virus, which is associated with liver cancer.

The first step in the process is to develop a therapeutic vaccine to treat women with breast cancer by stopping any recurrence of their disease or by shrinking their tumors, says Dr. Teresa Gilewski, a medical oncologist on the breast cancer service at Memorial Sloan-Kettering Cancer Center in New York City.

Once that goal has been reached, researchers can focus on preventive vaccines, she says.

SEVERAL APPROACHES UNDER INVESTIGATION

Using vaccines to treat breast cancer is still considered experimental, so there are several different approaches under review…

●**Vonderheide and his team are studying the effectiveness of an enzyme-based vaccine,** focusing on a peptide known as *telomerase*. Because tumor cells have more telomerase than normal cells, this vaccine is designed to generate a particular white blood cell to attack the telomerase in the cancer cells and kill off the tumor.

●**In other instances, vaccines are made by taking cells from a patient's own tumor** or from the tumor of other patients, and using those cells to bring about an immune response.

●**Another approach involves harvesting specialized white blood cells** from a patient through a process called leukapheresis. In a laboratory, these cells are stimulated with the patient's own cancer antigens, grown and then re-injected into the patient. The vaccine activates cancer-fighting T-cells in the immune system, causing them to multiply and attack tumor cells that produce the antigen.

info For more information on breast cancer vaccines, visit the University of Pennsylvania Web site at *www.uphs.upenn.edu/news/News_Releases/feb04/avonprint.htm*.

Hepatitis C Vaccine May Soon Be on Market

Robert B. Belshe, MD, director, Center for Vaccine Development, Saint Louis University School of Medicine, MO.

Adrian M. Di Bisceglie, MD, chief, hepatology, Saint Louis University School of Medicine, MO.

Researchers are taking a first step toward a vaccine for hepatitis C, the virus that destroys the liver, infects approximately 2.7 million Americans and kills an estimated 8,000 to 10,000 of them each year.

THE FIRST TRIAL

The vaccine is being tested on 45 healthy volunteers, whose reactions will be monitored for one year, says Dr. Robert B. Belshe, director of the Center for Vaccine Development at Saint Louis University School of Medicine in St. Louis, where the experiment is being done.

Blood samples will be taken periodically from the volunteers getting the vaccine to test for antibody and immune cell levels, Belshe says. If those responses are satisfactory, the next step will be a larger study, involving several hundred healthy volunteers. This will provide broader measures of safety and immune system response.

Scientists hope this first trial, which focuses on the vaccine's safety and whether it has the ability to arouse the body's immune defenses, will lead to a product that can be used to protect people at high risk of being infected by the virus, Belshe says.

A DIFFICULT TARGET

Dr. Adrian M. Di Bisceglie, chief of hepatology at the Saint Louis facility, says the hepatitis C virus is a very difficult target because "it mutates a lot and it is not a strong stimulator of the body's immune system."

"Only now, 15 years after the hepatitis C virus was identified, do we have vaccines that we hope can be effective," Di Bisceglie says.

"This vaccine is not expected to be the final vaccine," Belshe says. "But it is an important step along the way."

He hopes the hepatitis C vaccine program will follow the path of an earlier program that produced an effective vaccine against the hepatitis B virus. "That program also started with safety tests on healthy individuals, then moved to trials with people at high risk. The vaccine was so effective and so safe that it now is used routinely," Belshe says.

"This is really the first candidate for a hepatitis C vaccine for humans in the United States," says Di Bisceglie. The road ahead is a long one, Belshe warns, but he and other researchers are encouraged by the fact that the vaccine testing is now under way.

info Learn about hepatitis C at the Washington State Department of Health at *www.doh.wa.gov/topics/hepcfact.htm.*

Fast-Acting Vaccine Controls Ebola Virus

Peter Jahrling, PhD, senior research scientist, US Army Medical Research Institute of Infectious Diseases, Fort Detrick, MD.

Dennis Burton, PhD, professor of immunology, Scripps Research Institute, La Jolla, CA.

Nature.

A fast-acting version of the Ebola vaccine protects against the deadly virus in one month, instead of the usual six, and it could contain an outbreak of the virus more effectively, a study says.

Scientists have had success with a vaccine that stimulates the immune system against Ebola. But the battery of shots, which uses DNA from the virus along with boosters, takes more than six months to administer—too long a period of time to fight an outbreak.

The new vaccine is experimental and it hasn't been tested in people, but if it's approved, it could help public health workers control disease outbreaks faster and better.

A fast-working vaccine would not only benefit health workers, but it could corral an outbreak if used in a so-called "ring" vaccination—the process of inoculating contacts of infected people.

THE STUDY

In the study, researchers from the National Institutes of Health and the US Army's Medical Research Institute of Infectious Diseases tried to streamline the Ebola vaccine. They used a mix of crippled adenoviruses (a form of cold virus) carrying three genes for harmless proteins from the Ebola's Zaire strain.

Macaques (a kind of monkey) that received the vaccine quickly began producing blood proteins specific to Ebola, a key step in building immunity to the virus.

The resulting reaction was weaker than with the DNA-based vaccine, but it was faster. What's more, the single injection was strong enough to protect every animal from the virus only 28 days later, the researchers say. That's about the standard for vaccines against diseases such as measles and mumps.

RESULTS PROMISING

"It looks to be a very effective vaccine. A single shot protects the monkeys completely," says Dennis Burton, an immunologist at the Scripps Research Institute in La Jolla, California. "It's very impressive." Burton calls the chances the shot will work in humans "very high."

info To find out more about Ebola, try the National Center for Infectious Diseases (NCID) at *www.cdc.gov/ncidod*.

■ ■ ■ ■

What Is Ebola?

The Ebola virus was identified in 1976, and the disease it causes has plagued humans and nonhuman primates (monkeys, gorillas and chimpanzees) ever since. The onset of illness is abrupt and is characterized by fever, headache, joint and muscle aches, sore throat and weakness, followed by diarrhea, vomiting and stomach pain. A rash, red eyes, hiccups and internal and external bleeding may be seen in some people.

The virus kills roughly 80% of the people it infects, usually within one week. Its status as one of the world's deadliest and most gruesome viruses makes Ebola an obvious choice for bioterrorists.

West Nile Transmitted Through Transfusion

Dawn Wesson, PhD, associate professor, tropical medicine, Tulane University School of Public Health and Tropical Medicine, New Orleans.

News conference with Julie Gerberding, MD, director, Centers for Disease Control and Prevention.

Louis Katz, MD, president, America's Blood Centers, Washington, DC.

New England Journal of Medicine.

Morbidity and Mortality Weekly Report.

The *New England Journal of Medicine* has made official what many already believed—West Nile virus can be transmitted through blood transfusions. But screening the blood supply is greatly reducing the risk of such transmissions.

"Anybody who lives in the United States right now is concerned about the potential for virus transmission—and they should be—[but] the screening appears to be very effective," says Dawn Wesson, an associate professor of tropical medicine at Tulane University School of Public Health and Tropical Medicine in New Orleans.

The authors of the study confirmed that 23 patients had contracted West Nile through transfused blood or blood products in 2002. Ten of these people (43%) had suppressed immune systems due to an organ transplant or cancer, and eight (35%) were 70 years or older. The 23 cases were linked to 16 donors.

It's likely there were more than these 23 confirmed cases, say the study authors. "The presumption is that there were some cases without symptoms and some cases with symptoms where the relationship wasn't recognized," says Dr. Louis Katz, president of America's Blood Centers, in Washington, DC.

"We know that we're probably missing some cases," Katz says. Nevertheless, the chances of contracting West Nile from a blood donation are "microscopic," he says. "If you need a transfusion, West Nile should not deter you."

The first case of transmission of West Nile virus by blood transfusion was reported at the end of August 2002 in a woman who had received donated blood when she was undergoing an obstetrical procedure. Even before then, however, US health officials were looking into ways to screen the blood supply.

New tests to detect the virus in blood supplies became available in 2003 under FDA Investigational New Drug (IND) protocols. Blood supply experts have hailed the rapid development of the tests as an extraordinary achievement.

According to the study authors, as of July 14, 2003, all civilian blood donations collected in the United States and Puerto Rico had been screened for West Nile virus with the use of these tests. A total of 163 donations out of approximately 1 million that were screened were found to have West Nile virus and were removed from circulation.

Federal officials are quick to point out that blood testing has been largely successful. "[The test] is a major step forward in protecting the blood supply but it's not perfect," said Centers for Disease Control and Prevention director Dr. Julie Gerberding. "Transmission [of the West Nile virus through blood] represents a very low risk, but it's not zero risk."

'Down Under' Virus Provides West Nile Vaccine

Roy Hall, PhD, senior research officer, University of Queensland, Brisbane, Australia.

W. Ian Lipkin, MD, professor of pathology and neurology, College of Physicians and Surgeons, Columbia University, New York City.

Proceedings of the National Academy of Sciences.

Report on West Nile virus in the United States, Centers for Disease Control and Prevention.

An Australian strain of West Nile virus may provide a vaccine against its deadly cousin, the mosquito-borne West Nile infection that affects the United States.

Mice vaccinated with a weakened strain of the Kunjin virus don't contract West Nile even when injected with lethal amounts of the pathogen, Australian researchers say. Kunjin is endemic to Northern Australia, and although it can infect people, it rarely sickens them.

Widespread Kunjin activity in Northern Australia may help explain why that continent has seen no cases of transmitted West Nile so far, said Roy Hall, a microbiologist at the University of Queensland in Brisbane, and the leader of the research effort.

"Probably the next step will be to test it in horses, where there is also a demand for a safe, effective vaccine," Hall says.

Many scientists have been pushing hard for a West Nile vaccine. Dr. W. Ian Lipkin, an expert in West Nile virus at Columbia University in New York City, calls the new results from Australia significant. "Although studies in mice do not always translate to humans, this advance is likely to add to the armamentarium of candidate vaccines for the prevention of West Nile virus–associated disease."

■ ■ ■ ■

Few Symptoms, No Treatment

Almost 10,000 people in the United States have confirmed West Nile infections and hundreds have died of the disease, according to the Centers for Disease Control and Prevention (CDC).

Thankfully, most people who are infected with the virus will not develop any severe symptoms. The risk of severe illness and death is highest for people older than 50 years.

While much of the world's attention was focused on new health risks, such as *severe acute respiratory syndrome* (SARS) in 2003, West Nile virus reached epidemic levels in some western states and spanned the North American continent in record numbers.

According to the CDC, West Nile claimed the lives of 222 people in 2003, with 9,100 total cases reported. The disease was most prevalent in the southwest and western United States. Colorado recorded 45 deaths; Texas, 34; Nebraska, 24; and South Dakota, 14.

Of the 9,100 cases that were reported, 69% were reported as the milder form of the disease and 29% were reported as meningitis or encephalitis, the severe form of the disease, according to the CDC.

There is currently no specific treatment for West Nile infection. In mild cases, people experience symptoms such as fever and aches that pass on their own. In more severe cases, people usually require hospitalization where they can receive supportive treatment including intravenous fluids, help with breathing and nursing care.

Implanted Electrodes May Help Parkinson Patients

Anthony E. Lang, MD, professor, neurology, University of Toronto.
New England Journal of Medicine.

Deep-brain stimulation using implanted electrodes provides substantial, lasting benefits for patients with severe Parkinson's disease, according to a French study. But the implants are not a cure for the neurological condition.

Parkinson's disease occurs when a group of cells in an area of the brain called the *substantia nigra* begin to malfunction and eventually die. Those brain cells produce a substance called *dopamine,* a chemical transmitter that relays signals to the parts of the brain that control movement and coordination. When the cells in the substantia nigra begin to die, the amount of dopamine produced in the brain decreases.

Levodopa, the standard drug treatment for Parkinson's, increases levels of dopamine. It remains the gold standard for drug treatment of Parkinson's disease, says Dr. Anthony E. Lang, a professor of neurology at the University of Toronto. But the effects of levodopa can start to fluctuate in some patients, causing their condition to deteriorate. The implanted electrode technique was developed for these patients.

THE STUDY

Deep-brain stimulation requires a skilled surgical team and carries surgical risks that require the careful screening of patients. The French study included only relatively young Parkinson's patients, with an average age of 55 years, who were screened for dementia and psychiatric problems.

The optimistic result of the French study is that "it shows that excellent responses can be sustained over a course of five or more years" for patients with deteriorating conditions, says Lang, who reported similar results in a smaller study.

RESULTS SUGGEST IMPLANTS SHOULD BE USED MORE AGGRESSIVELY

The success of the electrode implant technique means it should be used more aggressively, before patients taking levodopa develop major disabilities that leave them bedridden and helpless.

"What you want to do is to prevent all those problems before they occur," Lang says, and implanted electrodes can accomplish that in many patients.

But, Parkinson's patients who take levodopa to control their tremors can also experience instability, speech problems, uncontrolled motions and other symptoms—and the implants do not prevent these problems.

IMPLICATIONS

"What we learn from the implant studies is that if you control all the dopamine-related problems, other things begin to become more evident," Lang says.

"This shows a need for refocusing attempts to develop new treatments for Parkinson's disease, treatments that affect not only the dopamine system, but other areas of brain function as well," he adds.

The real obstacle that is standing in the way of new treatments is that no one really knows what goes wrong in Parkinson's disease, Lang says. Attempts at gene therapy and stem cell implants have not been effective thus far.

info An overview of Parkinson's disease is given by the National Institute of Neurological Disorders and Stroke at *www.ninds. nih.gov.*

Possible Gene Cure On Horizon for Muscular Dystrophy

Thomas Rando, MD, PhD, associate professor, neurology, Stanford University School of Medicine and Medical Center and Palo Alto VA Medical Center, CA.

Sharon Hesterlee, PhD, director, research development, Muscular Dystrophy Association, Tucson.

Presentation, American Neurological Association annual meeting, San Francisco.

Researchers may be one step closer to an effective gene therapy for muscular dystrophy, the family of crippling and potentially deadly disorders marked by muscle wasting.

Instead of using a virus to deliver a missing or mutated gene, as is common with gene therapy, researchers at Stanford University School of Medicine turned to genetic material called *plasmids,* along with a protein called *integrase.*

THE STUDY

Study author, Dr. Thomas Rando, and his colleagues at Stanford used a gene called luciferase, which emits a light that can be detected by using a special camera. This way, the researchers could see if the gene was integrating into the cells.

The researchers injected plasmids containing the luciferase gene into one hind leg of lab mice and the luciferase gene plus integrase into the other leg.

Soon after the injection, both legs showed signs of the luciferase gene. Over time, however, the leg without integrase lost the luciferase gene. The leg with integrase continued to show signs of the luciferase gene, proving that the gene had integrated into the cells' DNA.

Although the technique was successful on lab mice, experiments are still in the early stages and it will be some time before human clinical trials could even be considered.

Because muscular dystrophy is caused by either a missing or malfunctioning gene that makes the protein *dystrophin,* Rando says the next step is to see if this technique works with the dystrophin gene.

DELIVERY A CHALLENGE

One of the biggest challenges that the researchers face, Rando says, is figuring out a way to deliver the corrective genes to every muscle cell in the body. Currently, they can only deliver the gene locally, by injecting it directly into the muscle.

Another concern is adverse effects, though Rando says he and his team haven't yet seen any using this technique.

One of the problems with standard gene therapy is that it uses viruses to deliver the gene. Although viruses are quite effective at getting into cells, the body is also primed to mount an immune response against viruses to eliminate them. Also, viruses are small and often can't hold larger, therapeutic genes, Rando explains.

Sharon Hesterlee, director of research development for the Muscular Dystrophy Association, calls the study "interesting" but "still in the very early stages."

info To learn more about the different types of muscular dystrophy and the available treatments for the disease, visit the Muscular Dystrophy Association at *www.mdausa. org/disease/40list.html*.

Extraordinary Device Uses Mind Power to Steer Wheelchairs

New Scientist.
New Scientist news release.

A system that "reads" the electrical activity of brain cells may some day allow severely disabled people to use their thoughts to steer a motorized wheelchair.

Unlike previous devices of this sort, this system does not require surgical implants. It utilizes a skullcap that is fitted with electrodes that monitor the electrical activity of a person's neurons.

THE TEST

Researchers have tested the device by having wearers try to control a steerable robot. It took two days of training for the volunteers to learn how to use their minds to control the robot.

In the robot tests, the electrodes in the skull-cap collected information about the brain's electrical activity and fed that information into a computer.

Software analyzed the person's brain activity and, using a wireless link, passed on commands to the robot.

The users can select three different commands for the robot—turn left, turn right and move forward. The software can interpret the specific command by identifying telltale brain activity associated with that command.

The scientists are working to expand the ability of the system to identify more commands from the brain.

The system was created by Swiss and Spanish scientists. If they ultimately succeed in developing the technology, it would be the first mind-controlled system that is able to operate something as complicated as a motorized wheelchair.

OTHER APPLICATIONS

Mind-controlled devices—or "brain–computer interfaces"—are the stuff of science fiction and science fact. Richmond, Virginia-based East3, Ltd., for example, is developing "advanced feedback technology" to help children develop attention and concentration skills.

The company's Attention Trainer system relies on a wireless headset that sends information about its wearer's brain activity to software in video games that the child plays. If the game involves driving, the software can modulate the player's performance depending on what the sensors perceive as his or her attention level. In the process, the child can learn to improve his focus on the game and filter out extraneous information.

The potential benefits of advanced feedback technology, whether increasing athletic performance, attention training or reducing stress, are truly amazing and are too important not to share," says John Berger, president and chief executive officer of East3.

info For information on different types of wheelchairs visit the Food and Drug Administration at *www.fda.org*.

Pavlov's Bell 'Rings' True With People, Too!

Jay Gottfried, MD, neurologist and neuroscientist, Wellcome Department of Imaging Neuroscience, London.
David Zald, PhD, assistant professor of psychology, Vanderbilt University, Nashville.
Science.

Pavlov trained his dogs to salivate at the sound of a bell. Humans, it seems, can be trained to crave certain foods just by seeing an abstract image on a computer.

What's more, if they've eaten their fill of, say, peanut butter, it doesn't mean that they won't start eating ice cream. This finding demonstrates people's natural "braking system" after eating certain foods.

THE STUDY

In the study, each participant was shown two abstract visual images together with the smell of either vanilla or peanut butter. As soon as the volunteers began to associate certain images with a certain smell, they were fed vanilla ice cream or peanut butter sandwiches. They were asked to eat until they were satisfied, but not uncomfortably full.

Participants who had eaten their fill of vanilla ice cream no longer responded to the visual cue associated with that flavor, but they did respond to the picture associated with peanut butter. Volunteers who had just finished eating peanut butter sandwiches only responded to the visual cue for vanilla ice cream.

The conclusion: Just because you're comfortably full from eating one food doesn't mean you won't eat something else. Consider the last time you gorged on a steak, convinced you had no more room in your stomach until someone suggested chocolate cake for dessert.

"The brain needs a way to put a brake on the system," says Dr. Jay Gottfried, lead author of a paper on the work and a neurologist and neuroscientist at the Wellcome Department of Imaging Neuroscience in London.

"These processes operate in a very food-specific fashion," Gottfried explains. "If what you need is a good balance of nutrients, vitamins and minerals, it's important to be sampling different foods." A braking effect is in place as long as it comes to the same food item.

David Zald, assistant professor of psychology at Vanderbilt University in Nashville, Tennessee, says, "We have to be able to modify how we respond relative to our current needs. If we didn't, we would respond the same way to food-related stimuli whether we were hungry or full, and probably all end up obese. The present study helps us start unraveling how our brains allow us to modify our responses based on our current needs."

IMPLICATIONS

What happens when the brake or updating mechanism doesn't work? "One could imagine a case where someone might have difficulty disengaging from this pattern of behavior, and this could lead to things like compulsive eating or other eating disorders," Gottfried says.

info Harvard Medical School at *www.med.harvard.edu/AANLIB/home.html* has information on different brain structures.

New Discovery May Cure Overactive Thyroid

Donald Bergman, MD, president, American Association of Clinical Endocrinologists, and clinical associate professor, medicine, Mount Sinai School of Medicine, New York City.

Kenneth Hupart, MD, chief, endocrinology, diabetes and metabolism, Nassau University Medical Center, East Meadow, NY.

The Lancet.

People who have Graves' disease have certain molecules that mistakenly attack their bodies, sending their thyroids into overdrive. But for 40 years, no one has been able to identify the particular molecule that causes the thyroid to overproduce. Now, British researchers say they've finally found it.

Although the molecule, called a *monoclonal antibody,* was isolated in only one patient—a 19-year-old man with Graves' disease—the discovery could hold significant promise for the future diagnosis and treatment of the disease.

CURRENT TREATMENTS

According to the National Graves' Disease Foundation (NGDF), there are three standard methods of treatment for Graves' disease—a patient may take drugs to inhibit the production of active thyroid hormone; he or she may be given radioactive iodine to destroy part or all of the gland; or the patient may have most of the thyroid gland surgically removed.

ONE LINE OF CELLS INVOLVED

"Monoclonal" means that the antibodies come from one line of cells. "It's thought to be one rogue cell that then multiplies itself," says Donald Bergman, president of the American Association of Clinical Endocrinologists. "It means a single clone of cells that's gone awry is producing this antibody that's causing all this damage. It's a very, very exciting discovery."

Because only one cell line appears to be involved, researchers may be able to find extremely targeted treatments for the disease. The more precisely targeted the therapy, the lower the risk of collateral damage to other cells in the body.

PROMISE OF NEW TREATMENTS

"The identification of this antibody and its availability to medical scientists represents a major step forward. Further studies will likely lead to a better understanding of Graves' disease," says Dr. Kenneth Hupart, chief of endocrinology, metabolism and diabetes at Nassau University Medical Center located in East Meadow, New York.

"More importantly, this report offers the promise of new therapies that may benefit patients with Graves' disease, such as reducing the incidence of disfiguring eye problems that they can develop. It can also give rise to new approaches to caring for patients with thyroid cancer," he adds.

But Hupart adds that the help won't come immediately. "These potential benefits will not be realized today or tomorrow, but they may help doctors lessen the burden of these thyroid diseases for patients in future years," he says.

■ ■ ■ ■

Facts About Graves' Disease

According to the National Graves' Disease Foundation, Graves' disease is more prevalent among females than males. It usually occurs in middle age, but also occurs in children and adolescents.

Symptoms of Graves' disease include fatigue, weight loss, restlessness, rapid heartbeat, changes in libido, muscle weakness, heat intolerance, tremors, enlarged thyroid gland, heart palpitations, increased sweating, blurred or double vision, increased appetite and nervousness and irritability.

info For more information on Graves' disease, visit the National Graves' Disease Foundation's Web site at *www.ngdf.org.*

Amazing Predictors Improve Transplant Success

Philip Marsden, MD, professor, medicine, University of Toronto, St. Michael's Hospital, Toronto.

Minnie Sarwal, MD, PhD, assistant professor, pediatrics, Stanford University School of Medicine, Palo Alto, CA.

New England Journal of Medicine.

One in 10 kidney transplant patients will reject the new organ. Faced with those odds, doctors have been eagerly looking for ways to improve the chances that transplant recipients will keep their new organs for as long as possible and with the fewest complications.

New research may help. The combination of ultrasound and computer chips that measure gene activity could help doctors better predict which kidney transplant patients are most likely to reject their new organs—and perhaps lead to genetically tailored ways to prevent this rejection.

THE STUDIES

German researchers showed that using a slightly new method of conventional ultrasound to measure blood flow in a transplanted organ they could accurately predict which transplant was most likely to fail in the short term. Patients whose blood flow was the most restricted three months after surgery were nine times more likely than those with freer blood flow to suffer serious rejection or die.

The average length of survival after surgery was 2.5 years in the group with restricted blood flow to the organ, but 23 years for patients without blood flow problems.

"Prior to this study it wasn't appreciated that this commonly used tool could predict outcomes," says Dr. Philip Marsden, a kidney specialist at the University of Toronto. "Now we recognize that [blood] flow within the kidney is telling us something about how the graft will do in the years ahead."

In another study, researchers at Stanford University in California used a gene chip to analyze the activity of more than 12,400 genes in the kidney cells of childhood transplant patients. Gene chips are slides that can read genes in a tissue sample to determine which tumors are highly aggressive.

The chip found clear differences between grafts that were healthy and those that were troubled, giving a genetic picture of the risk of organ rejection and the expected response to anti-rejection therapy.

"We're pretty excited by what the potential practical implications could be," says Dr. Minnie Sarwal, a Stanford pediatrician and kidney expert who led the research. "We could actually differentiate which rejection episodes may be the ones with the worst outcomes, which we currently can't do."

NO EASY FIX

Neither study holds all the answers to the problem of transplant rejection.

The German research gives doctors a fairly simple tool to predict severe rejection, but it offers nothing to stop it from occurring. The California study shows gene profiles can sort patients into groups depending on their rejection risk. But gene chip analysis isn't currently available to most doctors or patients.

■ ■ ■ ■

Transplant Facts

Approximately 15,000 kidney transplants will be performed in the United States this year, according to the United Network for Organ Sharing. And although advances in drugs that suppress the immune system have driven down rejection rates for kidney grafts—10% compared with 30% a decade ago—transplant failure remains a significant hurdle for patients. Failure is now the fourth leading cause of end-stage kidney disease in this country.

info Visit the United Network for Organ Sharing's Web site at *www.unos.org* for more on organ donation.

Sight Returns After 43 Years of Darkness

Ione Fine, PhD, research assistant professor, University of Southern California, Los Angeles.
Ivan Schwab, MD, professor of ophthalmology, University of California, Davis, and spokesman, American Academy of Ophthalmology.
Iqbal Ahmad, PhD, associate professor, ophthalmology, University of Nebraska Medical Center, Omaha.
Nature Neuroscience.

A chemical accident left Mike May completely blind at the age of three. But his real challenge began when he was finally able to see again.

In 2000, 43 years after May lost his sight, he had an experimental limbal stem cell transplant in his right eye that restored his vision. The procedure is rare, performed in perhaps 100 people each year in the United States.

Now that May, a California businessman, can see, he has found that sight is not that simple. His world consists of colors and abstract forms, not three-dimensional shapes.

He can't identify his wife from her face alone, nor can he tell the difference between male and female faces most of the time. Facial expressions remain a mystery.

May's experience represents an unprecedented opportunity to glean information about how vision works. Until now, scientists knew only that people blind for a long time whose vision returned had difficulties making sense of what they saw. But they didn't know why. Using advanced imaging techniques, researchers now have an idea of the effects of long-term blindness on various parts of the brain.

THE STUDY

Functional magnetic resonance imaging (fMRI) revealed that the parts of May's brain normally responsible for processing faces and objects were inactive. When he was shown something moving, however, that part of his brain showed high levels of activity.

"It's very much a wiring thing," says study author Ione Fine, who led the project while she was a researcher at the University of California at San Diego. "He can see. He just can't make sense of it."

Because he lost his sight at such a young age, May's brain never "learned" how to see. "Infants just out of the womb see poorly," says Dr. Ivan Schwab, professor of ophthalmology at the University of California, Davis and a spokesman for the American Academy of Ophthalmology. "The brain has to put it all together and the early years are very important."

"You might be able to go ahead and restore vision, but if the brain has not been conditioned to make sense of the information coming from the retina, then it will be very difficult for the patient," says Dr. Iqbal Ahmad, an associate professor of ophthalmology at the University of Nebraska Medical Center in Omaha.

A DIFFERENT LIFE

May says he's better now at guessing what he is seeing than he was when he first got his sight back. He has also become better and faster at figuring out what something is, in large part because he's amassing an internal library of information.

"I've built up the clues," he says. "I've seen lots of stuff and I now know what I missed."

May was a champion skier when he was blind (a guide skied ahead of him and shouted directions), but he had to close his eyes the first time he skied as a sighted person because the experience was so terrifying.

He still reads in Braille, only using his eyes as a "last resort." His wife joked that the best part of her husband's transformation was that he would be able to sort the laundry colors.

info For more on blindness and how people cope with it, visit the Prevent Blindness America Web site at *www.preventblindness.org.*

Painful Pelvic Disorder Linked to Small Adrenal Glands

Tony Buffington, DVM, PhD, professor, veterinary clinical sciences, Ohio State University, Columbus.
Richard Bercik, MD, associate director, urogynecology, and associate professor, obstetrics and gynecology, Yale University, New Haven, CT.
Journal of Urology.

Small adrenal glands may be an underlying risk factor for interstitial cystitis, according to a study, and these findings may offer a new direction to studying the disorder that can eventually lead to new treatments.

Interstitial cystitis is a chronic inflammatory condition of the bladder wall. Symptoms include urinary urgency and frequency, difficulty urinating, minimal urine output and pain in the bladder and the urethra that is temporarily relieved by voiding. In some patients, pain may radiate to the genitals, rectal area and thighs.

THE STUDY

In their study, Tony Buffington, a professor of veterinary clinical sciences at Ohio University, and his colleagues compared the adrenal glands of 13 cats that had interstitial cystitis with eight cats that did not have the disorder. The adrenal glands of the cats with interstitial cystitis were approximately half the size of those in the normal cats.

The researchers found that when cats were injected with *adrenocorticotropic hormone,* which normally causes the adrenal glands to secrete the stress hormone, *cortisol,* the cats who had interstitial cystitis produced lower levels of cortisol than would have been expected.

Despite their smaller size, the functioning of the adrenal glands in cats who have interstitial cystitis appears normal, Buffington says. "It is only under stress that it is abnormal," he adds.

Buffington believes this finding indicates that although there may not be adrenal insufficiency under normal circumstances, there may be an insufficient adrenal reserve during periods of stress. The decreased adrenal response may be the reason why interstitial cystitis gets worse during stressful periods, he adds.

STRESS CONNECTION

Dr. Richard Bercik, associate director of urogynecology at Yale University in New Haven, Connecticut, says that "physicians and lay people need to realize the connection between stress and interstitial cystitis."

"It is not just that stress exacerbates symptoms, but also that other diseases associated with stress disorders—for example, chronic fatigue syndrome, irritable bowel disease, fibromyalgia, endometriosis, chronic pelvic pain, anxiety, obsessive compulsive disorder, depression, neuralgia, temporomandibular joint (jaw joint) disease and many phobias—all can possibly interface with interstitial cystitis," Bercik adds.

info To learn more about interstitial cystitis, visit the National Kidney and Urologic Diseases Information Clearinghouse at *http:// kidney.niddk.nih.gov.*

15

Stroke Prevention

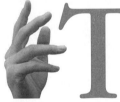

Astounding Treatment Gets Stroke Victims 'Back to Normal'

The combination of skin stimulation and stimulant drugs has been shown to help stroke victims or the elderly perform daily tasks that require deft fingers, like buttoning shirts and dialing telephones. Because of this, the treatment may even aid professional piano players or improve a blind person's ability to read Braille, according to recent research from Germany.

The study found that finger stimulation can temporarily reorganize parts of the brain. This process, called *coactivation,* reorganizes the brain synapses that link neurons. The stimulated brain area becomes more sensitive as more neurons are recruited to process tactile information relayed from the fingers.

Amphetamines doubled stimulation-induced gains in touching tasks, the study found.

"We are at the beginning of an era where we can interact with the brain," says researcher Hubert R. Dinse, a member of the study team.

"We can apply what we know about brain plasticity to train it to alter behavior. People are always trying to find ways to improve learning. What we tested was unconscious skill learning. How far could this carry to cognitive learning? That remains to be seen," Dinse says.

THE STUDY

In the study, participants wore a device that stimulated a patch of skin on the tips of their right index fingers for three hours. The researchers pressed two pins against the skin on either side of the tips of the participants' right index fingers.

The researchers were able to measure tactile acuity and perceptual learning by monitoring changes in the minimum distance required for the patients to detect two distinct pressure points on the tips of their index finger.

American Association for the Advancement of Science news release.
Science.

The coactivation method that was used in this study doesn't require active participation by the subject. That makes it an attractive treatment approach.

"In past experiments, we tested coactivation in people between 65 and 90 years old. The coactivation temporarily improved tactile acuity with little harassment to the subjects. According to our new findings, certain drugs can enhance the effects of coactivation. The drug component makes this coactivation approach even more promising," Dinse says.

info For more information on strokes visit the National Stroke Association's Web site at *www.stroke.org*.

New Therapy Helps Stroke and Brain Injury Patients Recover

Neurology.
American Academy of Neurology news release.

People who suffer a stroke or traumatic brain injury may benefit from a behavior-based therapy known as *shaping* that may help recovery more than other treatments.

In shaping therapy, patients are trained to perform specific and increasingly difficult tasks with their affected arm and they are rewarded for improvements. The tasks include activities such as pressing a light switch, moving a chair and pulling up socks. The rewards include encouragement and praise from clinical staff when the patients successfully perform a task.

THE STUDY

A recent study of shaping therapy included 13 people aged 17 to 21 years who had arm weakness or partial paralysis after a severe traumatic brain injury or stroke.

During the first phase of research, the patients underwent occupational therapy (in which a patient relearns everyday activities such as eating, drinking, dressing and bathing)

for 90 minutes per day. They showed no significant improvement in arm movement during that phase.

In the second phase, the patients received shaping therapy for 90 minutes each day. The result of the shaping phase was that arm movement improved in all the patients.

"In each patient, improvements were sustained for at least four weeks post-treatment," say the authors.

Study author Annette Sterr of the University of Liverpool adds, "The study shows that shaping—training, repetition and working with the affected limb—makes progress and helps the brain to adapt."

■ ■ ■ ■

What Happens During a Stroke

A stroke occurs when a blood clot blocks a blood vessel or artery, or when a blood vessel breaks, interrupting blood flow to an area of the brain. The stroke kills brain cells in the immediate area, creating an area of dead cells that doctors refer to as an *infarct*. These cells usually die within minutes to a few hours after the stroke starts.

It's crucial that a stroke victim get help within three hours of symptom onset. Beyond this window, reestablishment of blood flow and administration of appropriate medications may fail to help and can potentially cause further damage.

The five most common symptoms of a stroke include…

●**Sudden numbness or weakness** of face, arm or leg, especially on one side of the body.

●**Sudden confusion,** including trouble speaking or understanding.

●**Sudden trouble seeing** in one or both of the eyes.

●**Sudden difficulty walking,** dizziness, loss of balance or coordination.

●**Sudden severe headache** that is unusual for you.

If you experience any of those symptoms, you should call for help immediately.

Other important but less common stroke symptoms include sudden nausea, fever and vomiting. Stroke victims also could experience a brief loss of consciousness or such symptoms as fainting, confusion, convulsions or coma.

A stroke can forever damage a person's ability to define their world, according to the National Stroke Association. The skills of intellect, sensation, perception and movement, which are honed over the course of a lifetime and which so characterize our humanity are the very abilities most compromised by stroke. Stroke can rob people of the most basic methods of interacting with the world. But when stroke is diagnosed and treated in time, patients can make a full recovery.

info You can learn more about stroke and post-stroke rehabilitation from the National Institute of Neurological Disorders and Stroke at *www.ninds.nih.gov.*

Amazing! These Scans Speed Stroke Treatment

Jonathan H. Gillard, MD, lecturer and neuroradiologist, University of Cambridge, England.

A. Gregory Sorenson, MD, associate professor, radiology, Harvard Medical School, Boston.

Presentation, Radiological Society of North America annual meeting, Chicago.

A powerful, speedy way to perform magnetic resonance imaging (MRI) brain scans is proving to be valuable in the fast diagnosis and treatment of strokes, British radiologists report.

MRI produces images by beaming brief bursts of magnetic fields into the body. Older machines, using just two coils to create those magnetic fields, take 20 minutes to produce an image. Newer eight-coil machines give doctors a usable picture in just three minutes.

And that difference is vital because "stroke patients don't like being in an MRI very long," says study author Dr. Jonathan H. Gillard, a lecturer neuroradiologist at the University of Cambridge. Having an MRI scan can be a claustrophobic experience for patients, who must be sealed in a narrow tube, he notes. Someone who has suffered symptoms of a stroke is especially likely to fidget, movements that blur the MRI. For that reason, radiologists have preferred computed tomography (CT) scans, which are less detailed images, but are quickly available.

An ongoing study at the Cambridge Addenbrooke's Hospital shows the three-minute MRI is bearable for patients and gives better images than CT scans, says Gillard, who presented the findings to the Radiological Society of North America.

FASTER TREATMENT

The quicker test is also important because clot-dissolving treatment for some strokes must be administered within approximately three hours after the attack to be effective.

Used with 18 stroke patients, the three-minute MRI technique distinguished between those patients whose strokes were caused by burst blood vessels and those whose arteries were blocked by blood clots, Gillard reports—vital information for determining treatment.

If a blood clot causes a stroke, "giving clot-busting drugs means that the patient will most likely get fuller recovery and be less disabled," he says. However, if the cause of the stroke is a burst blood vessel, those drugs can cause further bleeding and more brain damage.

"If you give a clot-buster in the first three hours, the patient will benefit most," Gillard says. "This can tell you whether a blood vessel is blocked, and where the blockage is."

LEARNING NEW TRICKS

Eight-coil MRIs have been available for several years, but their use in diagnosing stroke "has been more delayed than I would like," says Dr. A. Gregory Sorenson, an associate professor of radiology at Harvard Medical School and a spokesman for the Radiological Society of North America.

"The major criticism of MRI has been that it takes too long," Sorenson says. "This report shows what many of us have known for a long time; that you can spend just a few minutes and get the information you need."

MORE POTENT SCANS ON HORIZON

And even more powerful MRI technology is on the way, he says. At least one major manufacturer is expected to announce availability of a 32-coil MRI device soon.

"You might be able to get an image in just one minute," Sorenson says. "As you push to more coils, you get a clear climb in clinical payoff."

info The American Stroke Association's Web site at *www.strokeassociation.org* has a section that is devoted to diagnosing and treating strokes.

New Substance Extends Stroke Treatment Time

Bioorganic and Medicinal Chemistry Letters.
Northwestern University news release.

Strokes may be debilitating, even deadly, but they don't have to be. Doctors can treat the attacks—provided they get to patients early enough for drugs to be effective.

Until recently, that time frame has been approximately three hours after the start of a stroke. But a new compound that was developed by Illinois researchers may double that "treatment window" for people who suffer a stroke or brain injury.

A study by researchers at Northwestern University in Evanston, Illinois, found that a single injection of the compound given up to six hours after the brain injury or stroke protects against additional brain cell death for one week or longer.

Currently, there is only one medication that is approved to improve blood flow to oxygen-deprived neurons near the affected area of the brain and this medication must be administered within three hours of the onset of a stroke. This helps minimize the potentially debilitating side effects of stroke or brain injury.

"Results of this study...could identify new therapeutic approaches to acute brain injury," says study leader Martin Watterson, a professor of molecular pharmacology and biological chemistry.

■ ■ ■ ■

Prevention Is Best

Every year, an estimated 750,000 Americans suffer strokes, and 160,000 die from the attacks, according to the National Stroke Association. Many of the survivors are left with permanent disability.

The National Stroke Association also offers the following guidelines that may be helpful for preventing strokes...

●**Know your blood pressure.** Hypertension is a strong risk factor for strokes.

●**Get checked for atrial fibrillation.** This heart rhythm anomaly is associated with stroke-causing blood clots. But drugs can control the condition and reduce the risk of stroke.

●**Stop smoking.** Smokers are at twice the risk of stroke as nonsmokers. Their risk starts returning to normal as soon as they quit.

●**Drink alcohol only in moderation.** The latest evidence suggests that a glass of wine or beer or one drink each day may lower the risk for stroke. But experts say nondrinkers shouldn't start drinking just to take advantage of the effect.

●**Know your cholesterol.** Lowering total cholesterol may reduce the odds of stroke. For some people, high cholesterol can be reduced through diet and exercise; others may require medication to bring it down.

●**Exercise more.** As little as 30 minutes of moderately vigorous activity every day might lower the risk for stroke. It will also improve all-around health.

●**Eat less salt, saturated fat and trans fats.** Cutting back on sodium and unhealthy fats can help lower blood pressure and, in turn, trim the risk of stroke.

●**Control circulation trouble.** If you have poor circulation, your doctor may be able to help improve it.

•**If you have diabetes, keep it in check.**
Having uncontrolled diabetes greatly increases the risk of stroke.

Antibiotics May Prevent Strokes

Paul Brassard, MD, MSc, clinical researcher, Department of Medicine and of Epidemiology and Biostatistics, McGill University Health Centre, Montreal.
Stroke.

A new study hints that antibiotics may prevent stroke in elderly people who have hypertension.

The findings bolster the theory that infections may contribute to inflammatory processes underlying strokes and heart attacks.

But both the authors of the study and outside experts caution that the results are preliminary and warrant further research.

"There are lots of residual things that we might not have accounted for that could have explained some of the findings," says study author Dr. Paul Brassard, a clinical researcher at McGill University Health Centre in Montreal.

Some studies have suggested that infections may be linked to heart disease and stroke and that, specifically, atherosclerosis (fatty buildup in the walls of arteries) may be a chronic inflammatory condition. Treating the cause, the theory holds, might prevent the onset of cardiovascular disease or slow its progression. Scientists know that inflammation is involved in vascular disease, it's just not clear what causes the inflammation or how the mechanism works.

"This just adds to the overall body of evidence that infection might contribute one way or another," Brassard says.

THE STUDY

The study team looked at the health records of 1,888 patients who had been treated for hypertension and had had a stroke. They were compared with 9,440 hypertensive individuals who had not had a stroke.

The researchers also looked to see which patients had taken antibiotics and when they used them.

Any antibiotic use was associated with a slightly decreased risk of stroke, but the relationship was not statistically significant except in the case of penicillin. The most striking results were in current penicillin users, who were 47% less likely to have a stroke than people who had not used antibiotics.

Even in the case of penicillin, the absolute numbers were low—1.1% of stroke patients were current users, versus only 1.7% of the control patients—and Brassard is not ruling out the possibility that this was a random occurrence.

Right now, researchers are awaiting the results of trials that are looking at antibiotic use in people who have already had a stroke or heart attack.

But even if those trials and others do show a cause-and-effect relationship between antibiotics and stroke prevention, it's not clear how this will affect treatment.

"It would open a big black box," Brassard admits. Before prescribing antibiotics to patients, doctors would have to seriously consider not only the individual but also the public health implications, as excessive antibiotic use contributes to bacterial resistance and makes future infections harder to treat.

Vitamin C May Stop Strokes —Even for Smokers

Monique Breteler, MD, PhD, Erasmus Medical Center, Rotterdam, The Netherlands.
Philip B. Gorelick, MD, MPH, head, cerebrovascular disease and neurological critical care, Rush University Medical Center, Chicago.
Neurology.

People who eat a diet rich in vitamin C may be at lower risk of suffering strokes, and smokers who do so may benefit the most. Antioxidants, including vitamin C, may protect cells from oxidative stress, which plays a role in stroke, Dutch researchers say.

Their study finds people with the lowest amount of vitamin C in their diets—less than 95 milligrams (mg) per day—were 30% more likely to have a stroke than people with the highest amount of it—more than 133 milligrams per day.

Smokers with diets high in vitamin C were more than 70% less likely to have a stroke than smokers with diets low in vitamin C.

The research "confirms that the healthy diet is good for you, one that is rich in antioxidants and vegetables, as we have seen over the last several years," explains study author Dr. Monique Breteler of Erasmus Medical Center in Rotterdam.

VITAMIN E HELPFUL

The study also found smokers benefited from high levels of vitamin E in their diets. They were approximately 20% less likely to have a stroke than smokers with diets low in vitamin E. But nonsmokers with high vitamin E levels didn't enjoy similar protection.

"This is not an excuse to continue smoking. There is more than enough medical evidence to show that smoking is extremely bad for you," Breteler cautions. "The effects of antioxidation are more than outweighed by other factors."

"But smoking causes damage because of increased oxidative stress. Then vitamin C has antioxidative properties, so we looked at [that] connection and saw that it was indeed the case," she says.

One possible explanation is that vitamin C enhances endothelial function, which inhibits artery clogging and lowers blood pressure.

But the link also could be that people who eat vitamin-rich fruits and vegetables may be more health-conscious than those who don't. Therefore, the study cautions that vitamin C alone may not be responsible for the results that were seen in this study.

The use of dietary supplements containing vitamins C and E and other antioxidants, however, did not seem to lower the risk of stroke more. But Breteler says this finding does not necessarily mean that supplements have no potential benefit.

SOURCES OF VITAMIN C

Rich sources of dietary vitamin C include oranges and other citrus fruits, strawberries, red and green peppers, broccoli and brussels sprouts. Good sources of vitamin E are vegetable oils such as sunflower seed, cottonseed, safflower, palm and wheat germ oils, margarine and nuts.

"I think it's important for the public to keep hearing the message about our diet and reducing stroke risk, and this study shows this quite very nicely," says Dr. Philip B. Gorelick, head of the cerebrovascular disease and neurological critical care department at Rush University Medical Center in Chicago.

Doctors Discover New Tool that Predicts Stroke

Thomas J. Wang, MD, instructor, medicine, Massachusetts General Hospital, Boston.
Albert L. Waldo, MD, professor, cardiology and medicine, Case Western Reserve University, Cleveland.
Journal of the American Medical Association.

Doctors have found a new tool to help predict strokes in people who have atrial fibrillation.

The tool, a risk scoring system, is important to people who have atrial fibrillation, a disorder in which the two upper chambers of the heart lose their ability to pump blood forcefully. Clots that form in these chambers can block blood vessels and cause strokes; 15% of all strokes occur in patients with atrial fibrillation, says the American Heart Association.

The risk scoring system—a simple calculation—can help doctors customize a treatment plan for every patient with atrial fibrillation, according to their individual risk score.

FIVE FACTORS PREDICT STROKE ODDS

The tool was derived from the results of the long-running Framingham Heart Study. It assigns a score to each of five major factors associated with a high risk of stroke—being older, being a woman, having high systolic blood pressure (the top number in a blood pressure reading), having a previous stroke or a short-term artery blockage, and having diabetes. A more complex analysis, including other factors such as smoking, can help determine the risk of death, says study author Dr. Thomas J. Wang, a Framingham researcher who is an instructor in medicine at Massachusetts General Hospital.

For example, using the scoring system, a 75-year-old man with a systolic reading of 150 and diabetes, but no previous stroke, gets a score of 16, indicating a 16% risk of a stroke in the next five years.

The risk scores were developed by following 705 patients with newly diagnosed atrial fibrillation who had not used the blood thinner warfarin for four years, Wang says.

The risk score is far from perfect, he acknowledges. "It still must be tested in the general population," Wang says. "But it raises the awareness of the risk of stroke in patients with atrial fibrillation."

Life-Saving Discovery Reduces Stroke Risk

Elaine M. Hylek, MD, MPH, assistant professor, medicine, Harvard Medical School, Boston.

Robert G. Hart, MD, professor, medicine, University of Texas Southwestern Medical Center, San Antonio.

New England Journal of Medicine.

Drug therapy that is used to prevent blood clots in people with the heart condition called atrial fibrillation can reduce stroke deaths and damage without increasing the risk of dangerous bleeding, a study finds. This is a finding of life-and-death importance to the growing number of Americans who have this condition.

ATRIAL FIBRILLATION AND STROKES

Atrial fibrillation reduces the heart's ability to pump blood, and the slower blood flow promotes the formation of clots that can block brain arteries, causing strokes.

Approximately 2.3 million Americans have atrial fibrillation, and it is the leading cause of stroke among the oldest Americans. The incidence of the condition increases with age. One of every 20 Americans 70 years or older has atrial fibrillation.

Blood-thinning therapy using aspirin or the more potent anticoagulant *warfarin* can prevent clots, but doctors fear that too-intensive treatment can cause bleeding in the brain, which does the same damage as a clot-caused stroke.

Clotting is measured by what is called the *international normalized ratio* (INR). A higher INR means freer-flowing blood with a lower risk of clots but a higher risk of dangerous bleeding. Physicians have known that an INR of 2.0 or higher can effectively reduce the risk of stroke, but there have been questions about the level at which a higher INR becomes dangerous.

THE STUDY

The study of more than 13,500 patients with atrial fibrillation shows that "the risk of hemorrhage does not increase until you reach an INR of about 4," according to Dr. Elaine M. Hylek, an assistant professor of medicine at Harvard Medical School and lead author of a paper on the study.

Not all atrial fibrillation patients get anticoagulant therapy. Those regarded as having a very low risk of stroke get no medication. Others, at some risk, are told to take aspirin. Warfarin is reserved for the patients with the highest risk, because it requires careful monitoring to achieve the desired INR and because of the risk of side effects.

One third of the 592 strokes reported in the study occurred in patients who were taking warfarin. Among those patients, an INR of less than 2 nearly doubled the risk of having a severe stroke and more than tripled the risk of dying from the stroke. Increased risk of bleeding in the brain was found only in INR readings of 3.9 or higher, Hylek says.

The study "reinforces that we do know the optimal range" of INR readings, says Dr. Robert

Hart, professor of medicine at the University of Texas Health Sciences Center at San Antonio.

A reading between 2 and 3 is optimal, not only for people who have atrial fibrillation but also for those people who are taking warfarin because they have mechanical heart valves, Hart explains.

"For people who are very elderly and who also have a high risk of bleeding, I would aim to be at the lower part of that range when possible," Hart advises.

info A primer on atrial fibrillation can be found from the American Heart Association at *www.americanheart.org*.

■ ■ ■ ■

What Is Atrial Fibrillation?

Atrial fibrillation is a serious heart condition that affects approximately 2 million people in the United States.

In this disorder, the heart's two small upper chambers—which are known as the *atria*—quiver instead of beating, causing ineffective pumping of the blood. The blood is not completely pumped out of the heart's chambers, so the blood that is left behind can clot. If a piece of the clot travels to an artery in the brain, it can cause a stroke.

Atrial fibrillation can affect both men and women, according to the National Institutes of Health.

The prevalence of atrial fibrillation increases with age and varies from one case for every 200 people younger than 60 years, to almost nine cases for every 100 people older than 80 years.

There are several symptoms of atrial fibrillation. These symptoms can include heart palpitations, racing or irregular pulse, dizziness, light-headedness, fainting, confusion, fatigue, shortness of breath, breathing difficulty or a sensation of tightness in the chest.

info For answers to some frequently asked questions about atrial fibrillation, visit the British Heart Foundation at *www.bhf.org.uk/questions/index.asp*. Click on "Medical."

High-Fat Diets Don't Increase Risk of Stroke

Ka He, MD, instructor, preventive medicine, Northwestern University Feinberg School of Medicine, Chicago.
Mark J. Albert, MD, director, stroke program, Northwestern University Feinberg School of Medicine, Chicago.
British Medical Journal.

A major study has found that a fat-rich diet, which clearly increases the risk of heart disease, doesn't seem to affect the risk of stroke.

"Right now, to be honest, we don't have a convincing explanation of what we found," says Dr. Ka He, who led the study while he was at the Harvard School of Public Health and now is an instructor in preventive medicine at Northwestern University's Feinberg School of Medicine in Chicago.

And the longstanding rules for a diet rich in vegetables and fiber and low in fatty foods still apply, He says.

"We don't want readers to misunderstand, and to think that they don't have to take care of their dietary fat intake," He says. "They still need to watch their diet because fat intake is an important indicator of the risk of heart disease."

Nevertheless, the results of a 14-year study of almost 44,000 middle-aged men are clear: "These findings do not support associations between intake of total fat, cholesterol, or specific types of fat and risk of stroke in men."

The researchers used questionnaires to assess diet measures, including consumption of selected foods, such as red meat, high-fat dairy products, nuts and eggs.

But after adjusting the results for the presence of two other known risk factors—age and smoking—the researchers concluded that there was no association between dietary fat intake and the incidence of stroke.

TWO EXPLANATIONS PROPOSED

The researchers offer two explanations for the puzzling result. One is that approximately 20% of strokes occur when a blood vessel bursts (these are known as hemorrhagic strokes) rather than when a clot blocks an artery in the brain (ischemic strokes). These hemorrhagic strokes are not necessarily related to the artery-clogging process of atherosclerosis, a condition often caused by heavy dietary fat intake, and that can result in a heart attack or ischemic stroke.

It's also possible that the consumption of unsaturated fatty acids that contribute to atherosclerosis may help to reduce inflammation. And they may have other favorable effects on the molecular events that can lead to ischemic stroke, the researchers speculate.

But that doesn't explain why cholesterol-lowering treatment for patients with heart disease has lowered the incidence of stroke in some trials, the report says.

In the end, all He can say is that "we think further research is needed."

ALL STROKES NOT THE SAME

According to Dr. Mark J. Albert, director of the stroke program at Northwestern, the study might miss a diet–stroke association because it does not distinguish between the different kinds of ischemic stroke that people might develop.

"Not all ischemic strokes have the same mechanism," Albert says.

"Studies that have distinguished carotid ischemic strokes, which tend to have the same mechanism as heart attacks, have found an association. Studies that lump all ischemic strokes tend not to find an association," Albert explains.

But whatever the scientific specifics may be, "the practical issue, even if you accept these results, is that no one is going to say, you had a stroke so it's okay to go ahead and eat a high-fat diet," Albert says.

"A significant percentage of stroke patients will die of heart disease, for which diet is a major risk factor," he says.

And in addition to eating properly, He says, "there are other factors to watch, such as exercising regularly, not smoking and controlling body weight. These are very important with respect to stroke prevention."

Air Pollution Tied to Stroke Risk

Marc R. Mayberg, MD, chairman, department of neurosurgery, Cleveland Clinic Foundation.
Thomas Johnson, MS, director, respiratory therapy, Long Island University, Brooklyn, NY.
Stroke.

When the air is dirty, you might worry about your lungs, but you should also worry about your stroke risk. A recent Taiwanese study found that hospital admissions for stroke increase with rising air-pollution levels.

Data compiled on more than 23,000 patients during the period between 1997 and 2000 shows a close relationship between the incidence of strokes and two major air pollutants—small particles and nitrogen dioxide, the study says.

The effect of the pollution was strongest on days when the temperature was higher than 68 degrees Fahrenheit.

"I am not surprised that there is a relationship between air pollution and stroke," says Dr. Marc R. Mayberg, chairman of the department of neurosurgery at the Cleveland Clinic Foundation and chairman of the American Heart Association stroke council.

A link between stroke and air pollution is to be expected because "there is pretty clear evidence that air pollution causes cardiovascular and respiratory disease," he says. "I am just surprised that they have been able scientifically to verify the relationship."

Previous studies trying to link air pollution to the risk of stroke have produced mixed results, Mayberg says. "It is a difficult thing to show because air pollution varies quite a bit, and it is not clear that air pollution on one day causes changes in the body that are evident a few days later. And different people have different stroke risks, so it is hard to isolate specific factors."

The Taiwanese researchers compared air pollution levels on the days when stroke patients entered the hospital with the levels one week before and one week after those admissions.

THE FINDINGS

Every 25% increase in the levels of fine particulate pollutants and nitrogen dioxide was associated with a 54% increase in hemorrhagic strokes, which occur when a blood vessel bursts. Hospital admissions for ischemic stroke, in which a clot blocks a blood vessel, increased by 55% for every 25% increase in nitrogen dioxide levels and 46% for every 25% increase in fine particulate pollutants in the air.

LESS EXPOSURE MAY MEAN LESS RISK

"When you do this kind of population study, you don't know anything about the patients, not even whether they are men or women," Mayberg says. "Also, you don't know what the link is between pollution and risk, what is it in air pollution that leads to stroke."

Thomas Johnson, director of respiratory therapy at Long Island University, suggests several mechanisms of damage. For example, "nitrogen dioxide alters arterial pressure and may stress already damaged blood vessels, especially in the brain," he says.

And pollutants can penetrate deeply enough to affect and attack the alveoli, the tiny sacs where air exchange occurs in the lungs, according to Johnson.

The people who should take the most precautions, Mayberg says, are those with known stroke risk factors such as diabetes, high blood pressure, heart disease and smoking. "They should try to avoid exposure to polluted air," he says.

Blood Molecule Tied to Hypertension Risk

Howard D. Sesso, ScD, MPH, epidemiologist, Brigham and Women's Hospital, Boston.
Robert A. Phillips, MD, chairman, department of medicine, Lenox Hill Hospital, New York City.
Journal of the American Medical Association.

An elevated blood level of an inflammation-related molecule is linked to high blood pressure, a study has found, but it's not clear if it is the cause or an effect of the process that leads to the condition.

"[C-reactive protein] may be an important marker for damage that occurs in the arteries," says study leader Howard D. Sesso, an epidemiologist at Brigham and Women's Hospital in Boston. "It is not perfectly clear whether it is the cause of high blood pressure or just reflects the damage being done to the arteries. Is it a direct link to the inflammatory process that is causing damage? Perhaps other processes are taking place."

THE FINDINGS

The findings are the latest in a series that have linked inflammation to heart attack, stroke and other cardiovascular problems. The inflammatory process that creates C-reactive protein is believed to attack blood vessels, causing damage that can interrupt the flow of blood and could eventually cause a heart attack or stroke.

The reported results come from the Women's Health Study, which has been following more than 20,000 female health professionals for years.

"This is the first observational study in which we have been able to demonstrate that high levels of C-reactive protein are associated with an increased risk of developing high blood pressure," Sesso says.

THE STUDY

The women were 45 years or older when the study began, and all had blood pressure no higher than 140/90. C-reactive protein levels were measured at the start. In an average follow-up period of almost eight years, those study subjects who had the highest levels of C-reactive protein in their blood were twice as likely to develop high blood pressure as those with the lowest levels.

The association between inflammatory markers such as C-reactive protein and the arterial damage that leads to heart attack and stroke "is now well-established," according to Dr. Scott C. Grundy, director of the Center for Human Nutrition at the University of Texas Southwestern Medical Center in Dallas.

"What is lacking is an adequate causal explanation for these associations," Grundy writes. "Undoubtedly, the causal connections are complex and, in many cases, undiscovered."

Dr. Robert A. Phillips, chairman of the department of medicine at Lenox Hill Hospital in New York City and an officer of the American Society on Hypertension, was skeptical of the marker's importance before this study.

Now he says, "Here is evidence that there might be something to it. We have data showing it can identify a group of people who are more likely to develop hypertension, something we did not have before."

A blood test for C-reactive protein is available, and Phillips has ideas for its use.

"You may want to use it as a screen for people at risk because of family history," he says. "If blood levels are high, you might be more aggressive with those people, getting them to lose weight and perhaps starting drug therapy earlier."

Stroke Patients Should Be Tested For Hidden Heart Risks

Circulation.
American Heart Association news release.

Doctors need to evaluate certain stroke patients for hidden heart risk even if those patients show no symptoms. This was one conclusion from a major study called the International Stroke Trial that included more than 20,000 patients.

Ischemic stroke, transient ischemic stroke (TIA; also called mini-stroke) and coronary heart disease all result from vascular disease, where there is restricted blood flow to the heart or brain. Experts found a link between silent heart disease and TIA and a link between silent heart disease and ischemic strokes originating in large blood vessels to the brain.

The researchers say that as many as 40% of patients who suffer ischemic strokes and mini-strokes have silent heart disease.

"Compared with patients with strokes caused by blockages in small vessels in the brain, patients with TIA or large-vessel strokes have a higher likelihood of also having coronary artery disease, whether or not they have a clear history of heart disease," says lead author Dr. Robert Adams. "There are data to indicate that some people already have significant heart disease by the time they have a stroke even though they don't have any recognized symptoms of heart disease."

info Learn more about stroke from the Mayo Clinic at *www.mayoclinic.com.* Click on "Diseases & Conditions."

Stroke Symptoms Are Different for Men and Women

Jaume Roquer, MD, PhD, physician-researcher, Servei de Neurologia, Hospital del Mar, Barcelona, Spain.

Lewis Morgenstern, director, stroke center, University of Michigan, Ann Arbor.

Rosabel Young, MD, MS, clinical assistant professor of neurology, David Geffen School of Medicine, UCLA, Los Angeles.

Some people consider stroke to be a men's health problem. Statistics prove that's not the case.

Strokes will kill an estimated 170,000 Americans this year—and about 97,000 of those cases will be women, according to the American Heart Association.

It is true, however, that women and men often experience markedly different symptoms. This may make it difficult to diagnose a stroke in women, and possibly delay treatment, new research says.

Most stroke patients describe roughly the same general collection of symptoms, including slurred speech, facial paralysis, dizziness and various sensory problems.

THE STUDY

Dr. Jaume Roquer, a researcher at the Servei de Neurologia at the Hospital del Mar in Barcelona, Spain, and his colleagues evaluated 722 women and 809 men admitted to a hospital for a first stroke between 1995 and 2000.

Women were more likely than men to have problems with speech and vision and have difficulties swallowing and chewing. Their hospital stays averaged 15.4 days, compared with 13.4 for men. Women were more disabled after the stroke, too.

However, women are about 60% more likely than men to report other symptoms not generally associated with strokes, such as limb pain, disorientation and fluctuations in consciousness, says Dr. Lewis Morgenstern, a stroke specialist at the University of Michigan.

In Rocquer's study, the women had higher rates of an irregular heart rhythm known as atrial fibrillation, in which the two upper chambers of the heart quiver rather than beat efficiently.

And women have more episodes of hemorrhagic—or bleeding—strokes than men, who are more prone to a blocked blood supply that triggers the attack. That may also partly affect the way each sex experiences the illness, Morgenstern says, but it doesn't fully explain the dichotomy.

WHAT IS A STROKE?

Strokes occur when a blood vessel that transports nutrients and oxygen to the brain either bursts or is blocked by a clot or atherosclerotic plaque. Either way, the area of the brain deprived of oxygen begins to die. And that, in turn, affects the part of the body that area controls.

Doctors have long known the two sexes often show dissimilar signs of other cardiovascular problems, most notably heart attack.

Recently they've found that a woman is likely to be older than a man when she has her first stroke, and that stroke is often more disabling and severe.

WOMEN SHOULD REDUCE RISKS

Health professionals may not always recognize underlying conditions that can lead to a woman's stroke, some doctors say. They may dismiss symptoms that might boost the risk of stroke in women.

Therefore, women should learn how best to reduce their risk of stroke and know when to ask for a thorough evaluation, experts say.

For instance, it might be especially important for women to keep blood pressure under control, says Dr. Roquer. Other preventive measures include not smoking, avoiding obesity and not abusing alcohol and drugs, he says.

Dr. Rosabel Young is another stroke expert who sees certain gender differences in her stroke patients. "Generally women seem to have more embolic than thrombolic" stroke, says Young, a clinical assistant professor of neurology at UCLA's David Geffen School of Medicine.

Embolic strokes are caused by clots that start in the heart or the neck's carotid artery and move to the brain. Thrombotic strokes involve stationery clots in blood vessels.

"[Usually], embolic strokes are worse," Young adds, "and have more complications."

For women, especially older women, heeding the physical symptoms they may experience is crucial. And they should try to reduce their cardiovascular risk factors by lowering blood cholesterol and quitting smoking, both Young and Roquer say.

Also, "if you have dizziness or panic attack symptoms and irregular heart rate, you should be checked out thoroughly for heart disease or stroke," Young adds.

Morgenstern says doctors should look for stroke in women complaining of unconventional symptoms because "time is of the essence" for effective treatments such as clot-busting drugs, which must be administered within the first few hours of symptom onset to be effective.

■ ■ ■ ■

The Statistics Prove It: Women Need to Be Aware of Stroke Risk

The American Heart Association offers the following information on strokes in women…

•**Stroke is the third leading cause of death for American women,** after heart disease and cancer. It claims more than twice as many lives as breast cancer alone.

•**Women account for more than three out of every five stroke deaths** in the United States.

•**The death rate for stroke in 2000** was substantially higher for black women than white women.

About 2.4 million American women are living with the aftermath of stroke.

For Women:
HRT Drug Combo
May Cause Stroke

JAMA/Archives of Neurology news release.

Women who have high blood pressure should think carefully before trying hormone replacement therapy to control the symptoms of menopause.

The hormone therapy could put them at increased risk for stroke, according to a recent study.

THE STUDY

The study, by Danish researchers, included 13,122 female nurses older than 44 years who had no major cardiovascular or cerebrovascular disease or cancer. The nurses were followed up for five years to check for occurrence of stroke.

During the study, 144 strokes (46 fatal) were recorded among the women. Overall, there was no association between hormone therapy use and risk of stroke. But the study did find that in a subgroup of 2,256 women with high blood pressure, the risk for stroke was more than twice as high for current hormone therapy users than for women who never used the treatment.

That risk of stroke was three times higher in hormone therapy users taking an estrogen-progestin combination.

When the study began, 28% of the women were current hormone therapy users, 14.3% were past users and 57.7% had never used it. The median length of time of hormone therapy use among current users was six years and among past users was two years.

Among the hormone therapy users, 35.5% used estrogen only (estradiol) and 59.2% used combination therapy (estrogen combined with norethisterone acetate).

"We discovered a consistent significantly increased risk of total stroke and various subtypes of stroke associated with the use of [hormone therapy] among hypertensive nurses," according to the study authors.

"This risk was most pronounced among nurses using estrogen–progestin therapy. Normotensive nurses using [hormone therapy] had no increased risk of stroke," they say.

■ ■ ■ ■

Hypertension and Stroke

High blood pressure is one of the leading risk factors for strokes. High blood pressure is considered a reading of 140/90 mmHg or greater. Roughly two of three Americans older than 65 years have high blood pressure by this definition.

People whose blood pressure falls between 120/80 mmHg and 139/89 mmHg are considered to have prehypertension. They are at significant risk of developing full-blown hypertension in the future.

High blood pressure isn't inevitable, however. Everyone can take steps to prevent the condition. For example, eating a healthy diet, reducing salt intake, exercising regularly, quitting smoking and limiting alcohol consumption are all proven ways of keeping blood pressure under control.

Stroke is the leading cause of disability among American adults, affecting an estimated 700,000 people a year in this country and killing more than 167,000. Between 15% and 30% of patients who survive strokes are left permanently disabled.

Early treatment of stroke with a drug that dissolves blood clots can dramatically increase the chances of a partial or full recovery from the attack. However, the majority of patients who have strokes don't reach the hospital in time to benefit from the drug.

info You can learn more about high blood pressure from the National Heart, Lung and Blood Institute at *www.nhlbi.nih.gov/health/index.htm*.

Women's Health

Great News, Girlfriend: Vitamin C Lowers Risk of Heart Disease

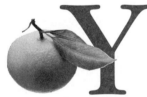 You might have heard many times that taking vitamin C can help you fight colds, but did you know that it also may be good for your heart? Researchers at the Harvard School of Public Health found that women who had a vitamin C intake of more than 360 milligrams (mg) per day had nearly a 30% reduction in their risk of heart disease.

Regular use of vitamin C supplements was associated with a lower incidence of coronary heart disease, says study author Dr. Stavroula Osganian, who is an assistant professor of pediatrics at Children's Hospital in Boston.

PREVENTABLE CONDITION

Cardiovascular disease, which includes heart disease and stroke, is responsible for 950,000 deaths in the United States every year. According to the American College of Cardiology, as many as two thirds of those deaths may be preventable with healthy lifestyle changes and medications.

THE STUDY

Osganian and her colleagues studied data from the large, ongoing Nurse's Health Study, which began in 1976.

In particular, they looked at food questionnaires completed in 1980 which detailed the diet and supplement habits of more than 85,000 female nurses between the ages of 30 and 55 years.

After 16 years of follow-up, the researchers compared the women's diets and use of supplements with their incidence of heart disease.

They considered other factors that affect heart disease risk, such as smoking, diabetes, exercise, vitamin E supplement use and aspirin.

Stavroula Osganian, MD, assistant professor, pediatrics, Children's Hospital, Boston, MA.

Balz Frei, MD, director, Linus Pauling Institute, Oregon State University, Corvallis.

Journal of the American College of Cardiology.

SUPPLEMENTS MORE EFFECTIVE THAN FOOD

The researchers found that dietary intake of vitamin C appeared to have little effect on the risk of developing coronary heart disease.

But if women used vitamin C supplements, their risk was reduced by 27%.

Osganian says the researchers didn't find a big difference between large and small doses of supplements, which means that taking more vitamin C isn't necessarily better.

The researchers cannot pinpoint why vitamin C supplements appear to be protective, but Osganian suspects it is because of their antioxidant properties.

She also points out that people who take vitamin C supplements just may lead healthier lives. That's one of the reasons she says more studies need to be done. In addition, these data were only from women.

THE IMPLICATIONS

So, should you take vitamin C supplements to protect yourself against heart disease?

Osganian says she doesn't take a vitamin C supplement specifically, but does take a multivitamin that contains C every day.

Other physicians recommend that people get up to 500 mg of vitamin C daily, either from their diet or from supplements. Vitamin C is abundant in red peppers, citrus fruits and broccoli.

OTHER FACTORS

"Supplemental vitamin C intake may lower your risk of heart disease, but it is equally important to eat a healthy diet and lead a healthy lifestyle," says Dr. Balz Frei, director of the Linus Pauling Institute at Oregon State University in Corvallis.

"Vitamin supplements are no magic bullet and always should be just that—supplements, not substitutes, for a healthy diet and a healthy lifestyle."

info For more information on vitamin C, visit the National Library of Medicine's MedlinePlus Web site at *www.nlm.nih.gov/medlineplus.* Click on "Medical Encyclopedia."

The Safe, Simple Tests That Find Heart Disease In Women

Presentation, American Heart Association's annual conference, Orlando.

University of Pittsburgh Medical Center news release.

A few safe and simple tests can help doctors identify—and possibly even prevent—heart disease in women who are middle-aged.

That's according to researchers at the University of Pittsburgh, who described their strategy at a meeting of the American Heart Association.

WEIGHT GAIN A FACTOR

"Most women gain 1 to 2 pounds per year as they approach and go through menopause, and a percentage of them will go on to develop heart disease as a result," according to Dr. Lewis H. Kuller, a professor of epidemiology at the University's School of Public Health.

"Keeping one's waist circumference from expanding is a good way to avoid a negative outcome, but more targeted monitoring of other predictors, such as insulin and coronary calcium, can give a more accurate indication of when a woman is entering the danger zone," Kuller says.

Kuller and his colleagues found a few simple tests can be used to monitor women and alert doctors to when they need to take action to prevent a heart attack.

THE TESTS

Insulin resistance can be measured by testing blood levels of insulin, glucose and adiponectin—a protein secreted by fat cells called adipocytes. Blood samples can also be used to measure levels of low-density lipoprotein (LDL) particles, which can lead to the development of coronary calcium deposits.

Coronary calcium deposits can be detected using electron beam tomography, a quick non-invasive scan.

"There are very effective therapies, both pharmacological and nonpharmacological, to prevent the progression of insulin resistance, the development of small and numerous LDL particles and, potentially, the progression of atherosclerosis," Kuller says.

He and his colleagues are currently testing these interventions.

■ ■ ■ ■

Women Less Likely to Survive Heart Disease

Heart disease is the nation's leading killer of women. One in three women in the United States dies of heart disease, according to the National Coalition for Women with Heart Disease.

The most common cardiac killer is heart attack, which claims 267,000 women per year —six times the number of those who die of breast cancer. Congestive heart failure accounts for nearly 32,000 lives a year, the group says.

The Coalition reports that women who have heart disease often face far worse odds for survival than men in several key measures. *Consider these facts…*

- **38% of women and 25% of men** will die within one year of a first recognized heart attack.

- **35% of female and 18% of male heart attack survivors** will have another heart attack within six years.

- **46% of female and 22% of male heart attack survivors** will be disabled with heart failure within six years.

- **Women are almost twice as likely as men** to die after bypass surgery.

- **Women are less likely than men to receive beta-blockers,** ACE inhibitors or even aspirin after a heart attack.

- **More women than men die of heart disease each year,** yet women receive only

  - 33% of angioplasties, stents and bypass surgeries.

  - 28% of implantable defibrillators.

  - 36% of open-heart surgeries.

- **Women make up only 25% of participants** in all heart-related research studies.

info You can learn more about how to prevent heart disease in women from the American College of Cardiology Foundation at *www.acc.org/media/patient/prevention.*

Hormone Therapy Increases Risk of Heart Disease

JoAnn Manson, MD, chief, preventive medicine, Brigham and Women's Hospital, and professor, medicine, Harvard Medical School, both in Boston.

Nieca Goldberg, MD, cardiologist, Lenox Hill Hospital, New York City.

New England Journal of Medicine.

Two studies that were conducted recently offer more evidence that hormone replacement therapy (HRT) does not treat or prevent heart disease.

THE STUDIES

In one study, HRT failed to slow the progress of atherosclerosis—a buildup of fatty deposits in the arteries—in women with the condition. And according to the second study, part of the Women's Health Initiative (WHI), hormone therapy puts women at great risk of heart attack during the first year of use.

HRT was originally prescribed to ease symptoms of menopause, including hot flashes, night sweats and disturbed sleep. When early data indicated it also might reduce the risk of coronary heart disease, doctors began to recommend the long-term use of HRT to prevent heart attacks.

Neither of these studies should be interpreted to mean that short-term HRT is not useful for treatment of menopausal symptoms such as hot flashes, the researchers say. Nor should the studies be interpreted to mean that women should only focus on heart health during and after menopause.

LIMITED USE OF HRT

But, "this means that the role of hormone therapy is much more limited than previously thought," says Dr. JoAnn Manson, one of the principal investigators of the WHI.

"Heart disease for women is not just a menopausal issue. It's about early diagnosis and early prevention, to ultimately make a woman healthy before she's in menopause so she'll be healthier as she goes through menopause," says Dr. Nieca Goldberg, a cardiologist at Lenox Hill Hospital in New York City and author of *Women Are Not Small Men*.

THE FIRST STUDY

The first study involved 226 postmenopausal women who had started to develop atherosclerosis. This condition, also called hardening of the arteries, can lead to heart attacks and strokes and is responsible for one of every two deaths in the United States.

Participants were randomly divided into three treatment groups: one group taking only estrogen, one group taking both estrogen and progestin and one group receiving "usual" medical care without hormones. On average, the participants were 64 years old, about 18 years past the typical onset of menopause.

After approximately three years' follow-up, the study authors found no significant differences in the progression of atherosclerosis (by measuring the narrowing of the coronary artery) between the three groups.

THE SECOND STUDY

The second study represents new analysis from the WHI. The WHI, designed by US researchers to look at potential approaches to the prevention of various diseases in 167,000 postmenopausal women, included a study devoted to HRT.

The HRT part of the trial involved 16,608 postmenopausal women aged 50 to 79. The participants were randomly assigned to receive estrogen plus progestin (HRT) or a placebo.

The women in the HRT group had an 81% increased risk of heart attack during the first year of use, compared with the women who did not take the hormonal regimen. Women

with higher LDL ("bad") cholesterol levels and women who were more than a decade beyond menopause seemed to have an even higher risk of heart disease, the study found. Although the women also had a lower risk of colorectal cancer and fractures related to osteoporosis, the researchers concluded that the benefits did not outweigh the risks.

info For more on the Women's Health Initiative, visit the National Heart, Lung and Blood Institute at *www.nhlbi.nih.gov/whi*.

Are Women Getting Enough Medicine to Control Blood Pressure?

Kristin Newby, MD, associate professor, medicine, Duke University Medical Center, Durham, NC.

Franz Messerli, MD, director, clinical hypertension, Ochsner Clinic Foundation Hospital, and clinical professor, medicine, Tulane Medical School, New Orleans.

Presentation, American Heart Association Scientific Sessions 2003, Orlando.

Hypertension, or high blood pressure, is a serious problem. As many as one in four Americans has high blood pressure, according to the American Heart Association. But nearly one third don't know it.

High blood pressure raises the risk of heart disease, stroke and kidney problems. And men and women are far from equal when it comes to hypertension.

Many women often receive more aggressive treatment for high blood pressure, but those medications don't lower their blood pressure readings as much as they do for men.

The National Heart, Lung, and Blood Institute reports that in women, approximately 75% know they have hypertension, but less than one in three have it under control.

"Women tended to be on more medications," says study author Dr. Kristin Newby, an associate professor of medicine at Duke

University Medical Center. "Instead of just a single agent, women tended to be on two to three drugs [to control hypertension]."

Despite this, "there was no measurable impact on blood pressure," Newby says.

The study raises new questions for researchers, including: Are women getting the medications in adequate doses, or is blood pressure harder to control in women?

THE STUDY

For this study, Newby and her colleagues gathered data from two other heart disease studies in progress. The subjects included 2,091 women and 5,084 men from across the United States.

Nearly two thirds of the women and half the men had high blood pressure. The women's average systolic blood pressure (the top number) was slightly higher than the men's, 150 versus 147. The women with high blood pressure tended to be older and more likely to have reduced kidney function, diabetes and a history of heart failure.

The researchers found that 16% of the women took three or more drugs every day to control their hypertension, while only 13% of the men took that much medication. Approximately 35% of women versus 30% of men were taking two medications for their high blood pressure.

The most common medications to treat high blood pressure include ACE inhibitors, beta-blockers, calcium channel blockers and diuretics. Only diuretics appeared to be prescribed to women more often than to men—33% of the time in women compared with 19% of the time in men.

Dr. Franz Messerli, director of clinical hypertension at Ochsner Clinic Foundation Hospital in New Orleans, finds it encouraging that although women's hypertension was not as well-controlled as men's, even after receiving intense antihypertensive therapy, "their outcomes are about the same."

"It's harder for women to get to the goals [normal blood pressure readings], but despite that, women do remarkably well," he says.

TAKE PRECAUTIONS

Newby says it's important for both men and women to have their blood pressure checked. It also is critical to maintain a healthy weight, quit smoking and exercise regularly.

And, if you've been diagnosed with high blood pressure, watch the amount of sodium in your diet and make sure that you take your medications as prescribed.

Finally, Good News About Menopause And Memory

Peter Meyer, PhD, assistant professor, preventive medicine, Rush University, Chicago.

Gary W. Small, MD, director, Aging and Memory Research Center and Memory Clinic, David Geffen School of Medicine, University of California, Los Angeles.

Neurology.

When women going through the "change of life" experience a memory lapse, they often blame it on a "menopausal moment." But researchers have found that the working memory and perceptual speed of women improve with age, even during menopause.

Peter Meyer, assistant professor of preventive medicine at Rush University in Chicago, and his colleagues tested the memories of 803 women each year for six years. The women were part of the large Study of Women's Health Across the Nation, sponsored by the National Institute on Aging, to record the natural history of the menopausal transition.

The women who were included in Meyer's study were aged 42 to 52 years and were tested annually on their working memory and perceptual speed. They also answered questions about their health, menopausal status, ethnicity and education.

The subjects were in different stages of pre- and post-menopause.

Premenopause is the reproductive stage of a woman's life. Perimenopause is the stage prior to menopause, when physical changes begin to accelerate due to declines in hormone production.

The working memory test asked the women to say backwards increasingly long lists of numbers. In the perceptual speed test, the women were shown a series of symbols and a corresponding number. They were asked to match as many symbols with their corresponding number as they could in 90 seconds.

Meyer found that perceptual speed and working memory improved slightly over time for women in premenopausal and early perimenopausal stages.

Only for the perceptual speed tests was there a decrease in scores, and that was for postmenopausal women.

Working memory scores for postmenopausal women did not change greatly over time, he reports.

Meyer says that, although the results are surprising, they do not indicate that women don't have problems with forgetfulness as they age.

WHAT CHANGE?

Women in the age group studied often say they have trouble remembering someone's name or coming up with the proper word, Meyer says. Why? "Verbal processing skills might be different, but not worse" with age, he says, somehow accounting for the forgetfulness. He hopes to find out more about that in future research.

Meyer also says that one explanation for the improvement on the perceptual speed and working memory tests might simply be a learning effect—the women got better at the tests with practice.

"I'm not surprised," says Dr. Gary W. Small, director of the Aging and Memory Research Center and Memory Clinic at the David Geffen School of Medicine at the University of California, Los Angeles.

At the clinic and in his book, *The Memory Bible,* Small proposes strategies to help people of any age improve their memories. "Mental activity is important to keep the brain healthy and young," he says.

info For tips on talking with your doctor about memory problems, visit the National Institute on Aging Web site at *www.nia publications.org/pubs/taking/p6.htm.*

Estrogen for Menopause Still Risky

Garnet L. Anderson, PhD, writing group chair, Women's Health Initiative Steering Group Committee, co-principal investigator, WHI Clinical Coordinating Center, and member, Fred Hutchinson Cancer Research Center, Seattle.
Stephen B. Hulley, MD, professor and chairman, department of epidemiology and biostatistics, University of California, San Francisco.
Journal of the American Medical Association.

Estrogen alone may be helpful in easing menopausal symptoms in women who have had a hysterectomy. However, it does not appear to be useful for preventing heart disease, and may in fact increase the risk of stroke.

That's the result of the estrogen-only arm of the Women's Health Initiative (WHI), the first major trial to look at this hormone alone. The increased risk of stroke was troubling enough to halt the trial approximately a year ahead of schedule.

THE STUDY

The study looked at the effects of conjugated equine estrogen (CEE), also known as PremarinT, on heart disease. PremarinT is the most widely used postmenopausal therapy in the United States.

In all, 10,739 postmenopausal women between the ages of 50 and 79 were randomly assigned to receive 0.625 milligrams (mg) per day of PremarinT or a placebo.

After an average of almost seven years of follow-up, the researchers found that PremarinT had no effect on reducing the risk of heart disease and no significant effect on pulmonary embolism or colorectal cancer, although it did increase the risk of stroke by 39%.

PremarinT was also found to cause a 39% reduction in the risk of hip fracture and a 23% reduction in the risk of breast cancer, although the researchers did not consider this statistically significant.

The study found that estrogen alone carried fewer risks than the combination of estrogen and progesterone.

This will be reassuring to women who have had a hysterectomy who need to manage their menopausal symptoms, says Garnet L. Anderson, co-principal investigator of the WHI Clinical Coordinating Center, which conducted the trial.

"The overall risk–benefit profile is really much more benign than it was for combined hormone therapy," Anderson says.

"This is not the best place to start for prevention, but if there [are menopausal symptoms] that need to be treated right now, then this probably is an acceptable trade-off," he adds.

NOT THE FIRST TRIAL TO BE STOPPED

This early halting is the latest in a string of abrupt endings to hormone trials. Two WHI trials using combination hormone therapy were halted because of unacceptably high risks of breast cancer, heart disease, stroke and blood clots.

In addition, a British trial and a Swedish trial, both looking at combination therapy, were also halted.

Experts largely agree that the estrogen use should be confined to treating menopausal symptoms.

"Don't use estrogen for prevention and, when treating menopausal symptoms, try other strategies [first]. Then, if the woman is properly informed and still wants to take hormone treatment, keep it at as low a dose as possible for as short a period as possible," says Dr. Stephen B. Hulley, professor and chairman of the department of epidemiology and biostatistics at the University of California, San Francisco.

Low Doses of Estrogen Build Bones

Karen Prestwood, MD, associate professor, medicine, University of Connecticut Center on Aging, Farmington.
Wulf Utian, MD, PhD, executive director, North American Menopause Society, and professor emeritus, Case Western Reserve University School of Medicine, Cleveland.
Journal of the American Medical Association.

Older women can get the bone-building benefits of estrogen by taking a fraction of the usual dose, which might minimize some of the potential dangers associated with hormone therapy, researchers have found.

Over the course of the three-year study, the lean dose—just a quarter of the conventional amount—led to substantial gains in bone mineral densities of the hip, wrist and spine.

Although the study was too small to determine if the treatment reduced a woman's risk of fractures, even slight increases in bone mass can prevent breaks. "Small increases in bone mineral density result in decreased fracture risk with other [drugs]," says study leader Dr. Karen Prestwood, a researcher on aging at the University of Connecticut. The lower dose may be beneficial to bones but carry a lower risk of side effects than stronger preparations, she adds.

ESTROGEN—FOR BETTER OR FOR WORSE

Estrogen has been the workhorse for the treatment and prevention of osteoporosis. The hormone helps prevent the body from cannibalizing the skeleton for calcium—the result of the loss of estrogen associated with menopause.

However, estrogen therapy, particularly in combination with progestin, has come into question lately. It's been well known that estrogen triggers uterine cancers, but several studies also have found the estrogen/progestin combination can cause breast cancer and may increase the risk of heart disease, stroke and blood clots.

Recently, newer drugs have arrived that also reduce the risk of fractures, though these have side effects many women can't tolerate, including breast tenderness, fluid retention, headaches and bloating.

If a lower dose of estrogen is effective, that's good news for the many women who worry about the cancer risks and other side effects that come from taking the usual dose.

THE STUDY

Prestwood's group followed 167 women who were at least 65 years old at the start of the study. About two thirds had low bone mass, a condition called *osteopenia,* and one third had osteoporosis. Roughly half the women were given 0.25 milligrams (mg) of 17-beta estradiol—the form of estrogen that circulates in the human body—and the rest were given a placebo.

By the end of the trial, women taking estrogen saw their bone mineral density rise by 1.2% compared with women on the sham treatment. The increase was 3.6% greater at the hip, 2.6% greater at the head of the femur and 2.8% greater in the spine. Blood markers of bone turnover—the skeleton consuming itself—declined in the women taking estrogen compared with women in the placebo group.

The findings support previous research indicating that lowering the dose of estrogen doesn't sacrifice its bone-saving effects. But this is the first long-term study to show the benefits of such a low dose of 17-beta estradiol.

RISKS UNCERTAIN

Although the study didn't find any increase in breast cancers among women taking estrogen, it wasn't large enough to detect such a risk if one existed, Prestwood says. The researchers did find that women taking low-dose estrogen had less incontinence, a frequent remnant of menopause.

Dr. Wulf Utian, executive director of the North American Menopause Society, says it's premature to assume that lower doses of estrogen will cause fewer side effects than higher amounts.

"The problem is that the expectation is that there will be fewer risks, but the only way we're ever going to prove that is with outcome studies," Utian adds.

info The Women's Health Initiative at *www. whi.org* has more information on the study's findings.

More Bad News: Hormone Therapy Hurts Your Bones

Jane A. Cauley, DrPH, professor, epidemiology, University of Pittsburgh.
Journal of the American Medical Association.

Hormone replacement therapy (HRT) helps prevent broken bones, but this benefit doesn't outweigh the long list of risks that accompany the regimen, research shows.

The latest in a series of studies has again found long-term use of HRT appears to cause more harm than good, at least for most women.

These results come from an arm of the Women's Health Initiative (WHI), which looked at the effects of the combination of estrogen and progestin.

TRIAL STOPPED

That trial was halted in July 2002—three years early—when researchers discovered a small but significant increase in the risk of breast cancer in women taking the two hormones. They concluded the benefits of the therapy, most notably its ability to prevent fractures, didn't outweigh the risks, including not just cancer, but also heart attacks, strokes and lung clots.

WORTH THE RISK?

HRT is a proven bone-builder, and as a result, it has been used for decades for the prevention and treatment of osteoporosis, a condition that puts 10 million American women at high risk of fractures. Are there some women for whom the risk of broken bones—and especially hip fractures—is so high that taking HRT makes sense?

The new study suggests the answer is "no."

"We did not see any evidence that there was a sub-group of women at high risk of fracture for whom the benefits [of HRT are substantial enough to ignore the perils]", says study author Jane A. Cauley, a bone expert at the University of Pittsburgh. The 8,500 women taking the hormones gained much more bone mass, a plus for skeletal strength, than the 8,100 women taking dummy pills in the WHI study. And their risk of fractures was approximately 25% lower than that of the other women.

But women at the highest risk of breaking a bone during the study didn't get more benefit from HRT than those at the lowest risk—while enduring the same odds of suffering a heart attack, stroke, breast cancer or other serious adverse effect.

However, Cauley warns women taking HRT for their bones to consult their doctor before stopping the drugs abruptly. Doing so can accelerate bone loss—by up to 5% a year —she says.

As an alternative to HRT for bone strength, women can take one of a variety of osteoporosis drugs that are on the market.

Some doctors believe HRT still has a role as a way for women to relieve symptoms of menopause, such as vaginal dryness and hot flashes. This therapy is generally only used for a number of months.

Size Matters—When It Comes to Bone Strength!

Henrik Ahlborg, MD, orthopedic surgeon, Malmö University Hospital, Malmö, Sweden.
New England Journal of Medicine.

When it comes to the strength of your bones, density is important—but don't forget about size.

So says recent research which suggests that doctors may want to rethink the way they calculate the risk of fractures in people who have a brittle skeleton.

Swedish and American researchers found that older women with broader bones are less vulnerable to age-related fractures. These fractures result from thinning bones, or osteoporosis, a condition that affects roughly 8 million women in the United States. Osteoporosis usually follows the drop in estrogen that occurs during menopause, though it also occurs to a lesser degree in men and in younger people who take certain bone-eroding steroids for long periods.

The standard way to measure bone strength —and thus, the risk of a fracture—is to examine its mineral density. Several devices can perform this test, but in general they use either X rays or ultrasound to read the mineral content of the interior (or cortical) section of bones in the spine, arm, heel and elsewhere.

Scientists have long known, however, that bone mineral density (BMD) is an imperfect gauge of strength and fracture odds. That's largely because other factors, including bone size and shape, also dictate its soundness under stress.

THE STUDY

Dr. Henrik Ahlborg, an orthopedic surgeon at Malmö University Hospital in Sweden, studied 108 postmenopausal women for an average of 15 years. The women, who were 48 years old when they began the study, had scans of the radius bone in their forearm every other year. They also had blood drawn to determine their estrogen levels.

Results showed that women who lost more bone in the interior of their radius over time tended to gain diameter there. This process, called *periosteal apposition,* makes bone stiffer, partially compensating for the loss of internal mass.

"The women with the lowest level of [estrogen] after menopause also had the most periosteal apposition," says Ahlborg.

BONE STRENGTH INDEX

Since both bone mass and bone structure (including size) are independently related to its risk of breaking, the researchers combined the two traits to create a strength index. Women with better scores on the strength index were less likely to suffer fractured arms over time than those with weaker bones.

Although the study looked only at women, men also undergo periosteal growth—indeed, more so than women. As a result, they may gain more protection from the widening.

Ahlborg's group is now trying to come up with a strength index for bones in the hip—a common and particularly devastating site of fractures in people with osteoporosis.

■ ■ ■ ■

Preventing Bone Loss

People with osteoporosis have several options to slow the pace of their bone loss, such as estrogen therapy and a variety of drugs. But these treatments don't build new bone or help bone grow in size. At the present time, parathyroid hormone injections are the only therapy shown to reduce fracture risk by bulking up the skeleton. Drug-free options for the prevention of bone loss include weight-bearing exercises, recommended daily amounts of calcium and vitamin D, and no smoking or alcohol.

info Try the National Osteoporosis Foundation at *www.nof.org* for more information on the brittle bone disease.

New Reason to Slim Down—It Could Prevent Osteoarthritis

Ray Fitzpatrick, PhD, professor, public health, University of Oxford, England.

Giles Scuderi, MD, chief, adult knee reconstruction, Beth Israel Medical Center, New York City.

Journal of Epidemiology and Community Health.

Recent research confirms that women who are overweight, especially when they are younger, are at greatly increased risk of developing osteoarthritis of the knee.

Approximately 2.4% of all adults older than 55 years have osteoarthritis of the knee, a condition in which the joint's cartilage breaks down and causes the bones to rub against each other.

By age 65, however, the condition is twice as common among women, a discrepancy that has led to speculation that birth control pills, socioeconomic status and high heels might be to blame.

THE STUDY

The researchers interviewed 29 women between the ages of 50 and 70 who were on a waiting list for knee replacement surgery, in addition to 82 women who had no known knee problems.

Each woman was asked about her height and weight at different stages of her life, about previous injuries, occupational activities and her use of hormones and birth control pills.

They also were subjected to a grueling series of questions on their shoe history: How old were they when they started wearing high heels? How often did they wear them? How high were the highest heels they wore? The women were shown 38 different styles and heights of shoes (front and profile) and life-size pictures of heels and asked to identify their preference. If they had worn any of the shoe styles, they were asked if they wore them for dancing, social events or work.

Some of the findings were not surprising: Knee osteoarthritis was associated with previous knee injury, arthritis of the feet, heavy smoking, certain occupational activities (such as lifting and bending) and, most important, being overweight.

MOST SIGNIFICANT

A body mass index of 25 or higher between the ages of 36 and 40 years of age was most significantly associated with osteoarthritis of the knee.

The researchers were not, however, able to find a connection between high heels and osteoarthritis. It's not entirely clear why some people thought that high heels contributed to osteoarthritis. "It was clinical speculation," hypothesizes study author Ray Fitzpatrick, a professor of public health at the University of Oxford in England. "One factor may have been that more women had osteoarthritis than men, but perhaps there was also a belief that there's something unnatural about high heels."

HEALTHY WEIGHT, HEALTHIER KNEES

Fitzpatrick counsels women—and men, for that matter—to turn their attention to the weight findings.

"We're not the first people to find that weight matters, and I think it's now quite clearly the single most preventable risk factor," he states. And by that he means overweight at any age, not just a younger age as was highlighted in this research. "This is a small study, and I wouldn't want you to think that current overweight is less important," Fitzpatrick cautions. "They are of similar importance, current overweight and overweight at an earlier stage."

"Weight is a major issue," confirms Dr. Giles Scuderi, chief of adult knee reconstruction at Beth Israel Medical Center in New York City. "Weight is a major cause of degenerative arthritis of weight-bearing joints."

info For more on osteoarthritis, visit the National Institute of Arthritis and Musculoskeletal and Skin Diseases at *www.niams. nih.gov/hi/topics/arthritis/oahandout.htm.*

Excess Pounds Double Risk of Cervical Cancer

James V. Lacey Jr., PhD, epidemiologist, National Cancer Institute, Bethesda, MD.

Margaret M. Madeleine, PhD, epidemiologist, Fred Hutchinson Cancer Research Center, Seattle.

Cancer.

Here's another reason for women to shed those extra pounds—being overweight doubles the risk of cervical cancer, according to a new study.

"Our study is not the first to look at obesity [and cervical cancer]," says James V. Lacey Jr., an epidemiologist at the National Cancer Institute and the lead author of the study.

Cervical adenocarcinomas account for about 10% to 15% of all cervical cancers, he says. According to the National Cancer Institute, every year in the United States, about 15,000 women are diagnosed with cancer of the cervix, the narrow, lower part of the womb that opens into the vagina. Most of those cancers are the more common squamous cell variety.

Lacey and his colleagues performed a study that controlled for human papilloma virus (HPV), a sexually transmitted virus that causes genital warts and is considered the primary risk factor for cervical cancer. "It showed us that when taking into account the role of HPV, obesity might be an important co-factor for cervical adenocarcinoma," Lacey says.

THE STUDY

In the study, Lacey and his team evaluated 124 women with adenocarcinoma, 139 with squamous cell cancer and 307 healthy control patients, ranging in age from 18 to 69 years. Researchers documented the women's height, weight and waist-to-hip ratio, another measure of obesity.

Women who had a body mass index (BMI) above 30, which is considered obese, were 2.1 times more likely to have adenocarcinoma, compared with women who had BMIs in the healthy range (under 25). Less consistent results were found for squamous cell cancers, Lacey says.

Other risk factors for cervical cancer include intercourse before age 18 years, multiple sex partners, or a partner with many previous partners. A Papanicolaou (Pap) test helps detect cervical cancers.

MAINTAIN WEIGHT

"The study emphasizes the need to avoid being overweight," Lacey continues. The link to cervical cancer was found "not just for obese women, but also for women who were overweight."

Exactly how excess weight may increase the risk of cervical cancer isn't known for sure. But it is thought that excess fat tissue can influence the levels of estrogen and other sex hormones, and that, in turn, can increase susceptibility to cancers.

The new study strengthens the argument for the role of hormones in the development of some cancers, says another expert, Margaret M. Madeleine. She is an epidemiologist at the Fred

Hutchinson Cancer Research Center in Seattle, and is familiar with the new research.

"No other study has been able to tease out as clearly the association between BMI and cervical cancer by histologic [tissue] type," Madeleine says.

info To learn more about cervical cancer, visit the National Cervical Cancer Public Education Campaign at *www.cervicalcancercampaign.org.*

■ ■ ■ ■

BMI Calculation

To calculate your body mass index (BMI), divide your weight (in pounds) by your height (in inches) squared, then multiply it by 703. Or use the calculator at the National Center for Chronic Disease Prevention and Health Promotion Web site at *www.cdc.gov/nccdphp/dnpa/bmi/calc-bmi.htm.*

Women Smokers Have Double the Risk Of Lung Cancer

Claudia Henschke, MD, PhD, professor, radiology, and division chief, chest imaging, Weill Medical College of Cornell University, New York City.

Frederic W. Grannis, MD, head, thoracic surgery, City of Hope Medical Center, Duarte, CA.

Presentations, Radiological Society of North America annual meeting, Chicago.

Being a woman appears to be a major risk factor for lung cancer. A 10-year study using *computed tomography* (CT) screening found women were twice as likely to develop lung cancer from using tobacco than men.

"The risk ratio of 2-to-1 is very high." says Dr. Frederic W. Grannis, head of thoracic surgery at City of Hope Medical Center in Duarte, California. "That's not good, particularly since so many young women are now smoking. That means that there is a potential for a worsening epidemic of lung cancer in women in coming years."

Years ago, Grannis adds, women were thought to have a lower susceptibility to lung cancer than men, but that may have been because they were simply not smoking as much. More recently, physicians have suspected women's susceptibility was higher, especially given the fact that women who have never smoked also develop lung cancer, something that rarely happens in men.

THE STUDY

The trial was part of a larger study, the Early Lung Cancer Project (ELCAP) in New York, which found that annual CT screening for both men and women could detect early tumors and reduce mortality rates. The trial on gender, which was partially funded by the National Institutes of Health, looked at 2,968 men and women aged 40 years and older who had some history of tobacco use.

Women who currently smoke or had smoked in the past had twice the risk of developing lung cancer as those who never smoked. Other risk factors included being older than 50, which conferred a 10 times greater risk, and having a heavier smoking habit, which increased the risk slightly.

The study did not address why women might be more vulnerable to the disease.

EARLY DETECTION IS POSSIBLE

According to the American Cancer Society, more people die every year of lung cancer than of breast, colon and prostate cancers combined. The tumors have few early symptoms and are often quite advanced by the time they are detected.

The good news is that in both men and women, CT scans managed to catch tumors much earlier than conventional screening methods.

This conclusion verified findings which were presented a few years ago. "Over 80% of cancers were found at the earliest stage," says lead author Dr. Claudia Henschke, division chief of chest imaging at Weill Medical College of Cornell University in New York City. "That's a dramatic change from 15% or less," the percentage of cancers found at the earliest stage in patients that aren't screened. The earliest stages, she adds, have a much higher cure rate, perhaps up to 50% as opposed to 10%. This means that people screened are more likely to have their cancer caught at a more treatable stage.

To reduce your risk of lung cancer, the message is simple: Quit smoking immediately. Once you've done that, get screened.

"If you're at risk of lung cancer, if you currently smoke or you're a former smoker and you're at least 50 years or older, you should consider having the scan," Henschke says.

"The evidence is accumulating rapidly that screening for lung cancer is highly effective in picking it up at an early stage," Grannis adds.

info For more on lung cancer, try the National Cancer Institute Web site at *www. cancer.gov.*

Hormone Therapy Raises Breast Cancer Risk

Walter Rosser, MD, head, department of preventive medicine, Queens University, Kingston, Ontario, Canada. *The Lancet.*

Not only does hormone replacement therapy (HRT) increase the risk of breast cancer for women who take the supplements, but those tumors also appear to be especially deadly.

That's the conclusion of a major, five-year study of more than 1 million British women, and it represents another major blow against HRT.

The researchers found that women taking combination HRT (estrogen and progestin) had a higher risk of developing breast cancer and a greater risk of dying from the disease than women not using the therapy.

Previous studies, including the Women's Health Initiative in the United States, have identified the link between breast tumors and HRT. But the British study is the first one to suggest that the tumors caused by hormone supplements are more aggressive.

THE STUDY

The Million Women Study was done between 1996 and 2001 by Cancer Research UK, an epidemiology unit based in Oxford, England. It followed almost 1.1 million British women who were 50 to 64 years old, half of whom had taken or currently took hormone supplements.

Current users of HRT were about two thirds more likely than nonusers—including those who'd once taken the therapy but dropped it—to develop breast cancer, the researchers say. Women taking HRT also were 22% more likely than those who'd never taken the drugs to die of breast cancer.

The work found that the breast cancer risks are magnified the longer women take hormone treatments—but also found that they fade with time after the therapy is stopped.

Over the last decade, the researchers estimate that the use of HRT in the United Kingdom has led to 20,000 extra cases of breast cancer among women ages 50 to 64 years.

TAKING HRT DESPITE THE RISKS

Dr. Walter Rosser, head of family medicine at Queens University in Kingston, Ontario, says that women who have severe menopausal symptoms may choose to take HRT despite the breast cancer risks.

"I would give it to them," he adds, "but probably for only six months at a time" to see how they feel when they stop the treatment.

Doctors in the United States may still prescribe HRT to women who have undergone menopause.

One reason is to control symptoms like hot flashes that are associated with the loss of estrogen that marks menopause.

Another reason is to prevent bone fractures from osteoporosis, another consequence of declining levels of the female sex hormone.

Until recently, many women had also been taking HRT to prevent heart and vessel disease. But new evidence shows that the therapy can harm the heart. One study showed that HRT doesn't slow the advance of atherosclerosis—a buildup of fatty deposits in the arteries—in women who already have the condition. Another study, part of the Women's

Health Initiative, found that HRT poses a great risk of heart attack during the first year of use.

Freezing Shrinks Benign Breast Tumors by 73%

Peter J. Littrup, MD, professor, radiology, urology and radiation oncology, Wayne State University, and director, image-guided therapy program, Karmanos Cancer Institute, Detroit.

George Hermann, MD professor, medicine, Mount Sinai Medical Center, New York City.

Presentation, Radiological Society of North America annual meeting, Chicago.

Doctors can sharply shrink the size of benign breast tumors by using a small probe that freezes abnormal breast cells.

The procedure, called *cryotherapy,* combines ultrasound and the probe in a type of image-guided therapy that is a painless, quick and noninvasive alternative to surgery, says Dr. Peter J. Littrup, a radiologist at Wayne State University and director of the image-guided therapy program at Karmanos Cancer Institute, both in Detroit.

"We can treat major tumors on an outpatient basis with minimum discomfort. It is a great boon for patients and patient care," says Littrup, who performed the procedure in 27 women, reducing the size of their noncancerous tumors by an average of 73%.

Benign breast lumps affect approximately 10% of women, most in their late teens and early 20s, and they are twice as common in black women as white women, Littrup says. Although most lumps aren't removed, approximately one million are excised annually because of their size, continued growth or for cosmetic reasons, he says.

Cryotherapy is currently used to treat cancerous tumors in the prostate, Littrup says. He is also involved in trials using the procedure to remove malignant tumors in the lung and kidney.

LETHAL ICE

To perform the procedure, doctors will first numb the area around the tumor, which is visible through ultrasound.

Next, they insert a cyroprobe—similar to a large needle—into the middle of the lesion and inject liquid nitrogen into it. An ice ball forms at the tip of the probe and continues to grow until the ultrasound confirms the entire lump has been engulfed, killing the tissue around the tumor, Littrup says.

The benefits of the procedure, according to Littrup, are that the ice is easily visible in the ultrasound so doctors can be precise in seeing the tumor; the method is painless; and it doesn't affect the collagen in the breast, so it keeps its shape. Also, there is no significant scarring.

Insurers don't automatically pay for the procedure for benign lumps, Littrup says—"it depends on the insurers." But because the patients don't have to stay overnight, the procedure is cost-effective, he says.

ANOTHER VIEW

Dr. George Hermann, a radiologist at Mount Sinai Medical Center in New York City, says the procedure is interesting, but he questions its use for benign breast lumps.

"You still have to do a biopsy, and then if it is benign, ask the question, 'Do you have to remove it?'" he says.

Further, he says, if cryotherapy is used to remove a cancerous tumor, it's impossible to evaluate the mass afterward because it's gone. When a lump is surgically removed, you can study it, which is important to treatment, Hermann says.

But Littrup says cryotherapy has already been shown effective in cancer treatment as a way to treat tumors without surgical intervention.

"We're seven years down the road with prostate cancer," he says, adding that improvements in technology such as new, smaller probes and better screening will only improve results with other cancers.

Women Are Not Getting The Whole Story On Hysterectomies

Obstetrics and Gynecology.

When your doctor recommends a hysterectomy, can you be sure he is offering you every surgical option? The answer may be an alarming "no"—at least according to a recent study.

Approximately 600,000 hysterectomies are performed each year in the United States. It is second only to caesarean delivery as the most frequently performed major abdominal surgery in women.

A recent survey of nearly 800 gynecologists in the Maryland, Virginia and Washington, DC, areas by researchers from Georgetown University Medical Center found that nearly 50% of respondents said they routinely perform a dramatic type of hysterectomy that removes the cervix.

And more than 60% said they didn't give their patients the option of considering a less drastic surgical choice, one that would keep the cervix intact.

"This, to our knowledge, is the first survey to be carried out in the United States of views of gynecologists regarding removal or conservation of the cervix at hysterectomy for benign disease," writes author Dr. Nadine Zakem, a physician at Georgetown University at the time of the study.

The researchers caution, however, that their findings may not be representative of practices and policies of gynecologists nationwide.

THE SURVEY

Hysterectomies can be performed in a number of ways. Dr. Zakem's survey focused on just two—the "total" hysterectomy, which removes the uterus and cervix through a major abdominal incision, and the subtotal or "supracervical" hysterectomy, which removes only the uterus, usually through the vagina.

For this study, an anonymous 18-question survey was mailed to 1,647 gynecologists, and 770 responded. A total of 45% of respondents said they routinely removed the cervix with every hysterectomy for benign uterine disease. Their reason for doing so, the study authors say, was "to eliminate the risk of cervical cancer," even though 88% of them acknowledged that the risk of cervical cancer in their patients was small.

And, although almost 18% of the doctors said they always counseled women regarding all their surgical options, 63% said they rarely or never did. Female doctors were as likely as male doctors not to tell women about their options.

The gynecologists in favor of the less drastic subtotal procedure point to recent studies showing that preserving the cervix may play an important role in preserving urinary, bowel and sexual activity—functions often damaged by a total hysterectomy.

Studies also show that the subtotal hysterectomy involves faster recovery, shorter hospital stay and reduced risk of postoperative complications, as well as no visible scar.

info For more information on hysterectomies and its alternatives, check with the US Food and Drug Administration at *www.fda. gov/fdac.*

Warning: These Painkillers May Cause Miscarriage

De-Kun Li, MD, research scientist, Kaiser Foundation Research Institute, Oakland, CA.
British Medical Journal.

Pregnant women who take aspirin or other painkillers known as NSAIDs may sharply increase their chances of miscarrying, a recent study has found.

The study of more than 1,000 pregnant women found the risk of miscarriage for those who took aspirin during pregnancy was 60% higher than for those who did not, and was 80% higher for those taking any NSAID (nonsteroidal anti-inflammatory drug) than for those who did not.

No increase in miscarriage was seen among users of acetaminophen, the active ingredient in Tylenol and related drugs, say researchers from the Kaiser Foundation Research Institute in California.

NSAIDs, widely used to treat arthritis, work by reducing production of molecules called prostaglandins in many organs of the body. Aspirin has the same action. Acetaminophen also inhibits prostaglandin production, but only in the central nervous system.

There are about a dozen NSAIDs on the market. Some are over-the-counter, such as *ibuprofen* (Advil) and *naproxen* (Aleve). Those that require prescriptions include Celebrex, Voltaren, Lodine, Nalfon and Indocin.

Animal studies indicate that prostaglandins are needed for fetal implantation in the wall of the uterus, say the researchers, led by Dr. De-Kun Li, a Kaiser Foundation research scientist. Suppressing prostaglandin production "can interrupt the natural process of implantation," Li says.

THE STUDY

The researchers interviewed 1,063 women in the San Francisco area who were in the Kaiser Permanente health program and who became pregnant between 1996 and 1998. They were asked about their use of NSAIDs and other painkillers.

There were 149 miscarriages among the 980 women who did not use NSAIDs, or approximately 15%. But 24.5% of the women (13 out of 53) who used the drugs miscarried, which means that the risk of miscarriage for users was 80% higher, the researchers say. The miscarriage rate was 60% higher for aspirin users than it was for nonusers.

There was a slight, statistically insignificant, increase in the miscarriage rate for women who took acetaminophen. The risk was highest when NSAIDs were taken around the time of conception or when they were taken for more than a week, the report says.

MORE RESEARCH NEEDED

Li says he hesitates to give advice to women on the basis of the study, because much more work is needed to prove a cause-and-effect relationship.

But he says that women with chronic conditions that require the use of NSAIDs should consult their doctors about what to do before and during pregnancy, and that other women would do well to use acetaminophen for headaches and other minor pains.

A similar study of more than 30,000 women in 2001 by researchers in Denmark found a comparable increase in miscarriage among NSAID users. As a result, the Royal College of Obstetrics and Gynecology in Britain has issued an advisory telling women to avoid NSAID use during pregnancy.

A spokesman for the American College of Obstetrics and Gynecology says his organization has not taken a stand on the issue.

info Get an introduction to NSAIDs from the American Academy of Orthopaedic Surgeons at *www.aaos.org*. The March of Dimes, at *www.modimes.org*, has more tips for a healthy pregnancy.

New Research May End Threat of Lupus

John Harley, MD, PhD, professor of medicine, Oklahoma Sciences Research Center and the University of Oklahoma Health Sciences Center, Oklahoma City. *New England Journal of Medicine.*

Patients with lupus, the autoimmune disorder that shows itself in a variety of ways, develop antibodies for the disease up to nine years before symptoms occur, researchers report.

The Lupus Foundation of America estimates that approximately 1.5 million Americans have the disease. Despite the fact that lupus can affect men and women of all ages, lupus occurs 10 to 15 times more frequently among adult women than adult men.

Fifty years ago, lupus had a mortality rate of 50%. Now the mortality rate is less than 10%, says Dr. John Harley, the lead researcher and a professor of medicine at the Oklahoma Sciences Research Center and the University of Oklahoma Health Sciences Center.

But although the mortality rate has fallen, lupus remains a life-threatening and life-altering disease.

THE STUDY

Harley and his colleagues looked for antibodies in blood samples from 130 patients. The blood samples had been collected years before symptoms of lupus appeared. Of the 130 patients, 115 had one or more of these antibodies up to nine years before symptoms appeared, the investigators report.

Harley believes that his findings indicate that patients who test positive for any of these antibodies are the ones most likely to develop lupus. However, these results should not be taken as a recommendation to test people for these antibodies, he adds. This is only preliminary data, he says.

What is needed, according to Harley, is a clinical trial that would treat people who have these antibodies with Plaquenil, a drug that inhibits lupus in patients with mild disease, to see if this treatment would prevent the onset of lupus.

The problem, Harley says, is that not all people with these antibodies develop lupus.

"There are people with positive tests who go on for years and years, if not decades and decades, without developing lupus. Right now, you can't tell which patients are at high risk for lupus and which are not, based on the test alone," he adds.

MORE RESEARCH

Harley's team continues to look into both genetic and environmental causes of lupus.

The researchers also have been doing immunochemical studies of the interaction of antibodies and antigens. Their findings have shown that the Epstein-Barr virus may play a role in the development of lupus. Right now, though, there is no implication for treating patients with lupus or those who are at risk for lupus, Harley says.

■ ■ ■ ■

Lupus: When the Immune System Attacks the Body

Lupus is chronic disease that, for unknown reasons, causes the immune system to attack the body's own tissue and organs, according to the Lupus Foundation of America. Lupus can affect the joints, kidneys, heart, lungs, brain, blood or skin.

Symptoms can include achy joints, frequent fevers, arthritis, skin rashes, anemia and chest pain.

Lupus develops most often between the ages of 15 and 44 years, and is two to three times more common among African-Americans, Hispanics, Asians and Native Americans than among Caucasians.

Only 10% of people with lupus will have a close relative who already has lupus or may develop lupus. Only approximately 5% of the children born to individuals with lupus will develop the illness.

info To learn more about lupus, visit the Lupus Foundation of America Web site at *www.lupus.org*.

The Best Hospitals In America

There are more than 6,000 hospitals in the US—but the doctors best suited to treating serious illness tend to be concentrated in a select few academic health centers and specialty hospitals. To identify these doctors, John Connolly, EdD, editor and publisher of *America's Top Doctors* surveyed more than 230,000 physicians and asked them to name the leaders in their field. The hospitals listed below are among those with the highest number of top physicians in nine different specialties...

CARDIOLOGY

- **Brigham and Women's Hospital (Boston)**

  Has the computer-enhanced da Vinci surgical system, a robotic technique that makes coronary bypass and other surgeries less invasive.

  617-732-5500

  www.brighamandwomens.org

- **Duke University Medical Center (Durham, North Carolina)**

  Has one of the nation's largest and most experienced interventional cardiology (angioplasty, angiogram, etc.) programs.

  919-684-8111

  www.mc.duke.edu

- **New York–Presbyterian Hospital (New York City)**

  Its surgeons have performed more heart transplants over the past 20 years than any other US hospital.

  877-697-9355

  www.nyp.org

- **Rush University Medical Center (Chicago)**

  The Rush Heart Institute provides the most comprehensive medical and surgical cardiac care in the Midwest.

  312-942-5000

  www.rush.edu.

- **St. Francis Hospital—The Heart Center (Roslyn, New York)**

  New York state's only specialty cardiac center. Approximately 15,000 cardiac catheterizations and 2,500 coronary bypass surgeries are performed here each year, three times the number done in many other centers.

  516-562-6000

  www.stfrancisheartcenter.com

GASTROENTEROLOGY

- **Cedars-Sinai Medical Center (Los Angeles)**

  Has pioneered various uses of the new video "capsule," a tiny camera that is swallowed in order to examine the gastrointestinal tract. Provides virtually every known gastroenterologic diagnostic procedure and treatment.

  310-423-3277

  www.csmc.edu

- **Mayo Clinic (Rochester, Minnesota)**

  One of the nation's largest gastroenterology departments with more than 70 full-time faculty members, including clinical experts in pancreatic disease, bowel disease and esophageal disorders.

  507-284-2511

  www.mayoclinic.org/rochester

Medical University of South Carolina (Charleston)

Its Digestive Disease Center emphasizes a coordinated team approach in diagnosing and treating digestive ailments.

843-792-2300

www.musc.edu

Mount Sinai Hospital (New York City)

A leader in diagnostic and treatment procedures for ulcerative colitis, inflammatory bowel disorder and other gastrointestinal conditions.

212-241-6500

www.mountsinai.org

University of Iowa Hospitals and Clinics (Iowa City)

Provides multidisciplinary, state-of-the-art medical care for gastrointestinal disease, liver disease and nutritional problems.

800-777-8442

www.uihealthcare.com

MEDICAL ONCOLOGY

Dana-Farber Cancer Institute (Boston)

Renowned for its scientific discoveries leading to major advances in treating cancer. Also recognized for its program focusing on women's cancers.

866-408-3324

www.dfci.harvard.edu

Fox Chase Cancer Center (Philadelphia)

Offers first-rate programs in patient care, research, cancer prevention and early detection.

888-369-2427

www.fccc.edu

Memorial Sloan-Kettering Cancer Center (New York City)

Widely respected as one of the world's leading cancer care centers.

212-639-2000

www.mskcc.org

University of Michigan Health System (Ann Arbor)

Has more than 200 cancer clinicians and researchers and treats more cancer patients than any other hospital in the state.

734-936-4000

www.med.umich.edu

University of Texas M.D. Anderson Cancer Center (Houston)

One of the nation's leading Comprehensive Cancer Centers. Nearly 70,000 persons with cancer are treated here annually.

800-392-1611

www.mdanderson.org

NEUROLOGY

Massachusetts General Hospital (Boston)

Its services include a brain tumor center, child neurology program and centers for genetic diseases, such as Gaucher's and Huntington's.

617-726-2000

www.mgh.harvard.edu

Mayo Clinic (Rochester, Minnesota)

Involved in cutting-edge studies on epilepsy, Parkinson's disease, molecular neurobiology and other neurological research.

507-284-2511

www.mayoclinic.org/rochester

New York University Medical Center (New York City)

Known for its evaluation and treatment of children and adults with neurological diseases. It has the largest epilepsy program in the eastern US.

212-263-7300

www.nyumedicalcenter.org

University of California–Los Angeles Medical Center

Offers comprehensive services for disorders of the brain, spinal cord, peripheral nerves and muscles, as well as neurobehavioral problems (psychiatric disorders with a neurological basis).

800-825-2631

www.healthcare.ucla.edu

University of California–San Francisco Medical Center

Has the only comprehensive memory disorders center and the largest Parkinson's center in northern California.

415-476-1000

www.ucsfhealth.org

OPHTHALMOLOGY

Bascom Palmer Eye Institute (Miami)

Recognized internationally as a leader in ophthalmic care, research and education. Its staff helped develop many advanced ophthalmic techniques, including innovative treatment of diabetic retinopathy.

800-329-7000

www.bpei.med.miami.edu

Johns Hopkins Hospital (Baltimore)

Its Wilmer Eye Institute is known worldwide as a leader in treating exceptionally complex and serious eye cases.

410-955-5000

www.hopkinsmedicine.org

Manhattan Eye, Ear and Throat Hospital (New York City)

Known internationally for its expertise in diagnosing and treating eye, ear, nose, throat and voice disorders.

212-838-9200

New York Eye and Ear Infirmary (New York City)

Founded in 1820, it is the nation's oldest continuously operating specialty hospital providing services for the diagnosis and treatment of disorders of the eyes, ears, nose and throat.

212-979-4000

www.nyee.edu

University of California–Los Angeles Medical Center

Last year, the Jules Stein Eye Institute had nearly 70,000 visits from patients with all categories of eye disorders and visual system diseases.

800-825-2631

www.healthcare.ucla.edu

ORTHOPEDIC SURGERY

Hospital for Joint Diseases (New York City)

One of the leading specialty hospitals in the country focused on orthopedics, rheumatology and musculoskeletal disorders.

212-598-6000

www.hjd.org

Hospital for Special Surgery (New York City)

The hospital's physicians have developed many advances in diagnosing and treating musculoskeletal conditions.

212-606-1000

www.hss.edu

New England Baptist Hospital (Boston)

One of the first artificial hip-replacement procedures in the US was performed here. It offers specialty services in musculoskeletal care, sports medicine and occupational medicine.

617-754-5800

www.nebh.org

New York–Presbyterian Hospital (New York City)

It is recognized for minimally invasive surgery of the shoulder joint and for its Center for Hip and Knee Replacement.

877-697-9355

www.nyp.org

Pennsylvania Hospital (Philadelphia)

Consistently ranked among the top hospitals in orthopedics, it offers services ranging from total joint replacement to pain management and sports medicine.

215-829-3000

www.pennhealth.com/pahosp

OTOLARYNGOLOGY

Barnes Jewish Hospital (St. Louis)

Offers various specialty programs to treat disorders of the ear, nose and sinus...throat and neck...and face, jaw and mouth.

314-867-3627

www.barnesjewish.org

Hospital of the University of Pennsylvania (Philadelphia)

Specialties include balance disorders, cochlear implantation, sinus disease, microsurgery of the ear, tumors of the head and neck, and vocal and speech disorders.

215-662-4000

www.pennhealth.com/upmc

Johns Hopkins Hospital (Baltimore)

Has one of the nation's largest otolaryngology-head and neck surgery departments. It treats a wide range of ear, nose and throat conditions, including hearing and balance disorders and laryngeal cancers.

410-955-5000

www.hopkinsmedicine.org

Lenox Hill Hospital (New York City)

Its Ames Vocal Dynamics Laboratory is considered one of the nation's foremost voice science research centers. It also has a specialty center for hearing, speech, language, oral-motor and swallowing disorders.

212-434-2000

www.lenoxhillhospital.org

Massachusetts Eye and Ear Infirmary (Boston)

Known for its specialized equipment and expert staff. Offers treatment for complex otolaryngologic

cases, including cancerous and noncancerous tumors of the head and neck.
617-573-5520
www.meei.harvard.edu

PHYSICAL MEDICINE AND REHABILITATION

■ **The Institute for Rehabilitation and Research (Houston)**
A world leader in rehabilitation and research. The institute's Spinal Cord Injury Program has been a model system for more than 30 years.
800-447-3422
www.tirr.org

■ **Rehabilitation Institute of Chicago**
Recognized for its expertise in treating cerebral palsy, spinal cord injury, stroke and traumatic brain injury.
800-354-7342
www.ric.org

■ **Spaulding Rehabilitation Hospital (Boston)**
Its specialty rehabilitation programs focus on vascular disease, amputations, brain injury and cardiac rehabilitation.
617-573-7000
www.spauldingrehab.org

■ **University of Texas Health Science Center (San Antonio)**
Facilities include the recently completed Reeves Rehabilitation Center, with a state-of-the-art clinic and 25-bed unit providing comprehensive rehabilitation programs and specialty inpatient and outpatient programs for brain-injured patients.
210-567-7000
www.uthscsa.edu

■ **University of Washington Medical Center (Seattle)**
Offers patients new treatments in pulmonary rehabilitation, rehabilitation psychology and neuropsychology—many developed through its own research programs.
206-598-3300
www.uwmedicine.org

THORACIC SURGERY

■ **The Cleveland Clinic (Cleveland, Ohio)**
Innovations include the Cyberknife (a 12-foot robotic arm used in surgery on lung cancer patients with unresectable lung tumors), minimally invasive surgical treatment procedures and lung transplants.
800-223-2273
www.clevelandclinic.org

■ **Massachusetts General Hospital (Boston)**
Has an international reputation in airway reconstructive surgery, esophageal cancer, advanced lung cancer and management of complex multi-system problems.
617-726-2000
www.mgh.harvard.edu

■ **Mount Sinai Hospital (New York City)**
Its division of thoracic surgery is known for its advancements in minimally invasive techniques, multidisciplinary treatment of difficult tumors and commitment to treating "incurable" conditions.
212-241-6500
www.mountsinai.org

■ **St. Luke's Episcopal Hospital (Houston)**
Home of the Texas Heart Institute, founded by Dr. Denton A. Cooley. Since 1962, the hospital has performed more than 100,000 open-heart procedures, including more than 900 heart transplants.
832-355-1000
www.sleh.com

■ **Stanford University Medical Center (Stanford, California)**
Specializing in rare and complex disorders, it offers comprehensive services for diseases of the lungs, esophagus, chest wall, airway and mediastinum (heart, aorta, trachea, esophagus and thymus gland).
650-723-4000
www.med.stanford.edu

Health Resources

- **Administration on Aging**
  Washington, DC 20201
  202-619-0724
  www.aoa.gov

- **Alzheimer's Association**
  225 North Michigan Ave., Suite 1700
  Chicago, IL 60601-7633
  800-272-3900, 312-335-8700
  www.alz.org

- **American Academy of Allergy, Asthma & Immunology**
  555 East Wells St.
  Milwaukee, WI 53202
  800-822-2762, 414-272-6071
  www.aaaai.org

- **American Academy of Dermatology**
  PO Box 4014
  Schaumburg, IL 60168-4014
  847-330-0230
  www.aad.org

- **American Academy of Neurology**
  1080 Montreal Ave.
  Saint Paul, MN 55116
  800-879-1960, 651-695-2717
  www.aan.com

- **American Board of Medical Specialties**
  1007 Church St., Suite 404
  Evanston, IL 60201-5913
  847-491-9091
  Board Certification Verification:
  866-ASK-ABMS (275-2267)
  www.abms.org

- **American Cancer Society**
  1599 Clifton Rd. NE
  Atlanta, GA 30329

800-ACS-2345 (227-2345)
www.cancer.org

- **American Chiropractic Association**
  1701 Clarendon Blvd.
  Arlington, VA 22209
  800-986-4636
  www.amerchiro.org

- **American Chronic Pain Association (ACPA)**
  PO Box 850
  Rocklin, CA 95677
  800-533-3231
  www.theacpa.org

- **American College of Obstetricians and Gynecologists**
  PO Box 96920
  Washington, DC 20090-6920
  800-673-8444, 202-638-5577
  www.acog.org

- **American College of Rheumatology**
  1800 Century Place, Suite 250
  Atlanta, GA 30345
  404-633-3777
  www.rheumatology.org

- **American Council for Headache Education**
  19 Mantua Rd.
  Mt. Royal, NJ 08061
  856-423-0258
  www.achenet.org

- **American Council on Alcoholism**
  1000 E. Indian School Rd.
  Phoenix, AZ 85014
  800-527-5344
  Alcoholism Treatment HelpLine: 800-527-5344
  www.aca-usa.org

■ **American Council on Exercise (ACE)**
4851 Paramount Dr.
San Diego, CA 92123
800-825-3636, 858-279-8227
www.acefitness.org

■ **American Dental Association**
211 E. Chicago Ave.
Chicago, IL 60611
312-440-2500
www.ada.org

■ **American Diabetes Association**
National Call Center
1701 North Beauregard St.
Alexandria, VA 22311
800-DIABETES (342-2383)
www.diabetes.org

■ **American Dietetic Association**
120 South Riverside Plaza, Suite 2000
Chicago, IL 60606-6995
800-877-1600
www.eatright.org

■ **American Foundation for Urologic Disease**
1000 Corporate Blvd.
Linthicum, MD 21090
800-828-7866, 410-689-3990
www.afud.org

■ **American Gastroenterological Association**
4930 Del Ray Ave.
Bethesda, MD 20814
301-654-2055
www.gastro.org

■ **American Geriatrics Society**
350 Fifth Ave., Suite 801
New York, NY 10118
212-308-1414
www.americangeriatrics.org

■ **American Heart Association**
7272 Greenville Ave.
Dallas, TX 75231
800-AHA-USA-1 (242-8721), 301-223-2307
www.americanheart.org

■ **American Liver Foundation**
75 Maiden Lane, Suite 603
New York, NY 10038
800-GO-LIVER (465-4837), 212-668-1000
www.liverfoundation.org

■ **American Lung Association**
61 Broadway, 6th Floor
New York, NY 10006
212-315-8700
www.lungusa.org

■ **American Lyme Disease Foundation, Inc.**
293 Route 100
Somers, NY 10589
914-277-6970
www.aldf.com

■ **American Macular Degeneration Foundation**
PO Box 515
Northampton, MA 01061-0515
888-MACULAR (622-8527), 413-268-7660
www.macular.org

■ **American Pain Foundation**
201 N. Charles St., Suite 710
Baltimore, MD 21201-4111
888-615-PAIN (7246)
www.painfoundation.org

■ **American Physical Therapy Association**
1111 North Fairfax St.
Alexandria, VA 22314-1488
800-999-APTA (2782), 703-684-APTA
TDD: 703-683-6748
www.apta.org

■ **American Psychological Association**
750 First St. NE
Washington, DC 20002-4242
800-374-2721, 202-336-5500
www.apa.org

■ **American Sleep Apnea Association**
1424 K St. NW, Suite 302
Washington, DC 20005
202-293-3650
www.sleepapnea.org

■ **American Society of Hypertension**
148 Madison Ave., 5th Floor
New York, NY 10016
212-696-9099
www.ash-us.org

■ **American Society of Plastic Surgeons**
444 E. Algonquin Rd.
Arlington Heights, IL 60005
888-4-PLASTIC (475-2784)
www.plasticsurgery.org

■ **American Speech–Language–Hearing Association**
10801 Rockville Pike
Rockville, MD 20852
800-498-2071, 800-638-8255
www.asha.org

■ **American Stroke Association**
7272 Greenville Ave.
Dallas, TX 75231
888-4-STROKE (478-7653)
www.strokeassociation.org

- **Anxiety Disorders Association of America**
  8730 Georgia Ave., Suite 600
  Silver Spring, MD 20910
  240-485-1001
  www.adaa.org

- **Arthritis Foundation**
  PO Box 7669
  Atlanta, GA 30357-0669
  800-283-7800
  www.arthritis.org

- **Centers for Disease Control and Prevention**
  1600 Clifton Rd.
  Atlanta, GA 30333
  800-311-3435, 404-639-3311
  www.cdc.gov

- **Colorectal Cancer Network (CCNetwork)**
  PO Box 182
  Kensington, MD 20895-0182
  301-879-1500
  www.colorectal-cancer.net

- **Council for Responsible Nutrition**
  1828 L St. NW, Suite 900
  Washington, DC, 20036-5114
  202-776-7929
  www.crnusa.org

- **The Crohn's & Colitis Foundation of America**
  386 Park Ave. S, 17th Floor
  New York, NY 10016
  800-932-2423
  www.ccfa.org

- **Deafness Research Association**
  1050 17th St., Suite 701
  Washington, DC 20036
  202-289-5850
  www.drf.org

- **Endocrine Society**
  The Hormone Foundation
  8401 Connecticut Ave., Suite 900
  Chevy Chase, MD 20815-5817
  800-HORMONE (467-6663)
  www.hormone.org

- **Herb Research Foundation**
  4140 15th St.
  Boulder, CO 80304
  303-449-2265
  www.herbs.org

- **The Leukemia & Lymphoma Society**
  1311 Mamaroneck Ave.
  White Plains, NY 10605
  800-955-4572, 914-949-5213
  www.leukemia-lymphoma.org

- **The Melanoma International Foundation**
  250 Mapleflower Rd.
  Glenmoore, PA 19343
  866-INFO-NMF (463-6663)
  www.nationalmelanoma.org

- **National Cancer Institute**
  Building 31, Room 11A-16
  9000 Rockville Pike
  Bethesda, MD 20892
  800-4-CANCER (422-6237)
  TTY: 800-332-8615
  www.cancer.gov

- **National Capital Poison Center**
  3201 New Mexico Ave. NW, Suite 310
  Washington, DC 20016
  202-362-3867
  Emergency Line: 800-222-1222
  www.poison.org

- **National Headache Foundation**
  820 N. Orleans, Suite 217
  Chicago, IL 60610
  888-NHF-5552 (643-5552)
  www.headaches.org

- **National Institute of Allergy and Infectious Diseases (NIAID)**
  Building 31, Room 7A-50
  31 Center Dr., MSC 2520
  Bethesda, MD 20892-2520
  301-496-1886
  www.niaid.nih.gov

- **National Institute of Arthritis and Musculoskeletal and Skin Diseases**
  One AMS Circle
  Bethesda, MD 20892-3675
  877-22-NIAMS (226-4267), 301-495-4484
  TTY: 301-565-2966
  www.niams.nih.gov

- **National Institute of Diabetes & Digestive & Kidney Diseases**
  Building 31, Room 9A04
  Center Drive, MSC 2560
  Bethesda, MD 20892-2560
  301-496-3583
  www.niddk.nih.gov

- **National Institute of Mental Health (NIMH)**
  6001 Executive Blvd.
  MSC 9663, Room 8184
  Bethesda, MD 20892-9663
  866-615-NIMH (6464), 301-443-4513
  TTY: 301-443-8431
  www.nimh.nih.gov

- **National Institute of Neurological Disorders and Stroke**
  PO Box 5801
  Bethesda, MD 20824
  800-352-9424, 301-496-5751
  TTY: 301-468-5981
  www.ninds.nih.gov

- **National Institute on Aging**
  Building 31, Room 5C27
  31 Center Dr., MSC 2292
  Bethesda, MD 20892
  301-496-1752
  www.nia.nih.gov

- **National Institute on Alcohol Abuse and Alcoholism (NIAAA)**
  5635 Fishers Lane, MSC 9304
  Bethesda, MD 20892-9304
  301-443-0796
  www.niaaa.nih.gov

- **National Kidney Foundation**
  30 East 33rd St., Suite 1100
  New York, NY 10016
  800-622-9010, 212-889-2210
  www.kidney.org

- **National Library of Medicine**
  8600 Rockville Pike
  Bethesda, MD 20894
  888-FIND-NLM (346-3656), 301-594-5983
  www.nlm.nih.gov

- **National Multiple Sclerosis Society**
  733 Third Ave.
  New York, NY 10017
  800-FIGHT-MS (344-4867)
  www.nmss.org

- **National Osteoporosis Foundation**
  1232 22nd St. NW
  Washington, DC 20037-1292
  202-223-2226
  www.nof.org

- **National Prostate Cancer Coalition**
  1154 15th St. NW
  Washington, DC 20005
  888-245-9455, 202-463-9455
  www.4npcc.org

- **The National Psoriasis Foundation**
  6600 SW 92nd Ave., Suite 300
  Portland, OR 97223-7195
  800-723-9166, 503-244-7404
  www.psoriasis.org

- **The National Safety Council**
  1121 Spring Lake Dr.
  Itasca, IL 60143-3201
  630-285-1121
  www.nsc.org

- **National Sleep Foundation**
  1522 K St. NW, Suite 500
  Washington, DC 20005
  202-347-3471
  www.sleepfoundation.org

- **National Spinal Cord Injury Association**
  6701 Democracy Blvd., Suite 300-9
  Bethesda, MD 20817
  800-962-9629
  www.spinalcord.org

- **National Stroke Association**
  9707 E. Easter Lane
  Englewood, CO 80112
  800-STROKES (787-6537), 303-649-9299
  www.stroke.org

- **The National Women's Health Information Center**
  8550 Arlington Blvd., Suite 300
  Fairfax, VA 22031
  800-994-WOMAN (9662)
  www.4women.gov

- **Parkinson's Disease Foundation**
  710 West 168th St.
  New York, NY 10032-9982
  800-457-6676
  www.pdf.org

- **The Skin Cancer Foundation**
  245 Fifth Ave., Suite 1403
  New York, NY 10016
  800-SKIN-490 (754-6490)
  www.skincancer.org

- **The Susan G. Komen Breast Cancer Foundation**
  5005 LBJ Freeway, Suite 250
  Dallas, TX 75244
  972-855-1600
  www.komen.org

- **United Network for Organ Sharing**
  PO Box 2484
  Richmond, VA 23218
  804-782-4800
  www.unos.org

- **US Food and Drug Administration**
  5600 Fishers Lane
  Rockville, MD 20857-0001
  888-INFO-FDA (463-6332)
  www.fda.gov

Index